Trends in Andrology and Sexual Medicine

This series will serve as a comprehensive and authoritative resource that presents state of the art knowledge and practice within the fields of Andrology and Sexual Medicine, covering basic science and clinical and psychological aspects. Each volume will focus on a specific topic relating to reproductive or sexual health, such as male and female sexual disorders (from erectile dysfunction to vaginismus, and from hypoactive desire to ejaculatory disturbances), diagnostic issues in infertility and sexual dysfunction, and current and emerging therapies (from assisted reproduction techniques to testosterone supplementation, and from PDE5i to SSRIs for premature ejaculation). In addition, selected new topics not previously covered in a single monograph will be addressed, examples including male osteoporosis and the approach of traditional Chinese medicine to sexual medicine. Against the background of rapid progress in Andrology and Sexual Medicine, the series will meet the need of readers for detailed updates on new discoveries in physiology and pathophysiology and in the therapy of human sexual and reproductive disorders.

Indexed in Scopus

This book series is published in partnership with the Italian Society of Andrology and Sexual Medicine SIAMS

Corresponding series editor and responsible for new book proposals: Emmanuele A. Jannini, eajannini@gmail.com

Mohamed Saeed Mohamed Hasan
Mohamed Lotfy Elsaie

Comprehensive MCQs in Andrology

A Review and Examination Guide

Springer

siams
Società Italiana di Andrologia
e Medicina della Sessualità

Mohamed Saeed Mohamed Hasan
Dermatology, Venereology and Andrology Department
Al Azhar University
Cairo, Egypt

Mohamed Lotfy Elsaie
Department of Dermatology, Venereology and Andrology
National Research Center
Cairo, Egypt

ISSN 2367-0088 ISSN 2367-0096 (electronic)
Trends in Andrology and Sexual Medicine
ISBN 978-3-032-20622-0 ISBN 978-3-032-20623-7 (eBook)
https://doi.org/10.1007/978-3-032-20623-7

This Springer imprint is published by the registered company Springer Nature Switzerland AG
The registered company address is: Gewerbestrasse 11, 6330 Cham, Switzerland

Contents

1 Embryology and Development of Male Genitalia

Learning Objectives

- Describe the timeline and key stages of male genital embryogenesis.
- Identify the roles of the SRY gene, testosterone, and DHT.
- Differentiate between Müllerian and Wolffian duct derivatives.
- Recognize congenital anomalies such as hypospadias and cryptorchidism.
- Apply embryological concepts to understand intersex disorders.

Select the Single Best Answer

1. Cranial to the cloacal membrane, cloacal folds unite to form:
   A. Genital swellings
   B. Genital tubercle
   C. Urogenital membrane
   D. Anal membrane
   E. Urethral folds
2. The anterior part of the cloacal membrane is called:
   A. Genital swelling
   B. Anal membrane
   C. Urogenital membrane
   D. Genital tubercle
   E. Urethral fold
3. Cloacal folds are embryologically derived from:
   A. Endoderm
   B. Ectoderm
   C. Mesoderm
   D. Urorectal septum
   E. Urethral folds

M. S. M. Hasan, M. L. Elsaie, *Comprehensive MCQs in Andrology*, Trends in Andrology and Sexual Medicine, https://doi.org/10.1007/978-3-032-20623-7_1

4. The mesoderm of the genital tubercle enlarges to form:
   A. Penile urethra
   B. Corpora cavernosa
   C. Penile skin
   D. Prepuce
   E. Crura of the penis
5. The endoderm of the genital tubercle tabularizes to form:
   A. Corpora cavernosa
   B. Glans penis
   C. Penile urethra
   D. Penile skin
   E. Prepuce
6. The ectoderm of the genital tubercle develops into:
   A. Penile skin
   B. Glans penis
   C. Penile urethra
   D. Corpora cavernosa
   E. Crura of the penis
7. The penile crura are continuous as:
   A. Corpus spongiosum
   B. Tunica albuginea
   C. Tunica vaginalis
   D. Corpus cavernosum
   E. Tunica vasculosa
8. The penile crura are covered by:
   A. Bulbospongiosus muscle
   B. Puborectalis muscle
   C. Ischiocavernosus muscle
   D. Superficial perineal muscle
   E. Levator ani muscle
9. The penile bulb continues as:
   A. Corpus spongiosum
   B. Tunica albuginea
   C. Tunica vaginalis
   D. Corpus cavernosum
   E. Tunica vasculosa
10. The penile bulb is covered by:
   A. Bulbospongiosus muscle
   B. Puborectalis muscle
   C. Ischiocavernosus muscle
   D. Transverse perineal muscle
   E. Levator ani muscle

11. The septum penis is formed by midline fusion of:
    A. Tunica vaginalis
    B. Tunica albuginea
    C. Colle's fascia
    D. Buck's fascia
    E. Tunica vasculosa
12. The most sensitive part of the penis is:
    A. Penile shaft
    B. Penile frenulum
    C. Penile root
    D. Foreskin
    E. Penoscrotal junction
13. The penile fundiform ligament arises from:
    A. Buck's fascia
    B. Colle's fascia
    C. Scarpa's fascia
    D. Fascia lata
    E. Dartos fascia
14. The penile suspensory ligament arises from:
    A. Buck's fascia
    B. Colle's fascia
    C. Scarpa's fascia
    D. Fascia lata
    E. Dartos fascia
15. The Colle's fascia of the penis:
    A. Is deep fascia
    B. Is caudal to Scarpa's fascia
    C. Dorsal vein, artery, and nerve pass through it
    D. Restricts penile hematoma
    E. Attached to the perineal membrane
16. Buck's fascia of the penis is:
    A. Superficial fascia
    B. The dorsal vein only passes through it
    C. Attached distally to the base of the glans penis
    D. Attached distally to the perineal membrane
    E. Cranial to Scarpa's fascia
17. The tunica albuginea of the penis:
    A. Its inner layer is orientated longitudinally
    B. Its outer layer is orientated circular
    C. It has a role in compression of emissary veins during erection
    D. Has the same thickness along its course
    E. Allows flexibility but reduces rigidity

18. The most common type of collagen in tunica albuginea:
    A. Type 1 and 2
    B. Type 1 and 3
    C. Type 2 and 3
    D. Type 1 and 4
    E. Type 1 and 5
19. Ischiocavernosus muscle:
    A. Originates from ischial tuberosity
    B. Inserts into midline raphe of penile bulb
    C. Responsible for ejaculation
    D. Relaxation causes detumescence
    E. Originates from central tendon
20. Arterial supply of the penis:
    A. Internal iliac artery
    B. Inferior external pudendal artery
    C. External iliac artery
    D. Inferior rectal artery
    E. Middle rectal artery
21. Venous drainage of the distal corpora cavernosa is:
    A. Superficial dorsal vein
    B. Deep dorsal vein
    C. Crural vein
    D. Saphenous vein
    E. Bulbar vein
22. Lymphatic drainage of penile skin is:
    A. Superficial inguinal nodes
    B. Deep inguinal nodes
    C. Femoral nodes
    D. Common iliac nodes
    E. External iliac nodes
23. The scrotum of a newborn is:
    A. Distinct raphe
    B. Base increases in width
    C. Infantile type
    D. Wrinkled
    E. Smooth
24. Arterial supply of the scrotum:
    A. Inferior external pudendal artery
    B. Internal pudendal artery
    C. Middle rectal artery
    D. Inferior rectal artery
    E. Bulbourethral artery

25. The penis is supported by suspensory ligament and:
    A. Deltoid ligament
    B. Fundiform ligament
    C. Penile ligament
    D. Cavernosal ligament
    E. Penoscrotal ligament
26. The corpus spongiosum develops from:
    A. Caudal genitourinary sinus
    B. Genital tubercle
    C. Urethral folds
    D. Genital swelling
    E. Cloacal membrane
27. Penis is derived from:
    A. Genital swelling
    B. Urogenital sinus
    C. Genital tubercle
    D. Cloacal membrane
    E. Urethral folds
28. The glans penis is homologous to:
    A. Clitoral hood
    B. Clitoris
    C. Clitoral glans
    D. Clitoral crura
    E. Clitoral bulb
29. The superficial dorsal veins drain into:
    A. Saphenous vein
    B. Retrocolonic plexus
    C. Circumflex system
    D. Pudendal plexus
    E. Vasal plexus
30. The following about Colle's fascia is false:
    A. It is the most superficial penile fascia
    B. It is continuous with dartos fascia
    C. It is formed of loose connective tissue with muscle fibers
    D. Tunica albuginea lies directly underneath
31. Lymphatic drainage from bulbar urethra travels:
    A. Via perianal nodes
    B. To deep pelvic nodes
    C. To superficial & deep inguinal nodes
    D. To prepubic nodes
    E. To para-aortic nodes

32. The glans penis is distal expansion of:
    A. Corpus cavernosum
    B. Corpus spongiosum
    C. Prepuce
    D. Urethra
    E. Buck's fascia
33. Major component of prepuce derives from:
    A. Frenulum
    B. Glans penis
    C. Penile shaft
    D. Glans stroma
    E. Corpora cavernosa
34. Which statement about scrotal rugae is false?
    A. They are transverse ridges
    B. Extend from scrotal raphe
    C. Attach laterally to inguinal region
    D. Wind dorsally to rejoin raphe
    E. In flaccid state curve upwards
35. Which is true about penile anatomy?
    A. Corpus spongiosum attaches to ischiopubic rami
    B. Cavernosal artery supplies urethra, glans, and spongiosum
    C. Buck's fascia continues with Colle's fascia
    D. Cavernosal nerve provides sensory supply
    E. Arcuate subpubic ligament maintains erection
36. A 1-year-old passes urine from underside of penis. Embryonic defect?
    A. Spongy urethra
    B. Labioscrotal folds
    C. Urethral folds
    D. Urogenital folds
    E. Genital tubercle
37. A 4-month-old passes urine from dorsum of penis. Defect?
    A. Spongy urethra
    B. Labioscrotal folds
    C. Cloacal membrane
    D. Urogenital folds
    E. Genital tubercle
38. A 25-year-old has fluid in tunica vaginalis. Diagnosis?
    A. Varicocele
    B. Rectocele
    C. Cystocele
    D. Hydrocele
    E. Hypospadias

39. Which two share same precursor tissue?
    A. Head of penis & clitoris
    B. Shaft of penis & clitoris
    C. Head of penis & labia minora
    D. Labia minora & majora
    E. Scrotum & clitoris
40. Which is true about genital differentiation?
    A. Urethral folds fuse in males to form penile urethra
    B. Urethral folds in females form labia minora
    C. Labioscrotal folds fuse in females to form vaginal opening
    D. Genital tubercle forms clitoris in females
    E. All of the above
41. The gubernaculum testis is essential for:
    A. Spermatogenesis
    B. Testicular descent
    C. Sperm motility
    D. Urethral development
    E. Penile erection
42. The prostate develops from:
    A. Mesonephric duct
    B. Urogenital sinus endoderm
    C. Cloacal membrane
    D. Paramesonephric duct
    E. Wolffian body
43. The seminal vesicles arise from:
    A. Paramesonephric duct
    B. Mesonephric duct outgrowth
    C. Cloaca
    D. Genital tubercle
    E. Allantois
44. Which part of urethra is derived from ectoderm?
    A. Penile glanular urethra
    B. Membranous urethra
    C. Prostatic urethra
    D. Bulbar urethra
    E. Penile shaft urethra
45. The genital swellings give rise to:
    A. Penis
    B. Testis
    C. Scrotum
    D. Prostate
    E. Glans

46. Homolog of labia majora in males is:
    A. Scrotum
    B. Penis
    C. Glans
    D. Testis
    E. Prostate
47. Epispadias results from:
    A. Failure of urethral folds fusion
    B. Malposition of genital tubercle
    C. Failure of cloacal division
    D. Persistence of urogenital sinus
    E. Abnormal mesonephric duct
48. Hypospadias is due to:
    A. Incomplete fusion of urethral folds
    B. Excess androgen stimulation
    C. Persistence of cloaca
    D. Failure of labioscrotal fusion
    E. Testicular agenesis
49. Cryptorchidism predisposes to all EXCEPT:
    A. Testicular torsion
    B. Testicular cancer
    C. Infertility
    D. Hydrocele
    E. Hormonal dysfunction
50. The urethral plate is derived from:
    A. Endoderm of urogenital sinus
    B. Mesoderm of genital tubercle
    C. Ectodermal ingrowth
    D. Neural crest
    E. Paramesonephric duct

✅ Key Takeaways

- Male genital development begins with the action of the **SRY gene** on the Y chromosome.
- **Testosterone** promotes Wolffian duct development; **Müllerian regression** is driven by AMH (anti-Müllerian hormone).
- **Dihydrotestosterone (DHT)** is essential for external genitalia differentiation.
- Disorders of sexual development may result from hormonal, genetic, or receptor pathway abnormalities.
- The **genital tubercle**, **urogenital folds**, and **labioscrotal swellings** form the phallus and scrotum.

- Clinical anomalies such as **hypospadias**, **epispadias**, and **cryptorchidism** often stem from disruptions in embryologic signaling.
- Understanding embryology is essential for **urological surgery**, **pediatric endocrinology**, and **genetic counseling**.

✅ Answer Key (1–50)

1. B
2. C
3. C
4. B
5. C
6. A
7. D
8. C
9. A
10. A
11. B
12. B
13. C
14. A
15. D
16. C
17. C
18. B
19. A
20. A
21. B
22. A
23. E
24. A
25. B
26. C
27. C
28. C
29. A
30. D
31. C
32. B
33. B
34. E
35. C
36. C
37. A

38. D
39. A
40. E
41. B
42. B
43. B
44. A
45. C
46. A
47. B
48. A
49. D
50. A

Explanations (1–50)

1. The **genital tubercle** forms cranial to the cloacal membrane from fused cloacal folds. It gives rise to phallus structures: penis in males, clitoris in females. Its formation is androgen-dependent in males.
2. The cloacal membrane has two parts: anterior is the **urogenital membrane**, posterior is the anal membrane. The urogenital membrane eventually ruptures to form the primitive urogenital opening.
3. Cloacal folds arise from **mesoderm** on either side of the cloacal membrane. They contribute to formation of urogenital folds, anal folds, and the genital tubercle.
4. The mesoderm of the genital tubercle proliferates to form **erectile tissue (corpora cavernosa)**. These structures form the bulk of the penis shaft and are critical for rigidity.
5. Endoderm of the genital tubercle contributes to the **penile urethra**, which is canalized to connect bladder to external meatus. Incomplete canalization may lead to hypospadias.
6. Ectoderm of the genital tubercle forms the **glans penis and penile skin**. It also invaginates at the tip to form the glandular urethra, which canalizes to meet endodermal urethra.
7. The penile crura are the proximal extensions of the **corpora cavernosa**. They attach to the ischiopubic rami and form the structural root of the penis.
8. The **ischiocavernosus muscle** covers the penile crura. Its contraction compresses venous drainage, helping maintain penile erection.
9. The **penile bulb** is the proximal expansion of the corpus spongiosum. It continues as corpus spongiosum along the shaft, surrounding the penile urethra.
10. The **bulbospongiosus muscle** covers the bulb of the penis. It contracts during ejaculation and urination, aiding expulsion of semen and urine.
11. The **septum penis** is formed by midline fusion of the **tunica albuginea** of each corpus cavernosum. This fibrous partition separates the erectile bodies while allowing some venous communication through perforations.

12. The **frenulum of the penis** is the most sensitive part due to dense innervation from the dorsal nerve of the penis (branch of pudendal nerve). It plays an important role in sexual stimulation and orgasm.
13. The **fundiform ligament** arises from **Scarpa's fascia** of the lower abdominal wall. It splits and encircles the penis like a sling, supporting it at the root.
14. The **suspensory ligament of the penis** originates from the **deep fascia of the anterior abdominal wall** and attaches to the pubic symphysis, providing central support.
15. **Colle's fascia** is a superficial fascia continuous with Scarpa's fascia. It attaches to the perineal membrane, restricting the spread of penile hematoma into thighs or abdomen.
16. **Buck's fascia** is the deep fascia of the penis. It encases the corpora cavernosa and corpus spongiosum, anchoring proximally to the perineal membrane and distally to the glans. It encloses dorsal vessels and nerves.
17. The **tunica albuginea** has an outer circular and inner longitudinal layer. This arrangement provides rigidity during erection by compressing emissary veins, preventing venous leakage, and maintaining tumescence.
18. The tunica albuginea is composed primarily of **type I and type III collagen**. This combination gives tensile strength and elasticity, allowing the penis to resist high intracavernosal pressures during erection.
19. The **ischiocavernosus muscle** originates from the ischial tuberosity and inserts on the crus penis. Its contraction stabilizes and compresses the crus, maintaining erection by reducing venous outflow.
20. The penis receives arterial supply mainly from the **internal pudendal artery** (branch of internal iliac). Its branches include dorsal, cavernosal, and bulbourethral arteries, all vital for erection and penile health.
21. The distal corpora cavernosa drain primarily via the **deep dorsal vein**, which empties into the prostatic venous plexus. Proper venous drainage is crucial for detumescence after erection.
22. The lymphatic drainage of penile skin goes to the **superficial inguinal nodes**. In contrast, glans and corpora drain deeper into external iliac and deep inguinal nodes, important in cancer staging.
23. In newborns, the scrotum appears **smooth** because rugae are not yet developed. With age and androgen exposure, scrotal rugae become more prominent, helping regulate testicular temperature.
24. The scrotum is supplied by branches of the **inferior external pudendal artery**, along with perineal branches of the internal pudendal artery. These vessels ensure thermoregulation for spermatogenesis.
25. The penis is supported by two ligaments: the **suspensory ligament** and the **fundiform ligament**, which stabilize the penile root during erection.
26. The **corpus spongiosum** develops from the **urethral folds**, enclosing the penile urethra. It prevents urethral compression during erection, ensuring semen and urine passage.
27. The **penis** develops from the **genital tubercle**, which elongates under testosterone stimulation. In females, the tubercle forms the clitoris.

28. The **glans penis** is homologous to the **clitoral glans** in females, both derived from the genital tubercle. This explains similar sensory innervation and sexual sensitivity.
29. The **superficial dorsal vein** drains penile skin and superficial fascia into the **saphenous vein**. This differs from the deep dorsal vein draining erectile tissues.
30. Colle's fascia is superficial and continuous with scrotal dartos fascia. It does not lie directly above tunica albuginea (that's Buck's fascia). Thus, the statement claiming otherwise is false.
31. Lymphatic drainage from the **bulbar urethra** goes first to **superficial and deep inguinal nodes**, then to pelvic nodes. This is clinically important in urethral cancer.
32. The **glans penis** is the distal expansion of the **corpus spongiosum**, forming the sensitive tip of the penis. It contains abundant sensory nerve endings.
33. The **prepuce** (foreskin) develops as a fold derived mainly from the **glans penis** and penile shaft epithelium. It provides protection and maintains mucosal lubrication.
34. Scrotal rugae are folds aiding in testicular thermoregulation. False statements include those suggesting abnormal lateral attachment or dorsal winding; these are incorrect anatomically.
35. **Buck's fascia** is continuous with **Colle's fascia** in the perineum, enclosing erectile tissues and vessels. This continuity helps confine infections or hematomas.
36. **Hypospadias** results from failure of **urethral folds** to fuse properly, leading to urethral opening on ventral penis. It's a common congenital anomaly, requiring surgical correction.
37. **Epispadias** results from malposition of the **genital tubercle**, leading to urethral opening on dorsal penis. It is often associated with bladder exstrophy.
38. **Hydrocele** is fluid accumulation in the **tunica vaginalis** surrounding the testis. It may be congenital (patent processus vaginalis) or acquired due to trauma or infection.
39. The **head of the penis and clitoris** share a common origin from the genital tubercle. This homology explains their structural and functional similarities.
40. All listed statements are true: in males, urethral folds fuse; in females, they form labia minora; labioscrotal folds remain separate as labia majora; genital tubercle becomes clitoris.
41. The **gubernaculum** guides testicular descent into the scrotum by shortening. Failure results in undescended testis (cryptorchidism).
42. The **prostate** develops from **endodermal outgrowths of the urogenital sinus**. These grow into surrounding mesenchyme and canalize to form prostatic ducts.
43. The **seminal vesicles** develop as lateral outgrowths from the **mesonephric (Wolffian) ducts** near the bladder trigone. They later join vas deferens to form ejaculatory ducts.
44. The **glandular urethra of the glans** is derived from ectodermal ingrowth at the tip, which canalizes and joins the endodermal urethra.

45. **Genital swellings** give rise to the **scrotum** in males and labia majora in females. Failure of fusion leads to bifid scrotum.
46. The **scrotum** is homologous to the **labia majora** in females, both derived from labioscrotal swellings.
47. **Epispadias** occurs due to abnormal positioning of the **genital tubercle**, resulting in urethral opening on the dorsum of penis.
48. **Hypospadias** arises from incomplete fusion of the **urethral folds**, producing a ventral opening. It may be associated with chordee (ventral curvature).
49. **Cryptorchidism** predisposes to torsion, infertility, and testicular cancer, but not hydrocele. Hydrocele has a different etiology.
50. The **urethral plate** is derived from the **endoderm of the urogenital sinus**, forming the penile urethra, later canalized to connect with ectodermal glandular urethra.

Further Reading

The explanations in this chapter are supported by the following key references:

1. Sadler TW. Langman's medical embryology. 14th ed. Philadelphia: Wolters Kluwer; 2023.
2. Moore KL, Persaud TVN, Torchia MG. The developing human: clinically oriented embryology. 11th ed. Elsevier; 2020.
3. Rey RA, Grinspon RP. Normal male sexual differentiation and aetiology of disorders of sex development. Best Pract Res Clin Endocrinol Metab. 2011;25(2):221–38.
4. Hughes IA, Davies JD, Bunch TI, et al. Androgen insensitivity syndrome. Lancet. 2012;380(9851):1419–28.
5. Hutson JM, Thorup J, Beasley SW. Mechanisms of testicular descent. Endocr Rev. 2013;34(5):725–52.
6. Achermann JC, Hughes IA. Disorders of sex development. In: Endocrinology: adult and pediatric. Elsevier; 2021.

Penile Anatomy and Variants

2

Learning Objectives

- Identify the key anatomical structures of the penis including corpora cavernosa, corpus spongiosum, and tunica albuginea.
- Describe the arterial and venous blood supply and its relevance to erectile physiology.
- Recognize the nerve supply and its role in sexual reflexes and sensation.
- Differentiate between normal anatomical variants and pathological anomalies.
- Apply anatomical principles in clinical scenarios involving trauma, Peyronie's disease, and congenital defects.

Select the Single Best Answer

1. The common site of pearly penile papule is:
   A. Glans penis
   B. Coronal sulcus
   C. Penile shaft
   D. Perineum
   E. Penile root
2. Pearly penile papule is usually:
   A. Single
   B. Arranged in rows
   C. Confluent
   D. Self limited
   E. Cockscomb-like

M. S. M. Hasan, M. L. Elsaie, *Comprehensive MCQs in Andrology*, Trends in Andrology and Sexual Medicine, https://doi.org/10.1007/978-3-032-20623-7_2

3. The most common cause of non-sclerosing lymphangitis:
   A. Diabetes mellitus
   B. Vigorous trauma
   C. Fracture penis
   D. Idiopathic
   E. Insect bite
4. The most common clinical presentation of sclerosing lymphangitis is:
   A. Pain through the penile shaft
   B. Complete edematous circle around coronal sulcus
   C. Serpiginous cord-like thickening around coronal sulcus
   D. Hematoma
   E. Penile edema
5. Peeper penis is a synonym of:
   A. Micropenis
   B. Micropothia
   C. Melgopenis
   D. Macropothia
   E. Congenital mega prepuce
6. Volcano penis is a synonym of:
   A. Micropenis
   B. Micropothia
   C. Melgopenis
   D. Macropothia
   E. Congenital mega prepuce
7. One of the following is a component of Smegma:
   A. Fishy odor
   B. Yellowish color
   C. Mixed bacterial and fungal flora
   D. Epithelial debris
   E. Carbohydrates
8. One of the following is a differential diagnosis of paraphimosis:
   A. Penile Mondor disease
   B. Acute angioedema
   C. Erythroplasia of Queyrat
   D. Penile wart
   E. Pearly penile papules
9. In phimosis, partial retraction with visible meatus is considered:
   A. Score 5
   B. Score 4
   C. Score 3
   D. Score 2
   E. Score 1

10. The normal size of the newborn stretched penis is:
    A. 1.5–2.5 cm
    B. 2.5–4.5 cm
    C. <1.5 cm
    D. 4–5 cm
    E. 1–2 cm
11. The newborn penile size is considered small if less than:
    A. 0.5 cm
    B. 1.2 cm
    C. 1.5 cm
    D. 1.9 cm
    E. 2.5 cm
12. The average size of an adult stretched penis is:
    A. 5–10 cm
    B. 7.5–12 cm
    C. 7.5–15 cm
    D. 10–18 cm
    E. 15–18 cm
13. Aphalia is caused by:
    A. Double genital tubercle
    B. Bifid genital tubercle
    C. Small genital tubercle
    D. Absent genital tubercle
    E. Large genital tubercle
14. Diphallia is caused by:
    A. Double genital tubercle
    B. Bifid genital tubercle
    C. Small genital tubercle
    D. Absent genital tubercle
    E. Large genital tubercle
15. Split median raphe of the scrotum is due to:
    A. Defective fusion of ectoderm
    B. Defective fusion of endoderm
    C. Defective fusion of mesoderm
    D. Subepithelial midline fistula
    E. Webbed penis
16. Which of the following is NOT associated with Igloo prepuce?
    A. Akroposthia
    B. Webbed penis
    C. Penile chordee
    D. Scrotal transposition
    E. Diphallia

17. Which of the following is NOT true about simple paraphimosis?
    A. It can occur at any age
    B. It presents with acute pain
    C. It is associated with late glans edema
    D. It is not associated with urinary retention
    E. It is not associated with ulceration
18. Which of the following is true about compound paraphimosis?
    A. It can occur at any age
    B. It is associated with late glans edema
    C. It is not associated with urinary retention
    D. It is not associated with ulceration
    E. It presents with acute pain
19. Which of the following is NOT a method for penile girth lengthening?
    A. Filler injection
    B. Biodegradable scaffolds
    C. Autologous fat injection
    D. Dermal fat grafts
    E. Ionophoresis
20. Which of the following is NOT true about Ram-horn penis?
    A. It is the most common type of penile edema
    B. Lymph accumulates more distally than proximally
    C. Penis buried in enlarging scrotum
    D. Swollen prepuce distorted like a snail shell
    E. Unequal fibrosis
21. Which of the following syndromes is associated with micropenis?
    A. Robinow syndrome
    B. Rud's syndrome
    C. Trisomy 21
    D. Klinefelter's syndrome
    E. All of the above
22. Which type of penile edema is seen in filarial lymphedema?
    A. Buried penis
    B. Straight hypertrophied penis
    C. Ram horn penis
    D. None of the above
    E. All of the above

Added Questions (23–50)

23. Penile Mondor's disease refers to thrombosis of:
    A. Cavernosal artery
    B. Deep dorsal vein
    C. Superficial dorsal vein
    D. Bulbar artery
    E. Circumflex vein

24. The most common site of penile fracture is:
    A. Corpus spongiosum
    B. Dorsal vein
    C. Tunica albuginea of corpora cavernosa
    D. Glans penis
    E. Bulbar urethra
25. Zoon's balanitis is also known as:
    A. Plasma cell balanitis
    B. Xerotic balanitis
    C. Circinate balanitis
    D. Diabetic balanitis
    E. Hypertrophic balanitis
26. The most common infectious cause of balanitis is:
    A. *Candida albicans*
    B. *Chlamydia trachomatis*
    C. *Neisseria gonorrhoeae*
    D. HSV
    E. HPV
27. The most common cause of penile carcinoma is:
    A. HPV infection
    B. Phimosis
    C. Poor hygiene
    D. Chronic balanitis
    E. All of the above
28. The usual histological type of penile carcinoma is:
    A. Adenocarcinoma
    B. Squamous cell carcinoma
    C. Basal cell carcinoma
    D. Melanoma
    E. Transitional cell carcinoma
29. Which HPV subtypes are most commonly associated with penile carcinoma?
    A. 6 and 11
    B. 16 and 18
    C. 31 and 33
    D. 42 and 43
    E. 51 and 52
30. The most common site of penile carcinoma is:
    A. Penile shaft
    B. Glans penis
    C. Penile root
    D. Urethra
    E. Perineum

31. The most common presenting symptom of penile carcinoma is:
    A. Ulcer or lump
    B. Pain
    C. Dysuria
    D. Hematuria
    E. Phimosis
32. The first lymph nodes affected in penile carcinoma are:
    A. Superficial inguinal nodes
    B. Deep inguinal nodes
    C. External iliac nodes
    D. Internal iliac nodes
    E. Para-aortic nodes
33. The classic triad of Peyronie's disease includes penile curvature, pain, and:
    A. Impotence
    B. Priapism
    C. Infertility
    D. Phimosis
    E. Penile edema
34. The most common cause of priapism is:
    A. Trauma
    B. Sickle cell disease
    C. Drugs
    D. Leukemia
    E. Idiopathic
35. The most common tumor of the penis in children is:
    A. Squamous cell carcinoma
    B. Rhabdomyosarcoma
    C. Yolk sac tumor
    D. Teratoma
    E. Kaposi's sarcoma
36. Epispadias is associated with which anomaly?
    A. Hypospadias
    B. Bladder exstrophy
    C. Cryptorchidism
    D. Chordee
    E. Varicocele
37. In hypospadias, the urethral opening is most commonly located at:
    A. Glans penis
    B. Penile shaft
    C. Penoscrotal junction
    D. Scrotum
    E. Perineum

38. The most important hormone in penile development during fetal life is:
    A. Estrogen
    B. Testosterone
    C. Progesterone
    D. DHT
    E. FSH
39. Congenital chordee is best defined as:
    A. Dorsal curvature
    B. Ventral curvature
    C. Lateral curvature
    D. Torsion
    E. Short penile shaft
40. Micropenis is defined as stretched penile length below:
    A. 2 SD of mean
    B. 1 SD of mean
    C. 3 SD of mean
    D. 5 cm
    E. 10th percentile
41. Buried penis is best described as:
    A. Penis hidden under pubic fat pad
    B. Penis with ventral curvature
    C. Penis covered by phimotic prepuce
    D. Penis with bifid raphe
    E. Penis with absent glans
42. The most common congenital anomaly of penis is:
    A. Phimosis
    B. Hypospadias
    C. Epispadias
    D. Chordee
    E. Aphalia
43. The first-line investigation in penile fracture is:
    A. X-ray
    B. Ultrasound
    C. MRI
    D. Retrograde urethrogram
    E. CT scan
44. The first-line management of penile fracture is:
    A. Conservative
    B. Surgical repair
    C. Radiotherapy
    D. Antibiotics only
    E. Observation

45. The most common benign penile tumor is:
    A. Fibroma
    B. Papilloma
    C. Leiomyoma
    D. Lipoma
    E. Angiokeratoma
46. The most common cause of megalourethra is:
    A. Urethral valves
    B. Congenital mesodermal defect
    C. Trauma
    D. Hypospadias
    E. Infections
47. Lichen sclerosus et atrophicus of penis is also called:
    A. Zoon's balanitis
    B. Balanitis xerotica obliterans
    C. Circinate balanitis
    D. Hypertrophic balanitis
    E. Plasma cell balanitis
48. The most common vascular lesion of penis is:
    A. Hemangioma
    B. Lymphangioma
    C. Angiokeratoma
    D. AV malformation
    E. Varix
49. Which imaging is best for penile vascular anomalies?
    A. X-ray
    B. Ultrasound Doppler
    C. CT
    D. MRI
    E. Retrograde urethrogram
50. The gold standard for penile carcinoma diagnosis is:
    A. MRI
    B. FNAC
    C. Biopsy
    D. Ultrasound
    E. CT

✅ Key Takeaways

- The penis comprises **two corpora cavernosa** and a **single corpus spongiosum**, enclosed by the tunica albuginea.
- **Buck's fascia** and **Colles' fascia** play key roles in structural support and compartmentalization.

- Penile erection depends on **cavernosal arterial inflow** and **venous occlusion**, governed by a neurovascular mechanism.
- The **dorsal nerve of the penis** is a branch of the pudendal nerve and is critical for sensory input.
- Anatomical variants like **penile curvature**, **webbed penis**, and **micropenis** must be differentiated from acquired pathologies.
- **Imaging techniques** such as penile Doppler ultrasound are useful in assessing vascular integrity.
- Knowledge of penile anatomy underpins safe and effective **andrological surgery** and **sexual medicine** practice.

✅ Answer Key (1–50)

1. B
2. B
3. B
4. C
5. B
6. E
7. D
8. B
9. C
10. A
11. C
12. C
13. D
14. A
15. A
16. E
17. C
18. B
19. E
20. A
21. E
22. C
23. C
24. C
25. A
26. A
27. E
28. B
29. B
30. B
31. A

32. A
33. A
34. B
35. B
36. B
37. A
38. D
39. B
40. A
41. A
42. B
43. B
44. B
45. B
46. B
47. B
48. A
49. B
50. C

Explanations (1–50)

1. Pearly penile papules are typically found around the **coronal sulcus**, appearing as small, dome-shaped papules. They are considered a normal anatomical variant and not a sexually transmitted disease.
2. Pearly penile papules are usually **arranged in rows** circumferentially around the coronal sulcus. They are multiple, symmetric, and benign, often mistaken for warts by patients.
3. Non-sclerosing lymphangitis most often follows **vigorous sexual activity or trauma**, causing lymphatic obstruction and swelling. It presents as a painless, cord-like lesion.
4. Sclerosing lymphangitis classically presents as a **serpiginous cord-like thickening around the coronal sulcus**. It results from inflammation and fibrosis of lymphatics.
5. "Peeper penis" is a synonym of **micropenis (micropothia)**, describing a true abnormally short penis with stretched length below −2.5 SD for age. It must be distinguished from *buried penis* or *congenital megaprepuce*, where penile size is normal but concealed by skin or fat. The term highlights underdevelopment due to endocrine or androgen defects.
6. "Volcano penis" is another term for **congenital mega prepuce**, due to ballooning of redundant foreskin. It is not a true micropenis.
7. **Smegma** consists of exfoliated epithelial debris and secretions. It may accumulate under the foreskin, predisposing to infection and penile carcinoma if hygiene is poor.

8. A key differential diagnosis of paraphimosis is **acute angioedema**, where swelling and trapping of foreskin mimic paraphimosis. Clinical context distinguishes them.
9. Phimosis grading: **Score 3** indicates partial retraction of foreskin with meatus visible. Higher scores show greater retractability.
10. A newborn stretched penile length is **1.5–2.5 cm**. This measurement helps identify micropenis and endocrinological abnormalities early.
11. Penile length <1.5 cm in newborns is considered **micropenis**. It warrants endocrine evaluation for androgen deficiency or pituitary problems.
12. The average adult stretched penile length is **7.5–15 cm**. This measurement is widely used to define normal versus micropenis in adulthood.
13. **Aphalia** (absence of penis) occurs due to failure of development of the genital tubercle. It is extremely rare and often associated with urinary anomalies.
14. **Diphallia** results from duplication of the genital tubercle. Patients may present with two partially developed or fully developed penises, usually with urinary anomalies.
15. **Split median raphe** of the scrotum is due to defective midline fusion of ectoderm during embryogenesis, sometimes associated with fistulas.
16. Igloo prepuce is associated with anomalies like akroposthia, webbed penis, chordee, and scrotal transposition. It is **not associated with diphallia**, making this the exception.
17. Simple paraphimosis occurs at any age, presents with pain and swelling, and is not typically associated with urinary retention or ulceration. **Late glans edema is less common**.
18. Compound paraphimosis is associated with **progressive glans edema**, urinary retention, and ulceration, unlike the simple type.
19. Ionophoresis is not a recognized method for penile girth enhancement. Established methods include **fillers, fat injections, and dermal grafts**, though complications are common.
20. Ram-horn penis is a type of penile edema where lymph accumulates distally, causing the prepuce to balloon and resemble a snail's shell. It is not the most common type.
21. Micropenis may be associated with **Klinefelter's syndrome, trisomy 21, Rud's syndrome, and Robinow syndrome**. Endocrine causes are also important.
22. Filarial infection causes **ram-horn type penile edema** due to lymphatic obstruction. Chronic filariasis leads to gross distortion and fibrosis.
23. Penile Mondor's disease is superficial dorsal vein thrombosis. It presents with a painful cord on the dorsal shaft, often resolving spontaneously.
24. Penile fracture usually involves rupture of the **tunica albuginea of corpora cavernosa** during trauma in intercourse. It requires urgent surgical repair.
25. Zoon's balanitis is **plasma cell balanitis**, a benign inflammatory condition presenting as shiny red patches on glans. It is not infectious or premalignant.
26. ***Candida albicans*** is the most common infectious cause of balanitis, especially in diabetics and uncircumcised men. Poor hygiene increases risk.

27. Penile carcinoma is multifactorial: **HPV, phimosis, poor hygiene, and chronic balanitis** are all major risk factors. Circumcision in infancy reduces risk.
28. The vast majority of penile cancers are **squamous cell carcinoma**, usually on glans or prepuce. Other types like melanoma are rare.
29. HPV **16 and 18** are the high-risk oncogenic types strongly linked to penile cancer. HPV 6 and 11 cause benign warts but not cancer.
30. The glans penis is the most common site of penile carcinoma. Lesions appear as ulcers, nodules, or fungating growths, often hidden under foreskin.
31. The most common presenting symptom of penile carcinoma is a **non-healing ulcer or lump**. Pain and urinary symptoms appear later.
32. Penile carcinoma spreads first to **superficial inguinal lymph nodes**, then to deeper iliac chains. Lymph node status determines prognosis.
33. Peyronie's disease presents with **penile curvature, pain, and erectile dysfunction** due to fibrous plaques in tunica albuginea.
34. The most common cause of priapism is **sickle cell disease** due to venous outflow obstruction by sickled RBCs. Drugs and trauma are other causes.
35. The most common penile tumor in children is **rhabdomyosarcoma**, a malignant mesenchymal tumor. It often arises in genitourinary tract.
36. Epispadias is strongly associated with **bladder exstrophy**. Both result from defective positioning of the genital tubercle.
37. In hypospadias, the urethral meatus is most often located at the **glans penis**, but can be more proximal in severe cases.
38. **Dihydrotestosterone (DHT)** is crucial for penile development in fetal life, mediating differentiation of genital tubercle.
39. Congenital chordee refers to **ventral curvature** of the penis, often associated with hypospadias or fibrous tissue tethering.
40. Micropenis is defined as a stretched length **below 2 SD of the mean** for age. It indicates inadequate androgen action in development.
41. A buried penis appears hidden under **pubic fat pad** despite normal length. It can be congenital or acquired with obesity.
42. The most common congenital penile anomaly is **hypospadias**, occurring in ~1/300 male births.
43. The first-line investigation for penile fracture is **ultrasound**, which detects tunical rupture. MRI is more detailed but less available.
44. The standard of care for penile fracture is **immediate surgical repair**, which preserves erectile function and reduces deformity.
45. The most common benign penile tumor is a **papilloma**, usually HPV-related. Other benign tumors are rare.
46. Congenital **megalourethra** arises from mesodermal defects causing deficient corpora support, leading to urethral ballooning.
47. Lichen sclerosus et atrophicus of penis is also known as **balanitis xerotica obliterans (BXO)**. It is chronic, sclerotic, and may cause phimosis.
48. The most common vascular lesion of penis is a **hemangioma**, usually presenting as a red-blue lesion at birth.

49. The best imaging for penile vascular anomalies is **ultrasound Doppler**, which shows flow characteristics non-invasively.
50. The gold standard for diagnosing penile carcinoma is **biopsy**, which confirms histology and guides management

Further Reading

The explanations in this chapter are supported by the following key references:

1. Standring S, editor. Gray's anatomy: the anatomical basis of clinical practice. 42nd ed. Elsevier; 2021.
2. Hsu GL, Brock G, von Heyden B, et al. Anatomy of the human penis: the relationship of the tunica albuginea, corpora cavernosa, and corpus spongiosum. J Androl. 2004;25(3):426–35.
3. Lue TF. Erectile dysfunction. N Engl J Med. 2000;342(24):1802–13.
4. Dean RC, Lue TF. Physiology of penile erection and pathophysiology of erectile dysfunction. Urol Clin N Am. 2005;32(4):379–95.
5. Baskin LS, Erol A, Li YW, et al. Anatomy of the neurovascular bundle of the penis. J Urol. 2000;163(3):925–8.
6. Santucci RA, Eisenberg L. Urethral anatomy and embryology. Urol Clin N Am. 2010;37(3):323–31.

Male Sexual Function and Response Cycle

3

Learning Objectives

- Describe the phases of the male sexual response.
- Identify the central and peripheral neural pathways involved in sexual function.
- Explain the hormonal influences on libido and arousal.
- Recognize the significance of vascular events in erection and detumescence.
- Understand clinical disorders associated with each phase of the response cycle.

Select the Single Best Answer

1. Which of the following occurs in the excitement stage of the male sexual response cycle?
   A. Vasocongestion of the penis
   B. Prosemen secretion
   C. Engorged testes with blood
   D. Blue balls
   E. Marked increase in penile diameter
2. Which of the following occurs in the excitement stage of the male sexual response cycle?
   A. Ischiocavernosus muscle contraction
   B. Accessory gland contraction
   C. Sacrospinal reflex activation
   D. Increase in arterial penile blood flow
   E. Increase in venous return

M. S. M. Hasan, M. L. Elsaie, *Comprehensive MCQs in Andrology*, Trends in Andrology and Sexual Medicine, https://doi.org/10.1007/978-3-032-20623-7_3

3. Which of the following occurs in the plateau stage of the male sexual response cycle?
   A. Blue balls
   B. Vasocongestion of the penis
   C. Intracavernosal pressure above systolic level
   D. Ejaculation
   E. Ischiocavernosus muscle contraction
4. In the latency phase of erection hemodynamics:
   A. Full tumescence and rigidity
   B. Pulsating penile shaft
   C. Increased cavernosal volume
   D. Decrease in penile volume
   E. Constant intracavernosal pressure
5. The sympathetic pathway of erection originates from:
   A. T10–T12
   B. T12–L2
   C. T10–L2
   D. S2–3
   E. S2–4
6. Excitatory erectile neurotransmitter includes:
   A. Oxytocin
   B. Opioids
   C. Endothelin-1
   D. Serotonin
   E. Norepinephrine
7. Inhibitory erectile neurotransmitter includes:
   A. Nitric oxide
   B. Dopamine
   C. Melanocortin
   D. Oxytocin
   E. Serotonin
8. The half-life of nitric oxide is:
   A. 25 s
   B. 20 s
   C. 15 s
   D. 10 s
   E. 5 s
9. Which of the following increases nitric oxide release?
   A. Castration
   B. Diabetes mellitus
   C. Hypercholesterolemia
   D. Androgens
   E. Penile denervation

10. Precursor of nitric oxide synthesis:
    A. Androgen
    B. Serotonin
    C. Oxytocin
    D. L-arginine
    E. Sildenafil
11. cGMP stimulates:
    A. Diacylglycerol
    B. Inositol triphosphate
    C. L-arginine
    D. Guanylate cyclase
    E. Protein kinase G
12. Endothelial nitric oxide stimulates:
    A. Guanylate cyclase
    B. Protein kinase G
    C. Adenylate cyclase
    D. Protein kinase C
    E. Diacylglycerol
13. Which of the following is required for erection?
    A. Sexual arousal
    B. Communication brain ↔ penile nerves
    C. Relaxation of penile blood vessels
    D. B + C
    E. A + B + C
14. Factors in normal erection:
    A. Hemodynamics of corpora cavernosa
    B. Biomechanical properties of tissues
    C. Geometry of the penis
    D. A + B + C
    E. B + C
15. Which condition may still permit erection?
    A. Mild arterial insufficiency with intact venous closure
    B. Severe arterial insufficiency with intact venous closure
    C. Normal arterial flow with venous leak
    D. A + B + C
    E. A + C
16. Why does relaxation of few cavernous fibers induce erection?
    A. Corpora cavernosa communicate
    B. Gap junctions among smooth muscle fibers
    C. Drug diffusion
    D. A + C
    E. B + C

17. pO_2 required for erection:
    A. <20 mmHg
    B. 40–50 mmHg
    C. 60–70 mmHg
    D. 70–80 mmHg
    E. >80 mmHg
18. Hemodynamic factors essential for erection:
    A. Intracavernosal resistance reduction
    B. Increased arterial inflow
    C. Restricted venous outflow
    D. A + B + C
    E. A + B
19. Which becomes engorged during erection?
    A. Corpora cavernosa
    B. Fibrous envelope
    C. Septum pectiniforme
    D. Integument
    E. Dorsal veins
20. Nitric oxide in cavernosal tissue is released from:
    A. Adrenergic nerve endings
    B. Cholinergic nerve endings
    C. Motor nerve endings
    D. Non-adrenergic nerve endings
    E. Non-adrenergic, non-cholinergic nerve endings
21. Essential substrate for nitric oxide synthesis:
    A. Endothelin-1
    B. ATP
    C. Oxygen
    D. Androgen
    E. Serotonin
22. FALSE about excitement stage of EPOR model:
    A. Tachycardia
    B. Increased blood pressure
    C. Increased respiratory rate
    D. Relaxation of facial muscles
    E. Sex flush
23. NOT true about erection neurophysiology:
    A. Spinal erection center S2–4
    B. Tactile input via dorsal penile nerve
    C. Hypothalamic projections to midbrain tegmentum
    D. Sacral center sends impulses via sympathetic cavernous nerves
    E. Prosemen secretion

24. FALSE about excitement stage of EPOR:
    A. Penile erection
    B. Scrotal lift
    C. Testes elevation
    D. Bladder neck closure
    E. Prosemen release
25. Role of glans penis in erection:
    A. Constricts urethral lumen
    B. Facilitates intromission
    C. Pumps blood distally
    D. Supports corpus spongiosum
    E. Veno-occlusive mechanism
26. NOT a pro-sexual neurotransmitter:
    A. Dopamine
    B. Acetylcholine
    C. Oxytocin
    D. Serotonin (5-HT)
    E. Nitric oxide
27. NOT true about NO signaling:
    A. NO stimulates cGMP production
    B. nNOS initiates erection, eNOS maintains it
    C. cGMP activates PKG → opens K^+, closes Ca^{2+} channels
    D. Low Ca^{2+} favors relaxation
    E. PDE degrades cGMP to maintain erection
28. NOT true about testosterone:
    A. Enhances libido
    B. Increases frequency of intercourse
    C. Increases nocturnal erections
    D. Increases visually stimulated erections
    E. Increases bone and lean mass
29. NOT true:
    A. NO is principal mediator
    B. Oxytocin induces erection in CNS
    C. Norepinephrine facilitates erection
    D. GABA-B is pro-erectile
    E. Cannabinoid CB1 inhibits erection
30. NOT true about smooth muscle contraction:
    A. MLCP holoenzyme structure
    B. MLCP inhibition enhances contraction
    C. Rho kinase phosphorylation enhances contraction
    D. Ca^{2+} entry via receptor-operated channels
    E. Latch state = relaxation phase

31. NOT true about NO:
    A. NOS converts arginine + O_2 → NO + citrulline
    B. nNOS upregulated in aging diabetic rats
    C. Three NOS isoforms: nNOS, iNOS, eNOS
    D. Gene transfer nNOS/eNOS augments erection
    E. iNOS gene transfer enhances erection
32. NOT true:
    A. CNP is most potent natriuretic peptide
    B. PKG-I induces relaxation via multiple mechanisms
    C. Low penile adenosine → priapism
    D. CGRP is potent vasodilator
    E. PGE1 erectogenic effects documented
33. Corpus spongiosum role:
    A. Compresses bulb to expel semen
    B. Pumps blood distally
    C. Constricts urethra
    D. Participates in veno-occlusive mechanism
    E. Regulates sinusoidal flow
34. TNF-α and erection, FALSE:
    A. Impairs NO-mediated vasodilation
    B. Endothelial dysfunction key in ED
    C. Oxidative stress predisposes ED
    D. Activates Rho-kinase pathway
    E. Upregulates nNOS expression
35. Which is NOT a male aphrodisiac?
    A. Grapes
    B. Watercress
    C. Ambrein
    D. Saltpeter
    E. Tribulus terrestris
36. Penile erection results from:
    A. Decrease in cAMP
    B. Upregulation of fibrotic cytokines
    C. Cavernosal smooth muscle contraction
    D. Increased prostaglandins
37. Which erectogenic drug can cause false-positive opiate test?
    A. Avanafil
    B. Papaverine
    C. Phentolamine
    D. Trazodone
38. Factors in normal erection:
    A. Corpora cavernosa hemodynamics
    B. Tissue biomechanics
    C. Penile geometry
    D. All of the above

39. NO in cavernosal tissue is released from:
    A. Adrenergic endings
    B. Cholinergic endings
    C. Motor endings
    D. NANC nerve endings
40. Essential mediator for smooth muscle relaxation:
    A. Endothelin-1
    B. ATP
    C. cGMP
    D. GMP
41. During sexual stimulation, FALSE:
    A. Scrotal wall thickens
    B. Testes elevate
    C. Testes enlarge
    D. Erection by parasympathetic dilation
    E. Ejaculation always before detumescence
42. Intracavernosal drugs causing erection, EXCEPT:
    A. Phenoxybenzamine
    B. Clonidine
    C. Papaverine
    D. Prostaglandins
    E. Phentolamine
43. Sexual dysfunction links, FALSE:
    A. ED in diabetes
    B. Orgasmic dysfunction in diabetic women
    C. ED and ejaculatory dysfunction in hypertension
    D. Low libido in renal failure
    E. Increased libido in multiple sclerosis

Added Questions (44–50)

44. Emission phase of ejaculation is mediated mainly by:
    A. Parasympathetic S2–4
    B. Sympathetic T12–L2
    C. Pudendal motor nerves
    D. Hypogastric plexus only
    E. Dorsal penile nerve
45. Expulsion phase of ejaculation is mediated by contraction of:
    A. Bulbospongiosus and ischiocavernosus
    B. Levator ani
    C. Detrusor
    D. Dartos
    E. Cremaster

46. The refractory period after orgasm is primarily due to:
    A. Prolactin release
    B. Testosterone surge
    C. Elevated dopamine
    D. Persistent cGMP levels
    E. Estrogen activity
47. Which hormone is most important for libido?
    A. Cortisol
    B. Testosterone
    C. LH
    D. Prolactin
    E. FSH
48. Which neurotransmitter is anti-erectile?
    A. Serotonin
    B. Dopamine
    C. Oxytocin
    D. Nitric oxide
    E. Melanocortin
49. Which PDE is inhibited by sildenafil?
    A. PDE-2
    B. PDE-3
    C. PDE-4
    D. PDE-5
    E. PDE-6
50. The most common vascular cause of ED is:
    A. Cavernosal arterial insufficiency
    B. Venous leakage
    C. Peyronie's disease
    D. Varicocele
    E. Deep dorsal vein thrombosis

✅ Key Takeaways

- The male sexual response includes libido, erection, orgasm, and resolution.
- Penile erection is mediated by parasympathetic activation and nitric oxide-induced vasodilation.
- Sympathetic discharge facilitates emission and ejaculation.
- Testosterone plays a central role in maintaining libido and erectile function.
- Neurological integrity is essential; spinal cord injuries at different levels can impair specific sexual phases.
- Psychological factors and interpersonal context profoundly influence arousal and satisfaction.
- Disorders include hypoactive sexual desire, erectile dysfunction, delayed orgasm, and anorgasmia.

✅ Answer Key (1–50)

1. A
2. D
3. C
4. D
5. C
6. A
7. E
8. E
9. D
10. D
11. E
12. A
13. E
14. D
15. E
16. B
17. C
18. D
19. A
20. E
21. C
22. D
23. D
24. E
25. B
26. D
27. E
28. D
29. C
30. E
31. B
32. A
33. C
34. E
35. D
36. D
37. B
38. D
39. D
40. C
41. E
42. B

43. E
44. B
45. A
46. A
47. B
48. A
49. D
50. A

Explanations (1–50)

1. During the excitement phase, **vasocongestion of the penis** occurs as penile arteries dilate, increasing blood inflow and initiating erection. Other listed events occur later.
2. Early in arousal, **arterial penile inflow increases**, leading to tumescence. Ischiocavernosus contraction happens in plateau/orgasm.
3. In plateau, **intracavernosal pressure exceeds systolic pressure** due to full rigidity. This maintains erection until ejaculation.
4. Latency phase means post-detumescence, with **penile volume reduced** and cavernosal pressure normalized.
5. The sympathetic outflow important in erection/ejaculation is from **T10–L2** segments, contributing to emission and detumescence.
6. **Oxytocin** facilitates erections centrally. Endothelin and norepinephrine are inhibitory.
7. **Serotonin** is inhibitory to erection, explaining why SSRIs cause ED.
8. Nitric oxide has a very short half-life, about **5 seconds**, enabling rapid local action.
9. **Androgens** increase NO activity; castration, diabetes, and hyperlipidemia reduce it.
10. **L-arginine** is the amino acid precursor for NO synthesis.
11. cGMP acts via **protein kinase G**, leading to smooth muscle relaxation.
12. NO activates **guanylate cyclase**, raising cGMP.
13. Erection requires **arousal, intact neural communication, and vascular relaxation**. All three must work in concert.
14. Normal erection depends on **hemodynamics, tissue biomechanics, and penile geometry**.
15. ED can occur even with mild arterial insufficiency or venous leakage. **Both arterial inflow and venous occlusion must be intact** for rigidity.
16. Relaxation spreads via **gap junctions between smooth muscle cells**, so even localized relaxation can propagate.
17. Cavernosal pO_2 must rise to **60–70 mmHg** to sustain erection.
18. Essential hemodynamics: **arterial inflow increase, intracavernosal resistance drop, and venous restriction**.
19. Erection fills **corpora cavernosa**, the erectile bodies.
20. NO in corpora is released by **NANC nerves** (non-adrenergic, non-cholinergic).

21. Substrates for NO synthesis include **oxygen and L-arginine**.
22. In excitement, HR, BP, and respiration rise; sex flush may occur. **Facial relaxation is false**.
23. Erection is parasympathetic (S2–4). Sympathetic cavernous fibers regulate ejaculation, not erection initiation.
24. Excitement includes erection, scrotal lift, and testis elevation. **Bladder neck closure and prosemen release happen later**.
25. The glans facilitates **intromission** by lubrication and shape.
26. **Serotonin** is inhibitory, not pro-erectile.
27. PDE degrades cGMP to end erection. Saying "PDE maintains erection" is false.
28. Testosterone increases libido and nocturnal erections but **not visually triggered erections**.
29. **Norepinephrine is anti-erectile** (vasoconstrictive). Claiming it facilitates erection is false.
30. The "latch state" is a **sustained contraction**, not relaxation.
31. iNOS gene transfer does not improve erections.
32. CNP is not the most potent NP. ANP/BNP are stronger. So this statement is false.
33. Corpus spongiosum primarily **keeps urethra open under pressure** for semen expulsion.
34. TNF-α impairs NO, increases oxidative stress. **It downregulates nNOS**, not upregulates.
35. **Saltpeter** is not an aphrodisiac. Grapes, watercress, ambrein, tribulus have roles.
36. Erection involves **prostaglandins** raising cAMP and cGMP, not decreases.
37. **Papaverine** may give false opiate positives.
38. Normal erection needs **hemodynamics, biomechanics, geometry**—all factors.
39. NO arises from **NANC nerve endings** in corpora.
40. cGMP is the **main mediator** of smooth muscle relaxation.
41. Ejaculation does not always precede detumescence. That statement is false.
42. **Clonidine** is not erectogenic. Others are.
43. Multiple sclerosis usually causes **reduced libido**, not increased.
44. Emission is sympathetic (T12–L2), propelling semen into urethra.
45. Expulsion uses **bulbospongiosus and ischiocavernosus** contractions.
46. Refractory period is prolonged by **prolactin release** post-orgasm.
47. **Testosterone** is the hormone most vital for libido.
48. **Serotonin** is the main inhibitory neurotransmitter for erection. Elevated serotonin reduces penile tumescence and delays ejaculation, explaining why SSRIs cause sexual side effects. In contrast, dopamine, oxytocin, NO, and melanocortins are all pro-erectile.
49. **Sildenafil** inhibits **PDE-5**, preventing the breakdown of cGMP. This prolongs smooth muscle relaxation, enhancing cavernosal blood flow and sustaining erection. Its selectivity for PDE-5 explains efficacy, though mild PDE-6 inhibition explains visual side effects.
50. The most common vascular cause of erectile dysfunction is **arterial insufficiency of cavernosal arteries**, typically due to atherosclerosis, hypertension,

diabetes, or smoking. Venous leak is also possible, but less common. This is why ED is considered an early marker of cardiovascular disease.

Further Reading

The explanations in this chapter are supported by the following key references:

1. Masters WH, Johnson VE. Human sexual response. Boston: Little, Brown; 1966.
2. Bancroft J. Human sexuality and its problems. 3rd ed. Churchill Livingstone; 2009.
3. Giuliano F, Rampin O. Neural control of erection. Physiol Rev. 2000;80(2):537–76.
4. Andersson KE. Mechanisms of penile erection and basis for pharmacological treatment of erectile dysfunction. Pharmacol Rev. 2011;63(4):811–59.
5. Waldinger MD. The neurobiological approach to premature ejaculation. J Sex Med. 2015;12(4):123–35.
6. Corona G, Rastrelli G, Maggi M. The physiology of male sexual function. Endocr Rev. 2019;40(4):108–32.

Male Reproductive Anatomy and Physiology

4

Learning Objectives

- Describe the hormonal control of the HPG axis.
- Understand the cellular role of Sertoli and Leydig cells in the testis.
- Trace the process of spermatogenesis from spermatogonia to mature spermatozoa.
- Explain sperm maturation and storage in the epididymis.
- Recognize the feedback mechanisms regulating testosterone and gonadotropins.

Select the Single Best Answer

1. Which of the following structures is responsible for sperm production?
   A. Epididymis
   B. Vas deferens
   C. Rete testis
   D. Seminiferous tubules
   E. Prostate gland
2. The hormone that primarily stimulates Leydig cells to produce testosterone is:
   A. FSH
   B. LH
   C. Prolactin
   D. Inhibin
   E. GnRH
3. Sertoli cells are involved in all of the following EXCEPT:
   A. Formation of the blood-testis barrier
   B. Nourishment of developing sperm
   C. Secretion of inhibin
   D. Testosterone production
   E. Phagocytosis of residual cytoplasm

M. S. M. Hasan, M. L. Elsaie, *Comprehensive MCQs in Andrology*, Trends in Andrology and Sexual Medicine, https://doi.org/10.1007/978-3-032-20623-7_4

4. The acrosome of the sperm is derived from which organelle?
   A. Nucleus
   B. Mitochondria
   C. Golgi apparatus
   D. Rough endoplasmic reticulum
   E. Lysosome
5. The pampiniform plexus plays an essential role in:
   A. Sperm capacitation
   B. Nutrient absorption
   C. Thermoregulation of the testis
   D. Testosterone storage
   E. Spermatid adhesion
6. The tunica albuginea is:
   A. The inner lining of seminiferous tubules
   B. A connective tissue capsule surrounding the testis
   C. A muscle sheath of the scrotum
   D. The fibrous lining of the epididymis
   E. The lining of the tunica vaginalis
7. The prostate secretes which of the following components into semen?
   A. Spermatozoa
   B. Fructose
   C. Alkaline phosphatase
   D. Acid phosphatase
   E. Progesterone
8. Which part of the epididymis is primarily responsible for sperm storage?
   A. Head
   B. Neck
   C. Body
   D. Tail
   E. Vas deferens
9. The ejaculatory duct is formed by the union of:
   A. Epididymis and urethra
   B. Seminal vesicle and prostate
   C. Vas deferens and seminal vesicle
   D. Prostate and urethra
   E. Urethra and Cowper's gland
10. Which layer of the testis is derived from the peritoneum?
   A. Tunica vaginalis
   B. Tunica albuginea
   C. Dartos fascia
   D. Cremasteric fascia
   E. Colles' fascia

11. The dartos muscle is responsible for:
    A. Sperm propulsion
    B. Thermoregulation by skin wrinkling
    C. Blood flow regulation to testis
    D. Sperm capacitation
    E. Penile erection
12. Spermatogenesis is regulated by:
    A. Testosterone alone
    B. FSH and testosterone
    C. LH and prolactin
    D. Estrogen
    E. Inhibin
13. The blood-testis barrier is formed by:
    A. Leydig cells
    B. Spermatogonia
    C. Sertoli cells
    D. Myoid cells
    E. Peritubular capillaries
14. The structure that carries sperm from the epididymis to the ejaculatory duct is:
    A. Seminal vesicle
    B. Urethra
    C. Vas deferens
    D. Cowper's gland
    E. Prostate
15. Which of the following is NOT a component of semen?
    A. Sperm
    B. Seminal fluid
    C. Prostatic secretions
    D. Urine
    E. Secretions from Cowper's glands
16. Fructose in semen is primarily secreted by:
    A. Prostate
    B. Epididymis
    C. Seminal vesicles
    D. Cowper's glands
    E. Testis
17. Testosterone is converted to DHT in target tissues by:
    A. Aromatase
    B. 17β-HSD
    C. 5α-reductase
    D. 3β-HSD
    E. FSH

18. The enzyme responsible for sperm motility regulation is:
    A. Hyaluronidase
    B. Phosphodiesterase
    C. Tyrosine kinase
    D. cAMP-dependent protein kinase
    E. Acrosin
19. Which testicular cell type produces inhibin?
    A. Leydig cells
    B. Sertoli cells
    C. Myoid cells
    D. Spermatogonia
    E. Spermatocytes
20. Capacitation of sperm occurs in:
    A. Seminiferous tubules
    B. Epididymis
    C. Vas deferens
    D. Urethra
    E. Female reproductive tract
21. Which zone of the prostate is most commonly involved in BPH?
    A. Central zone
    B. Peripheral zone
    C. Transitional zone
    D. Anterior fibromuscular zone
    E. Posterior zone
22. Which of the following structures secretes mucus during ejaculation?
    A. Prostate
    B. Seminal vesicles
    C. Cowper's glands
    D. Testes
    E. Epididymis
23. The prostate is histologically classified as a:
    A. Simple tubular gland
    B. Compound tubuloalveolar gland
    C. Compound acinar gland
    D. Serous gland
    E. Mucous gland
24. The tunica vaginalis consists of:
    A. Smooth muscle
    B. Fibrous tissue
    C. Parietal and visceral layers
    D. Only a visceral layer
    E. Epithelial folds

25. Which of the following is derived from the mesonephric duct?
    A. Uterus
    B. Fallopian tubes
    C. Epididymis
    D. Urethra
    E. Vagina
26. The gubernaculum is responsible for:
    A. Testicular hormone production
    B. Testicular descent
    C. Sperm production
    D. Sperm motility
    E. Spermatid formation
27. The Leydig cells are located in:
    A. Within seminiferous tubules
    B. Interstitial space between tubules
    C. Basement membrane
    D. Tunica albuginea
    E. Epididymis
28. The muscle responsible for testicular elevation is:
    A. Dartos
    B. Cremaster
    C. Internal oblique
    D. External oblique
    E. Puborectalis
29. The spermatic cord contains all of the following EXCEPT:
    A. Vas deferens
    B. Pampiniform plexus
    C. Testicular artery
    D. Ureter
    E. Cremasteric muscle
30. The zona pellucida reaction is triggered by:
    A. Sperm motility
    B. Acrosome reaction
    C. Hormonal surge
    D. Penetration of corona radiata
    E. Flagellar movement
31. Sperm maturation occurs primarily in the:
    A. Testis
    B. Epididymal head
    C. Epididymal tail
    D. Rete testis
    E. Vas deferens

32. The chromosomal sex of a male is:
    A. XX
    B. XY
    C. YY
    D. XO
    E. XXY
33. The process of sperm development is known as:
    A. Spermiogenesis
    B. Spermatocytogenesis
    C. Spermatogenesis
    D. Fertilization
    E. Oogenesis
34. What is the ideal temperature for spermatogenesis?
    A. 35 °C
    B. 37 °C
    C. 33 °C
    D. 39 °C
    E. 30 °C
35. Which testicular hormone provides negative feedback to FSH secretion?
    A. Testosterone
    B. Estrogen
    C. Inhibin
    D. DHT
    E. Activin
36. Spermiation refers to:
    A. Formation of spermatids
    B. Differentiation of spermatocytes
    C. Release of mature sperm into lumen
    D. Fertilization
    E. Maturation in epididymis
37. Sperm gain full motility in the:
    A. Testis
    B. Vas deferens
    C. Ejaculatory duct
    D. Epididymis
    E. Seminal vesicle
38. The enzyme facilitating sperm penetration of zona pellucida is:
    A. Hyaluronidase
    B. Acrosin
    C. Trypsin
    D. Lipase
    E. Helicase

39. The epididymis connects the testis to the:
    A. Seminal vesicle
    B. Prostate
    C. Vas deferens
    D. Urethra
    E. Ejaculatory duct
40. The most posterior part of the male urethra is the:
    A. Spongy
    B. Membranous
    C. Penile
    D. Bulbar
    E. Prostatic
41. Which cell organelle is most abundant in the sperm midpiece?
    A. Nucleus
    B. Ribosomes
    C. Golgi apparatus
    D. Mitochondria
    E. Rough ER
42. Spermatogonia are located:
    A. Within the lumen of seminiferous tubules
    B. Between Sertoli cells
    C. Adjacent to the basement membrane
    D. In the rete testis
    E. In the epididymis
43. Which of the following is NOT a function of the seminal vesicles?
    A. Secretion of fructose
    B. Prostaglandin secretion
    C. Fibrinogen-like protein secretion
    D. Sperm motility inhibition
    E. Acid phosphatase secretion
44. Which of the following testicular cells is diploid (2n)?
    A. Spermatids
    B. Spermatocytes (primary)
    C. Spermatogonia
    D. Sertoli cells
    E. Both B and C
45. Which segment of the male urethra passes through the urogenital diaphragm?
    A. Prostatic
    B. Membranous
    C. Bulbar
    D. Penile
    E. Spongy

46. The urethral glands of Littre are located in the:
    A. Prostatic urethra
    B. Membranous urethra
    C. Spongy urethra
    D. Bladder neck
    E. Ejaculatory duct
47. Which phase describes the conversion of spermatids to mature spermatozoa?
    A. Spermatogenesis
    B. Spermatocytogenesis
    C. Spermiogenesis
    D. Fertilization
    E. Capacitation
48. The most common type of epithelium in the male reproductive tract is:
    A. Simple squamous
    B. Stratified squamous
    C. Simple columnar
    D. Pseudostratified columnar
    E. Transitional
49. The terminal part of the vas deferens widens to form the:
    A. Ejaculatory duct
    B. Ampulla
    C. Epididymal duct
    D. Spermatic sinus
    E. Tunica vaginalis
50. Which of the following contributes the largest volume to semen?
    A. Prostate
    B. Cowper's glands
    C. Testes
    D. Seminal vesicles
    E. Urethral glands

✅ Key Takeaways

- The **HPG axis** regulates testosterone production and spermatogenesis via **GnRH, LH, and FSH**.
- **Leydig cells** produce testosterone under LH stimulation; **Sertoli cells** support spermatogenesis under FSH.
- **Spermatogenesis** takes approximately 74 days and involves mitosis, meiosis, and spermiogenesis.
- The **epididymis** is crucial for sperm maturation, motility acquisition, and storage.
- Testosterone and inhibin B exert **negative feedback** on the hypothalamus and pituitary.
- Disruptions in hormonal balance can lead to **infertility** or **hypogonadism**.
- Understanding this physiology informs diagnosis and treatment of **male infertility** and **androgen disorders**.

✅ Answer Key (1–50)

1. A
2. B
3. E
4. C
5. D
6. A
7. C
8. B
9. B
10. A
11. D
12. C
13. A
14. D
15. B
16. E
17. D
18. A
19. B
20. C
21. D
22. B
23. C
24. A
25. E
26. D
27. A
28. E
29. B
30. C
31. A
32. C
33. D
34. B
35. C
36. E
37. A
38. D
39. C
40. A
41. E
42. B

43. A
44. C
45. D
46. A
47. C
48. E
49. B
50. D

Explanations (1–50)

1. Seminiferous tubules are the sites of spermatogenesis. These coiled structures in the testis house germ cells and Sertoli cells responsible for the development and maturation of sperm.
2. LH (Luteinizing hormone) stimulates Leydig cells to produce testosterone, essential for spermatogenesis and male secondary sexual characteristics.
3. Sertoli cells do many things—form the blood-testis barrier, secrete inhibin, and support germ cells—but do not produce testosterone, which is done by Leydig cells.
4. The acrosome originates from the Golgi apparatus and contains enzymes (like acrosin) that help the sperm penetrate the egg during fertilization.
5. The pampiniform plexus is a venous network that regulates temperature by cooling arterial blood entering the testes, critical for optimal sperm production.
6. The tunica albuginea is a dense connective tissue capsule surrounding the testes and providing structural integrity.
7. The prostate secretes acidic fluid rich in enzymes like acid phosphatase and PSA, which helps in liquefying semen post-ejaculation.
8. The tail of the epididymis stores mature sperm until ejaculation. It is functionally distinct from the head and body regions.
9. The ejaculatory duct forms from the union of the vas deferens and seminal vesicle, transporting sperm to the urethra.
10. The tunica vaginalis is a serous membrane derived from peritoneum, covering the testes except at the posterior border.
11. The dartos muscle, located in the scrotal wall, wrinkles the scrotal skin to conserve heat during cold temperatures.
12. FSH and testosterone work together to stimulate Sertoli cells and complete the process of spermatogenesis.
13. The blood-testis barrier, formed by tight junctions between Sertoli cells, protects developing sperm from immune attack.
14. The vas deferens is a muscular tube that transports sperm from the epididymis to the ejaculatory ducts.
15. Urine is not a component of semen; presence of urine indicates pathology. Normal semen includes sperm, prostatic, and seminal vesicle secretions.
16. Fructose, a major energy source for sperm, is secreted by the seminal vesicles.

17. 5α-reductase converts testosterone to dihydrotestosterone (DHT), which has a higher affinity for androgen receptors in target tissues.
18. cAMP-dependent protein kinase is key to regulating sperm motility by modifying flagellar beat.
19. Sertoli cells produce inhibin, which provides negative feedback to the anterior pituitary to reduce FSH levels.
20. Capacitation is the final maturation step of sperm that occurs in the female reproductive tract and enables fertilization.
21. The transitional zone of the prostate is most commonly involved in benign prostatic hyperplasia (BPH).
22. Cowper's glands secrete a mucus-like pre-ejaculate that lubricates and neutralizes urethral acidity during sexual arousal.
23. The prostate is a compound tubuloalveolar gland, with multiple ducts opening into the prostatic urethra.
24. The tunica vaginalis is made up of a parietal and visceral layer and functions to reduce friction between testis and scrotum.
25. The epididymis develops from the mesonephric (Wolffian) duct during embryogenesis.
26. The gubernaculum guides testicular descent from the abdomen into the scrotum during fetal development.
27. Leydig cells are found in the interstitial spaces between seminiferous tubules and secrete testosterone.
28. The cremaster muscle, derived from the internal oblique, elevates the testes in response to temperature or tactile stimuli.
29. The ureter is not part of the spermatic cord. The cord contains vas deferens, arteries, veins, lymphatics, and nerves.
30. The zona pellucida reaction is triggered by the acrosome reaction, facilitating sperm penetration into the oocyte.
31. Sperm maturation—acquiring motility and fertilizing capability—occurs in the epididymis, especially in the tail.
32. The male chromosomal sex is XY, with the Y chromosome determining male differentiation.
33. Spermatogenesis is the overall process of sperm production from spermatogonia to spermatozoa.
34. The optimal temperature for spermatogenesis is 2–4 °C below body temperature, i.e., around 34–35 °C.
35. Inhibin, secreted by Sertoli cells, selectively inhibits FSH release, regulating spermatogenesis.
36. Spermiation is the final step of spermatogenesis where mature spermatozoa are released into the lumen of seminiferous tubules.
37. Sperm gain full motility in the epididymis, assisted by secretions and structural maturation.
38. Acrosin, released from the acrosome, digests the zona pellucida, allowing sperm to penetrate the ovum.
39. The epididymis connects the testis to the vas deferens, facilitating transport and maturation of sperm.

40. The membranous urethra is the shortest and most posterior segment of the male urethra, passing through the urogenital diaphragm.
41. The midpiece of sperm contains numerous mitochondria to generate ATP required for flagellar movement.
42. Spermatogonia, the earliest germ cells, are diploid and reside near the basement membrane of seminiferous tubules.
43. Seminal vesicles secrete fructose, prostaglandins, and fibrinogen-like proteins—but not acid phosphatase, which is a prostatic product.
44. Both primary spermatocytes and spermatogonia are diploid (2n) cells involved in the early stages of spermatogenesis.
45. The membranous urethra passes through the urogenital diaphragm and is surrounded by the external urethral sphincter.
46. The glands of Littre are mucous-secreting glands located along the spongy (penile) urethra.
47. Spermiogenesis is the transformation of spermatids into mature spermatozoa, involving nuclear condensation and flagella formation.
48. Most of the male reproductive tract is lined by pseudostratified columnar epithelium, suited for absorption and secretion.
49. The ampulla is the dilated terminal part of the vas deferens, which joins the seminal vesicle to form the ejaculatory duct.
50. The seminal vesicles contribute ~60–70% of semen volume, making them the largest contributor.

Further Reading

The explanations in this chapter are supported by the following key references:

1. Guyton AC, Hall JE. Textbook of medical physiology. 14th ed. Elsevier; 2021.
2. Plant TM, Zeleznik AJ. Knobil and Neill's physiology of reproduction. 4th ed. Academic Press; 2015.
3. Walker WH. Molecular mechanisms of testosterone action in spermatogenesis. Steroids. 2009;74(7):602–7.
4. Sharpe RM. Regulation of spermatogenesis. In: Endocrinology: adult and pediatric. Elsevier; 2021.
5. Ramasamy R, Stahl PJ, Schlegel PN. Medical therapy for spermatogenic dysfunction. Nat Rev Urol. 2012;9(1):56–65.
6. Aitken RJ, Baker MA. Oxidative stress, sperm survival and fertility control. Mol Cell Endocrinol. 2006;250(1–2):66–9.

Male Sexual Orientation, Identity, and Behavior Disorders

5

Learning Objectives

- Define sexual orientation and distinguish it from sexual behavior and identity.
- Examine theories regarding the origins of sexual orientation.
- Discuss neurobiological and genetic findings related to male sexual orientation.
- Appreciate sociocultural and psychological factors influencing orientation.
- Recognize the implications for medical care and psychological support.

Select the Single Best Answer

1. In sexual medicine, "gender" refers to:
   A. Socially defined roles and norms
   B. Composite of sex plus personal traits
   C. Identity matching assigned sex
   D. Identity different from assigned sex
   E. Living as identified gender
2. "Cisgender" means:
   A. Social rules for men/women
   B. Composite of biology and traits
   C. Identity aligns with assigned sex
   D. Identity differs from assigned sex
   E. Social transition to affirmed gender
3. "Transgender" means:
   A. Social rules for men/women
   B. Composite of sex + traits
   C. Identity aligns with assigned sex
   D. Identity differs from assigned sex/expectations
   E. Social transition to affirmed gender

M. S. M. Hasan, M. L. Elsaie, *Comprehensive MCQs in Andrology*, Trends in Andrology and Sexual Medicine, https://doi.org/10.1007/978-3-032-20623-7_5

4. The essence of gender dysphoria is:
   A. Non-sexual identity incongruence
   B. Physical abnormalities
   C. Primarily sexual arousal
   D. Arousal-dependent
   E. Attraction to desired gender only
5. “Gender expression” describes:
   A. Social rules
   B. Outward communication of gender (dress/voice/behavior)
   C. Identity aligns with assigned sex
   D. Identity different from assigned sex
   E. Process of living as identified gender
6. Most accurate single cause of gender dysphoria:
   A. Genetic only
   B. Hormonal imbalance only
   C. Psychological only
   D. Idiopathic/multifactorial
   E. Faulty bonding/child-rearing alone
7. Kinsey score **0** indicates:
   A. Exclusively homosexual
   B. Predominantly homosexual, incidental heterosexual
   C. Predominantly homosexual, more than incidental hetero
   D. Exclusively heterosexual
   E. Predominantly heterosexual, incidental homosexual
8. Kinsey score **1** indicates:
   A. Exclusively homosexual
   B. Predominantly homosexual, incidental hetero
   C. Predominantly homosexual, > incidental hetero
   D. Exclusively heterosexual
   E. Predominantly heterosexual, incidental homosexual
9. Kinsey score **6** indicates:
   A. Exclusively homosexual
   B. Predominantly homosexual, incidental hetero
   C. Predominantly homosexual, > incidental hetero
   D. Exclusively heterosexual
   E. Predominantly heterosexual, incidental homosexual
10. Kinsey score **5** indicates:
   A. Exclusively homosexual
   B. Predominantly homosexual, incidental hetero
   C. Predominantly homosexual, > incidental hetero
   D. Exclusively heterosexual
   E. Predominantly heterosexual, incidental homosexual

11. Kinsey score **4** means:
    A. Exclusively homosexual
    B. Predominantly homosexual, incidental hetero
    C. Predominantly homosexual, > incidental hetero
    D. Exclusively heterosexual
    E. Predominantly heterosexual, incidental homosexual
12. Enteric/STI proctitis historically labeled “gay bowel syndrome” is commonest in:
    A. Heterosexual men
    B. MSM (gay/bisexual men)
    C. Lesbians
    D. Cisgender broadly
    E. Gender dysphoria
13. **Exhibitionism** is:
    A. Arousal from being humiliated/bound
    B. Attraction to prepubescent children
    C. Touching/rubbing non-consenting persons
    D. Use of inanimate objects for arousal
    E. Exposing genitals to unsuspecting persons
14. **Fetishism** is:
    A. Arousal from being humiliated
    B. Attraction to prepubescent children
    C. Non-consensual rubbing
    D. Arousal from inanimate objects
    E. Exposing genitals to strangers
15. **Frotteurism** is:
    A. Arousal from suffering
    B. Attraction to prepubescents
    C. Non-consensual touching/rubbing
    D. Arousal from objects
    E. Public exposure
16. **Pedophilia** is:
    A. Arousal from suffering
    B. Attraction to prepubescent children
    C. Non-consensual rubbing
    D. Arousal from objects
    E. Exposing genitals
17. **Masochism** is:
    A. Arousal from being humiliated or in pain
    B. Attraction to prepubescents
    C. Non-consensual rubbing
    D. Arousal from objects
    E. Public exposure

18. Face masking/blowing as a sexual focus best fits:
    A. Masochism
    B. Pedophilia
    C. Frotteurism
    D. Exhibitionism
    E. Fetishism
19. **Necrophilia** is sexual interest in:
    A. Adults
    B. Enemas
    C. Corpses
    D. Body parts
    E. Vomiting
20. **Teleiophilia** is sexual interest in:
    A. Adults
    B. Enemas
    C. Corpses
    D. Body parts
    E. Vomiting
21. **Partialism** is sexual interest in:
    A. Adults
    B. Enemas
    C. Corpses
    D. Specific body parts
    E. Vomiting
22. **Klismaphilia** is sexual interest in:
    A. Adults
    B. Enemas
    C. Corpses
    D. Body parts
    E. Vomiting
23. **Emetophilia** is sexual interest in:
    A. Adults
    B. Enemas
    C. Corpses
    D. Body parts
    E. Vomiting
24. Main mimic of infantile masturbation (gratification disorder):
    A. Dyskinesia
    B. Dystonia
    C. Child abuse
    D. Epilepsy
    E. Parasitosis

25. "Idiosyncratic" masturbation often refers to:
    A. Inflatable dolls/artificial vaginas
    B. Circular clitoral massage
    C. Insertion of fingers/phallic objects vaginally
    D. Prone rubbing against sheets
    E. Manual penile stimulation
26. The most common basic sexual position:
    A. Missionary
    B. Viennese oyster
    C. Butterfly
    D. Riding high
    E. Cowgirl
27. **Fellatio** is:
    A. Intercrural rubbing
    B. Foreskin-to-glans mutual masturbation
    C. Circular group oral acts
    D. Oral sex on female genitals
    E. Oral sex on male genitals
28. **Cunnilingus** is:
    A. Intercrural rubbing
    B. Foreskin docking
    C. Group circular oral acts
    D. Oral sex on female genitals
    E. Oral sex on male genitals
29. **Bukkake** refers to:
    A. Group of males ejaculating on one person
    B. Intercrural rubbing
    C. Mutual foreskin "sheathed" masturbation
    D. Group circular oral sex
    E. Simultaneous oral sex by two people
30. **Frottage** (consensual male-male) is:
    A. Group male ejaculation on one person
    B. Mutual penile rubbing between two males
    C. Foreskin docking
    D. Group circular oral sex
    E. Simultaneous oral sex
31. **Tribadism** is:
    A. Group male ejaculation
    B. Male-male penile rubbing
    C. Female-female vulvar rubbing
    D. Group circular oral sex
    E. Simultaneous oral sex

32. **Docking** is:
    A. Group male ejaculation
    B. Male-male penile rubbing
    C. Female-female vulvar rubbing
    D. Group circular oral sex
    E. Glans inserted into another's foreskin
33. **Daisy chain** describes:
    A. Group male ejaculation
    B. Male-male penile rubbing
    C. Female-female vulvar rubbing
    D. Chain of partners each doing oral sex on the next
    E. Mutual foreskin docking
34. Freud's **oral stage**:
    A. 1–3 y
    B. 3–6 y
    C. Birth–1 y
    D. 6–puberty
    E. Puberty–adult
35. Freud's **genital stage**:
    A. 1–3 y
    B. 3–6 y
    C. Birth–1 y
    D. 6–puberty
    E. Puberty–adult
36. Freud's **phallic stage**:
    A. 1–3 y
    B. 3–6 y
    C. Birth–1 y
    D. 6–puberty
    E. Puberty–adult
37. Freud's **anal stage**:
    A. 1–3 y
    B. 3–6 y
    C. Birth–1 y
    D. 6–puberty
    E. Puberty–adult
38. Most accurate statement about gender dysphoria:
    A. A person's own sense of gender identity
    B. Always fixed early in childhood
    C. Static after puberty
    D. Entirely culturally determined
    E. Localized to cerebrum alone

39. A key biological factor in gender development:
    A. Psychological only
    B. Prenatal hormones
    C. Prenatal social context
    D. Postnatal social context
    E. Post-pubertal hormones only
40. Before genital gender-affirming surgery, standards typically include:
    A. ≥18 years of age
    B. Daily opposite-gender undergarments
    C. ~12 months real-life experience + continuous hormones
    D. A + C
    E. B + C
41. **Sexual orientation** best defined as:
    A. Knowledge about sex topics
    B. School sex-ed activities
    C. A chosen decision to prefer same-sex encounters
    D. Pattern of erotic/romantic attraction by others' gender(s)
    E. Most frequent sexual behavior
42. Orientation vs behavior—most accurate:
    A. Behavior directly equals orientation
    B. Heterosexual orientation precludes homosexual behavior
    C. Behavior is more variable than orientation; mismatches occur
    D. Homosexual orientation precludes heterosexual behavior
    E. Orientation is a direct function of behavior
43. The term **MSM**:
    A. Refers to the homosexual community
    B. Describes behavior, not identity
    C. Does not apply if not gay/bisexual
    D. Absent in some societies
    E. Replaces sexual orientation
44. Which statement on frequencies is NOT true?
    A. Kinsey reported ~37% of men with ≥1 same-sex orgasm
    B. Orientation estimates range ~1–10%
    C. ~8% males exclusively homosexual ≥3 years (Kinsey)
    D. Researchers often use 4–5% (men), 2–3% (women)
    E. Gay activism reduces true prevalence
45. Genetic contributions to orientation—best statement:
    A. Disproven
    B. X-linked region (e.g., Xq28) implicated in a subgroup; complex genetics
    C. No genome screens done
    D. Xq28 linkage uniformly confirmed across all studies
    E. Most gay men attribute it to dysfunctional families

46. INAH-3 findings—best statement:
    A. Always larger in homosexual men
    B. Human nuclei do not match animal models
    C. May parallel MPOA/anterior hypothalamus regulating male sexual behavior
    D. Definitively regulates orientation
    E. Fully disproved
47. Traits linked with higher homophobia:
    A. Similar to other phobias only
    B. Frequent prosocial contact with gay people
    C. Authoritarian and conservative attitudes
    D. Never any same-sex attraction
    E. Positive mental health marker
48. **Sex therapy** is best described as:
    A. Weekly ≥1 year mandatory
    B. Only for couples
    C. Solely behavioral drills
    D. Specialized psychotherapy (with behavioral/medical integration)
    E. Only targets performance anxiety
49. For ED, combining medical + psychological care:
    A. Improves medical efficacy
    B. Improves satisfaction
    C. Reduces drop-outs
    D. Improves sexual outcomes
    E. All of the above
50. **Mindfulness** is:
    A. Core for conduct disorder therapy
    B. Present-focused, non-judgmental awareness of thoughts/feelings
    C. Requires lotus posture
    D. Requires mantra chanting
    E. Heightens colors/emotions by itself
51. Mindfulness shows particular benefit for:
    A. Men with PE
    B. Women with anorgasmia
    C. Women with HSDD
    D. Women with HSDD or arousal disorder + childhood sexual abuse history
    E. Men with ED + depression
52. Tele-sex therapy:
    A. Outperforms in-person consistently
    B. Universally accepted standard
    C. Improves access/anonymity; reduces embarrassment
    D. Gives therapists deeper emotional read
    E. Always needs new certification/insurance

53. "Paraphilic disorder" (vs paraphilia) requires:
    A. Any atypical interest
    B. Only legal involvement
    C. Distress/impairment or non-consent/risk of harm
    D. Partner displeasure only
    E. >6 months duration without distress
54. **Voyeuristic disorder** involves:
    A. Watching consenting adults
    B. Observing unsuspecting persons naked/undressing/sexual activity
    C. Exposing genitals
    D. Using objects
    E. Non-consensual rubbing
55. **Zoophilia** refers to:
    A. Corpses
    B. Animals
    C. Enemas
    D. Body parts
    E. Vomiting
56. **Compulsive sexual behavior** (hypersexuality) is characterized by:
    A. High desire without consequences
    B. Persistent, uncontrolled sexual impulses with impairment/distress
    C. Only frequent masturbation
    D. Exclusively paraphilic interests
    E. Always due to mania
57. **Minority stress** model posits:
    A. Stigma and discrimination contribute to adverse mental/sexual health
    B. Genetics only explains disparities
    C. Access solves all disparities
    D. Orientation is pathologic
    E. Conversion efforts are effective
58. **Conversion therapy** (sexual orientation/gender identity "change"):
    A. Evidence-based and safe
    B. Improves mental health
    C. Ineffective and associated with harm
    D. First-line for teens
    E. Legal requirement in many countries
59. In consensual BDSM, the ethical frame is often:
    A. SSC/RACK emphasizing consent, risk awareness, and aftercare
    B. Assumed consent within relationships
    C. Medical supervision mandatory
    D. Always pathological
    E. Invariably non-consensual

60. **Autonomic arousal + anxiety** commonly worsen:
    A. Desire
    B. Premature ejaculation and erectile dysfunction
    C. Penile size
    D. Testosterone levels
    E. Sex orientation

✅ Key Takeaways

- Sexual orientation is a multidimensional construct involving attraction, behavior, and self-identification.
- Theories include hormonal, genetic, neuroanatomical, and psychosocial contributions.
- The INAH-3 nucleus and prenatal androgen exposure have been studied in relation to orientation.
- Sexual orientation is not a pathology and requires affirming, inclusive care.
- Clinicians should approach discussions with cultural sensitivity and confidentiality.
- Stigma can negatively affect mental health outcomes in non-heterosexual individuals.

✅ Answer Key (1–60)

1. A
2. C
3. D
4. A
5. B
6. D
7. D
8. E
9. A
10. B
11. C
12. B
13. E
14. D
15. C
16. B
17. A
18. E

19. C
20. A
21. D
22. B
23. E
24. D
25. D
26. A
27. E
28. D
29. A
30. B
31. C
32. E
33. D
34. C
35. E
36. B
37. A
38. A
39. B
40. D
41. D
42. C
43. B
44. E
45. B
46. C
47. C
48. D
49. E
50. B
51. D
52. C
53. C
54. B
55. B
56. B
57. A
58. C
59. A
60. B

Explanations (1–60)

1. Gender in sexual medicine refers to **socially defined rules, roles, and expectations** linked to being male, female, or another identity. It is distinct from biological sex and from personal gender identity. The best choice is **A**.
2. Cisgender describes individuals whose **gender identity matches the sex they were assigned at birth**. They may have any sexual orientation, but their internal and external identity align with the assigned sex. Correct is **C**.
3. Transgender is an umbrella term for people whose **gender identity or expression differs** from the sex assigned at birth. This may or may not involve medical transition or social expression. Correct answer **D**.
4. Gender dysphoria is **non-sexual in nature**, involving incongruence between experienced gender and assigned sex. It causes distress but is not dependent on sexual arousal. Correct is **A**.
5. Gender expression is how people **externally communicate gender identity**, through clothing, hairstyle, voice, or behaviors. It is independent of assigned sex and orientation. Best answer is **B**.
6. The etiology of gender dysphoria is **idiopathic and multifactorial**, including biological, hormonal, psychological, and social influences. No single cause explains all cases. Thus **D** is correct.
7. Kinsey 0 reflects **exclusive heterosexuality**, with no homosexual attraction or behavior reported. It defines one end of the Kinsey spectrum. Correct is **D**.
8. Kinsey 1 means **predominantly heterosexual with incidental homosexual attraction or behavior**. It reflects minor same-sex experiences but overall heterosexuality. Correct answer **E**.
9. Kinsey 6 indicates **exclusive homosexuality**, representing the other extreme of the Kinsey continuum. Correct is **A**.
10. Kinsey 5 means **predominantly homosexual with only incidental heterosexual attraction/behavior**. The pattern is almost entirely homosexual. Best answer is **B**.
11. Kinsey 4 describes **predominantly homosexual with more than incidental heterosexual activity**. It shows bisexuality with a strong homosexual leaning. Correct is **C**.
12. Historically, "gay bowel syndrome" was used (now outdated) to describe **enteric STIs in MSM**. Today, specific infections like proctitis are named directly. Correct is **B**.
13. Exhibitionism involves **exposing genitals to unsuspecting strangers** for arousal. It becomes a disorder when recurrent, distressing, or impairing. Correct answer **E**.
14. Fetishism means **sexual arousal from inanimate objects** (e.g., shoes, fabrics). It differs from partialism, which focuses on body parts. Best answer is **D**.
15. Frotteurism is the act of **touching or rubbing against a non-consenting person** in crowds for arousal. It is criminal when acted on. Correct is **C**.
16. Pedophilia refers to **sexual attraction to prepubescent children**. Acting on it constitutes abuse, making it harmful and illegal. Correct answer **B**.

17. Masochism is arousal from **humiliation, binding, or pain**. It may be consensual in BDSM but is disordered when causing distress or harm. Correct is **A**.
18. Masking or blowing on the face reflects **fetishism**, because arousal is focused on a specific non-genital stimulus. Correct answer **E**.
19. Necrophilia means **sexual attraction to corpses**. It is extremely rare, pathological, and unlawful. Correct answer **C**.
20. Teleiophilia refers to **sexual attraction to adults**, considered the normative pattern of human sexuality. Correct is **A**.
21. Partialism is **sexual focus on specific body parts** like feet or hair, instead of whole partners. Correct is **D**.
22. Klismaphilia is arousal from **enema use**, often involving insertion of liquids for erotic stimulation. Best answer is **B**.
23. Emetophilia is arousal linked to **vomiting acts**, either self or partner. It is uncommon but classified among paraphilias. Correct is **E**.
24. Infantile masturbation (gratification disorder) can mimic **epileptic seizures** with rhythmic movements. EEG may be needed for distinction. Correct answer **D**.
25. Idiosyncratic masturbation often means **prone rubbing against sheets**, which may later hinder satisfaction with partner sex. Correct is **D**.
26. The **missionary position** is the most widely used sexual position across cultures. It is considered the basic sexual position. Correct is **A**.
27. Fellatio is **oral stimulation of male genitals** (penis/scrotum). Correct answer **E**.
28. Cunnilingus is **oral stimulation of female genitals** (vulva, clitoris). Correct is **D**.
29. Bukkake is a practice involving **multiple men ejaculating on one person**, originally a pornography term. Correct is **A**.
30. Frottage among consenting males means **mutual rubbing of penises**. It differs from non-consensual frotteurism. Correct answer **B**.
31. Tribadism is **mutual vulvar rubbing between two females**, sometimes called "scissoring." Correct is **C**.
32. Docking is **inserting the glans into another male's foreskin**, practiced among uncircumcised men. Correct is **E**.
33. Daisy chain refers to **a group sequentially performing oral sex on each other in a circle**. Correct is **D**.
34. Freud's oral stage covers **birth–1 year**, with gratification via feeding/sucking. Correct is **C**.
35. Freud's genital stage is from **puberty to adulthood**, involving mature sexuality and relationships. Correct is **E**.
36. The phallic stage (ages **3–6 years**) focuses on genital curiosity and role identification. Correct is **B**.
37. The anal stage (**1–3 years**) centers on toilet training and control issues in Freud's theory. Correct is **A**.
38. Gender dysphoria involves a person's **internal sense of gender identity**, not just culture or anatomy. Correct answer **A**.
39. **Prenatal hormones**, particularly androgen exposure, play a major role in gender development. Correct is **B**.

40. Standards before gender surgery require **age ≥18** and **real-life experience plus hormone use**. Correct answer **D**.
41. Sexual orientation = **pattern of erotic and romantic attraction** toward genders. Correct is **D**.
42. Sexual behavior is **more variable** than orientation; mismatches can occur. Correct is **C**.
43. MSM means **men who have sex with men**, describing behavior regardless of identity. Correct is **B**.
44. Activism changes visibility but not innate prevalence, so "reduces frequency" is false. Correct is **E**.
45. Genetics: evidence suggests **Xq28 involvement in a subgroup**, but orientation is multifactorial. Correct is **B**.
46. INAH-3 may parallel animal hypothalamic regions regulating male sexual behavior. Correct is **C**.
47. High homophobia correlates with **authoritarian and conservative traits**. Correct is **C**.
48. Sex therapy is **specialized psychotherapy combining behavioral and medical approaches**. Correct is **D**.
49. Combining medical + psychological ED treatment improves outcomes across **efficacy, satisfaction, and adherence**. Correct is **E**.
50. Mindfulness is a **practice of present-focused, non-judgmental awareness** of thoughts and sensations. Correct is **B**.
51. Mindfulness is especially effective for **women with desire/arousal disorders and CSA history**. Correct is **D**.
52. Online sex therapy improves **accessibility and reduces embarrassment**, but is not yet universal standard. Correct is **C**.
53. Paraphilic disorder requires **distress/impairment or non-consent/harm**, not just atypical interest. Correct is **C**.
54. Voyeuristic disorder = **watching unsuspecting people naked or sexual**. Correct is **B**.
55. Zoophilia = **sexual attraction to animals**. Correct is **B**.
56. Compulsive sexual behavior = **uncontrolled impulses causing distress/impairment**, not just high desire. Correct is **B**.
57. Minority stress model: **stigma/discrimination harm mental and sexual health** in minorities. Correct is **A**.
58. Conversion therapy is **ineffective and harmful**, condemned by health bodies. Correct is **C**.
59. Consensual BDSM uses frameworks like **SSC/RACK**, stressing consent and safety. Correct is **A**.
60. Sympathetic overactivation worsens **premature ejaculation and erectile dysfunction**. Correct is **B**.

Further Reading

The explanations in this chapter are supported by the following key references:

1. American Psychiatric Association. Diagnostic and statistical manual of mental disorders (DSM-5-TR). 5th ed. Washington, DC: American Psychiatric Association; 2022.
2. World Health Organization. ICD-11: international classification of diseases. Geneva: WHO; 2019.
3. Bancroft J. Human sexuality and its problems. 3rd ed. Elsevier; 2009.
4. Zucker KJ, Lawrence AA. Epidemiology of gender identity disorder. Int Rev Psychiatry. 2009;21(5):397–409.
5. Kafka MP. Hypersexual disorder: a proposed diagnosis for DSM-5. Arch Sex Behav. 2010;39(2):377–400.
6. Levine SB. Clinical practice with sexually atypical patients. J Sex Marital Ther. 2018;44(3):197–209.
7. Di Cristofaro A, Jannini TB, Colonnello E, Limoncin E, Mollaioli D, Ciocca G, Sansone A, Jannini EA. XYGO: proposing a new holistic measure of gender identity and sexual orientation. Nat Rev Urol. 2025;22(6):387–405.

Disorders of Sexual Desire and Arousal—50 MCQs

6

Learning Objectives

- Define and classify male sexual desire and arousal disorders.
- Explore endocrine, psychological, and iatrogenic causes.
- Utilize validated tools for assessment.
- Evaluate pharmacologic and psychosexual therapy options.
- Apply a biopsychosocial model in management.

Select the Single Best Answer

1. The term satyriasis means:
   A. Hypoactive sexual desire
   B. Hyperactive sexual desire
   C. Sexual aversion
   D. Castration
   E. Decrease arousal state
2. Hypoactive sexual desire in males is mainly due to:
   A. Increase estrogen
   B. Decrease prolactin
   C. Increase testosterone
   D. Decrease testosterone
   E. Decrease nitric oxide level
3. Which of the following drugs is NOT associated with male desire apathy?
   A. Tramadol
   B. Isotretinoin
   C. SSRIs
   D. H2 blockers
   E. Beta blockers

M. S. M. Hasan, M. L. Elsaie, *Comprehensive MCQs in Andrology*, Trends in Andrology and Sexual Medicine, https://doi.org/10.1007/978-3-032-20623-7_6

4. Which of the following is NOT a symptom of sexual aversion?
   A. The need for intimacy before starting sexual activity
   B. Intense antipathy to different forms of sexual contact
   C. Specific aversion to erect penis or semen
   D. The wish to end every sexual contact as quickly as possible
   E. Hypoactive sexual desire and anorgasmia
5. Hypersexuality is a pattern of sexual behaviors that is marked by:
   A. Obsessive thoughts
   B. Compulsive behaviors
   C. Inability to stop the behaviors despite negative consequences
   D. B + C only
   E. A + B + C
6. Hypersexuality is NOT related to:
   A. Kluver Bucy syndrome
   B. Bipolar disorders and mania
   C. Addiction
   D. Brain injuries
   E. Polycythemia
7. Sexual apathy refers to:
   A. Hypoactive sexual desire
   B. Hyperactive sexual desire
   C. Sexual aversion
   D. Castration
   E. Decrease arousal state
8. Hypoactive Sexual Desire Disorder is described as:
   A. Persistent deficiency/absence of desire and fantasies causing distress
   B. Persistent strong desire causing distress
   C. Persistent recurrent headache
   D. Use of pornography causing distress
   E. Fear of intimacy without desire loss
9. Sexual Aversion Disorder is described as:
   A. Aversion and avoidance of genital sexual contact causing distress
   B. Aversion to partner in general causing distress
   C. Aversion to masturbation causing distress
   D. Aversion to oral sex only
   E. Aversion to pornography
10. Lack of desire is reported by:
    A. 1 in 3
    B. 1 in 5
    C. 1 in 4
    D. 1 in 2
    E. 1 in 10

11. Immediate causes directly influencing sexual performance include:
    A. Performance anxiety
    B. Communication problems
    C. Clumsy technique
    D. All of the above
    E. None of the above
12. Which of the following is NOT a hormone affecting desire/arousal?
    A. Testosterone
    B. Estrogen
    C. Prolactin
    D. Prostaglandin
    E. Dopamine
13. Which is NOT a component of sexual desire?
    A. Cultural component
    B. Drive component
    C. Hormonal component
    D. Motivation component
    E. Emotional bonding
14. Which of the following is NOT true about hypersexuality?
    A. ≥7 orgasms/week
    B. Due to lack of masturbation
    C. Persistent ≥6 months
    D. Causes social/functional impairment
    E. Associated with distress
15. Nymphomania refers to:
    A. Excessive sexual desire in women
    B. Excessive sexual desire in men
    C. Low sexual desire in women
    D. Arousal disorder in women
    E. Sexual apathy
16. A common psychological cause of sexual aversion disorder is:
    A. Childhood sexual trauma
    B. Excess testosterone
    C. High prolactin
    D. Relationship satisfaction
    E. Dopamine excess
17. Which of the following brain regions is linked to sexual desire regulation?
    A. Prefrontal cortex
    B. Amygdala
    C. Hypothalamus
    D. All of the above
    E. None of the above

18. A neurochemical strongly enhancing sexual desire is:
    A. Serotonin
    B. Dopamine
    C. Prostaglandin
    D. Histamine
    E. Cortisol
19. A neurochemical strongly inhibiting sexual desire is:
    A. Dopamine
    B. Oxytocin
    C. Serotonin
    D. Testosterone
    E. Adrenaline
20. Male hypoactive desire prevalence increases most after which age?
    A. 20
    B. 30
    C. 40
    D. 50
    E. 60
21. Persistent sexual thoughts interfering with daily life are best described as:
    A. Sexual apathy
    B. Hypersexuality
    C. Arousal disorder
    D. Sexual aversion
    E. Libido loss
22. Which medical condition is most often linked with low desire in men?
    A. Diabetes mellitus
    B. Hypertension
    C. Rheumatoid arthritis
    D. Asthma
    E. Hyperthyroidism
23. Female sexual arousal disorder differs from hypoactive desire by:
    A. Lack of genital swelling/lubrication despite desire
    B. Lack of sexual fantasies
    C. Aversion to contact
    D. Excessive desire
    E. None of the above
24. Which hormone decline in women contributes to arousal disorder?
    A. Estrogen
    B. Progesterone
    C. Cortisol
    D. FSH
    E. LH

25. Arousal disorder in men is most often clinically equivalent to:
    A. Premature ejaculation
    B. Erectile dysfunction
    C. Priapism
    D. Peyronie's disease
    E. Phimosis
26. A couple presenting with mismatched sexual desire is best described as:
    A. Hypoactive sexual desire disorder
    B. Sexual aversion disorder
    C. Desire discrepancy
    D. Dyspareunia
    E. None of the above
27. A validated tool for assessing sexual desire is:
    A. IIEF
    B. FSFI
    C. Kinsey Scale
    D. SHIM
    E. A + B
28. Kinsey scale score of 0 means:
    A. Exclusively homosexual
    B. Exclusively heterosexual
    C. Bisexual
    D. Asexual
    E. Hypersexual
29. Persistent genital arousal disorder (PGAD) is characterized by:
    A. Ongoing arousal without desire
    B. Desire without arousal
    C. Complete loss of libido
    D. Hypersexuality
    E. Anorgasmia
30. A common antidepressant linked to desire loss is:
    A. SSRI
    B. TCA
    C. MAOI
    D. Bupropion
    E. Lithium
31. A drug that may enhance desire by dopamine stimulation is:
    A. Bromocriptine
    B. Fluoxetine
    C. Cimetidine
    D. Spironolactone
    E. Methyldopa

32. The DSM-5 merged “Hypoactive Sexual Desire” and “Female Arousal Disorder” into:
    A. HSDD
    B. Sexual Interest/Arousal Disorder
    C. Sexual Aversion Disorder
    D. Orgasmic Disorder
    E. Hypersexual Disorder
33. Which chronic illness is most associated with hypoactive desire?
    A. Diabetes
    B. Asthma
    C. Cancer
    D. COPD
    E. Migraine
34. Which marital factor is a strong risk for low desire?
    A. Poor communication
    B. Infidelity
    C. Conflict and stress
    D. All of the above
    E. None of the above
35. The most common medication-induced cause of hypersexuality is:
    A. Dopamine agonists (e.g., for Parkinson’s)
    B. SSRIs
    C. Antihistamines
    D. H2 blockers
    E. Antipsychotics
36. Hypoactive desire in men can be evaluated first by checking:
    A. Testosterone
    B. Prolactin
    C. LH/FSH
    D. Thyroid
    E. All of the above
37. The best initial therapy for hypoactive desire due to low testosterone is:
    A. PDE5 inhibitors
    B. Testosterone replacement
    C. SSRIs
    D. Dopamine agonists
    E. Psychotherapy
38. The “dual control model” of sexual response includes:
    A. Excitation and inhibition systems
    B. Dopamine and serotonin only
    C. Testosterone and estrogen
    D. Hypothalamic and cortical regulation
    E. Desire and arousal only

39. Excess prolactin in men causes:
    A. Increased libido
    B. Reduced libido
    C. Erectile dysfunction
    D. B + C
    E. None
40. A frequent comorbidity of hypersexuality is:
    A. Anxiety disorders
    B. Depression
    C. OCD
    D. Substance abuse
    E. All of the above
41. Female sexual aversion disorder is often associated with:
    A. Dyspareunia
    B. Vaginismus
    C. PTSD
    D. A + C
    E. All of the above
42. A psychotropic that improves sexual desire is:
    A. Bupropion
    B. Fluoxetine
    C. Sertraline
    D. Paroxetine
    E. Citalopram
43. Persistent distressing lack of interest in sex despite normal physiology is:
    A. HSDD
    B. Aversion disorder
    C. Arousal disorder
    D. Hypersexuality
    E. Asexuality
44. Which hormone is central to female libido?
    A. Estrogen
    B. Progesterone
    C. Testosterone
    D. Oxytocin
    E. Prolactin
45. Which psychological intervention is most effective for desire disorders?
    A. Psychoanalysis
    B. Cognitive behavioral therapy
    C. Hypnosis
    D. Couples therapy
    E. CBT + couples therapy

46. A rare syndrome where sexual desire emerges after frontal lobe injury is:
    A. Kluver–Bucy syndrome
    B. Frontal disinhibition syndrome
    C. McCune–Albright
    D. Prader–Willi
    E. Leriche syndrome
47. The ICD-11 term for compulsive sexual behavior is:
    A. Hypersexual disorder
    B. Compulsive sexual behavior disorder
    C. Sexual addiction
    D. Impulse control disorder
    E. Nymphomania
48. Which factor does NOT reduce sexual desire?
    A. Diabetes
    B. Stress
    C. Obesity
    D. Alcohol in moderation
    E. Antidepressants
49. The most common presentation of HSDD in women is:
    A. Loss of sexual fantasies
    B. Loss of sexual thoughts and receptivity
    C. Complete aversion to partners
    D. Anorgasmia
    E. Genital pain
50. Which treatment is FDA-approved for female hypoactive desire disorder?
    A. Sildenafil
    B. Flibanserin
    C. Testosterone patches
    D. PDE5 inhibitors
    E. Estrogen cream

✅ Key Takeaways

- Desire disorders include hypoactive sexual desire disorder (HSDD) and sexual aversion.
- Arousal disorders may involve failure to achieve or maintain sexual excitement.
- Causes range from hypogonadism, depression, SSRIs, relationship discord, and chronic illness.
- Treatment options include testosterone replacement, psychotherapy, behavioral techniques, and couple therapy.
- Differentiating primary from secondary disorders guides therapy.

✅ Answer Key (1–50)

1. B
2. D
3. E
4. E
5. E
6. E
7. A
8. A
9. A
10. A
11. D
12. D
13. C
14. B
15. A
16. A
17. D
18. B
19. C
20. D
21. B
22. A
23. A
24. A
25. B
26. C
27. E
28. B
29. A
30. A
31. A
32. B
33. A
34. D
35. A
36. A
37. B
38. A
39. D
40. E
41. E
42. A

43. A
44. C
45. E
46. B
47. B
48. D
49. B
50. B

Explanations (1–50)

1. **Satyriasis**—Refers to hyperactive sexual desire in men, often associated with compulsive sexual behavior and sometimes psychiatric illness.
2. **Hypoactive desire in men**—Low testosterone is the most common biological cause, leading to reduced libido and fantasies.
3. **Drugs and desire apathy**—Beta blockers primarily affect erections, while SSRIs, isotretinoin, tramadol, and H2 blockers reduce libido.
4. **Sexual aversion symptoms**—Aversion is characterized by fear and disgust at sexual contact, not by general hypoactive desire or anorgasmia.
5. **Hypersexuality**—Defined by obsessive thoughts, compulsive acts, and inability to stop despite harm, aligning with behavioral addiction.
6. **Not related to hypersexuality**—Polycythemia has no role; hypersexuality is seen in mania, brain injury, Kluver–Bucy syndrome, and addiction.
7. **Sexual apathy**—Refers to low desire or hypoactive sexual desire, not aversion or hypersexuality.
8. **HSDD**—DSM-5 defines it as persistent lack of fantasies/desire causing distress or interpersonal problems.
9. **Sexual Aversion Disorder**—Defined as avoidance of genital contact with a partner, producing significant distress.
10. **Prevalence of low desire**—Surveys suggest up to one-third of adults report low desire, though not always clinically significant.
11. **Immediate causes**—Performance anxiety, poor communication, and poor technique all directly impact desire and arousal.
12. **Hormones**—Testosterone, estrogen, and prolactin influence libido. Prostaglandins play no primary role in desire.
13. **Components of desire**—Drive, motivation, and cultural influences are core. "Hormonal component" is not a formal classification.
14. **Hypersexuality myths**—It is not due to lack of masturbation; rather it's persistent excessive sexual activity causing distress.
15. **Nymphomania**—Refers to compulsive or excessive sexual desire in women, analogous to satyriasis in men.
16. **Psychological cause of aversion**—Childhood trauma and sexual abuse are strongly linked to later aversive responses.

17. **Brain regions**—Sexual desire regulation involves hypothalamus, amygdala, and prefrontal cortex. Thus, all listed regions are involved.
18. **Dopamine**—A key neurotransmitter stimulating sexual motivation and reward pathways.
19. **Serotonin**—High serotonin activity inhibits sexual desire, explaining SSRI-associated low libido.
20. **Male desire decline**—Hypoactive desire becomes more common after age 50 due to hormonal and metabolic changes.
21. **Hypersexuality**—Persistent intrusive sexual thoughts interfering with life define hypersexuality, not apathy or aversion.
22. **Chronic illness**—Diabetes mellitus is most associated with low desire through hormonal and vascular mechanisms.
23. **Female arousal disorder**—Defined as inability to achieve genital arousal despite normal desire, differentiating it from HSDD.
24. **Estrogen**—Estrogen decline post-menopause causes vaginal dryness and impaired arousal.
25. **Male arousal disorder**—Clinically manifests as erectile dysfunction in the presence of preserved desire.
26. **Desire discrepancy**—When partners have mismatched levels of sexual desire, it often leads to relational conflict.
27. **Tools**—The IIEF (men) and FSFI (women) both assess desire domains, making them validated tools.
28. **Kinsey scale 0**—Represents exclusively heterosexual orientation.
29. **PGAD**—A rare condition of persistent genital arousal without associated sexual desire or relief after orgasm.
30. **SSRIs**—Strongly linked with loss of libido as a side effect.
31. **Bromocriptine**—A dopamine agonist used in hyperprolactinemia, can improve libido.
32. **DSM-5**—Combined female hypoactive desire and arousal disorders under "Female Sexual Interest/Arousal Disorder."
33. **Chronic illness**—Diabetes is the most common systemic cause of HSDD in both sexes.
34. **Marital risk factors**—Conflict, stress, and poor communication all strongly impair desire.
35. **Hypersexuality cause**—Dopamine agonists (e.g., pramipexole in Parkinson's) are notorious for causing compulsive sexual behavior.
36. **Initial tests**—Serum testosterone is the first-line investigation for male hypoactive desire.
37. **Therapy**—Testosterone replacement is the treatment of choice when deficiency is confirmed.
38. **Dual control model**—Desire and arousal are regulated by an excitation system (dopamine-driven) and inhibition system (serotonin-driven).
39. **Prolactin**—Excess leads to reduced libido and erectile dysfunction, often due to pituitary adenomas.

40. **Comorbidities of hypersexuality**—Commonly linked to anxiety, depression, OCD, and substance use disorders.
41. **Female aversion disorder**—Associated with dyspareunia, vaginismus, and trauma-related PTSD.
42. **Bupropion**—An antidepressant that enhances dopamine/noradrenaline and often improves libido.
43. **HSDD**—Persistent lack of sexual interest or fantasies causing distress defines hypoactive sexual desire disorder.
44. **Testosterone**—While estrogen influences arousal, testosterone is central to female libido.
45. **Best therapy**—Combination of CBT and couples therapy addresses psychological and relational factors in desire disorders.
46. **Frontal lobe injury**—Disinhibition syndromes after frontal injury can cause pathological hypersexuality.
47. **ICD-11**—Officially recognizes "Compulsive Sexual Behavior Disorder" as a diagnosis, not "sexual addiction."
48. **Alcohol**—While heavy alcohol lowers desire, moderate intake is not typically inhibitory, unlike obesity, stress, and antidepressants.
49. **Female HSDD**—Typically presents as loss of sexual thoughts, fantasies, and receptivity to initiation by partner.
50. **Flibanserin**—FDA-approved for premenopausal women with HSDD, acting on serotonin and dopamine pathways.

🎯 Further Reading

The explanations in this chapter are supported by the following key references:

1. American Psychiatric Association, editor. Diagnostic and statistical manual of mental disorders (DSM-5-TR). 5th ed. Washington, DC: American Psychiatric Association; 2022.
2. World Health Organization. ICD-11: international classification of diseases. Geneva: WHO; 2019.
3. Corona G, Isidori AM, Buvat J, et al. Testosterone supplementation and sexual desire: a meta-analysis. J Sex Med. 2014;11(6):1577–92.
4. Bancroft J, Janssen E. The dual control model of male sexual response. Neurosci Biobehav Rev. 2000;24(5):571–9.
5. Clayton AH, Juarez EM. Hypoactive sexual desire disorder in men. Sex Med Rev. 2017;5(3):285–94.
6. Hackett G. The role of testosterone in male sexual desire. Trends Urol Mens Health. 2018;9(2):17–22.

Male Erectile Dysfunction

7

Learning Objectives

- Understand the classification and prevalence of ED.
- Examine underlying mechanisms: vascular, neurological, hormonal, and psychological.
- Apply diagnostic tools such as IIEF-5 and penile Doppler ultrasound.
- Compare treatment modalities.
- Assess the impact of comorbid conditions like diabetes, hypertension, and depression.

Select the Single Best Answer

1. Psychogenic erection is:
   A. Induced by tactile stimulation of the genitals
   B. Poorly controlled
   C. Short duration
   D. Centrally stimulated
   E. Occurs during rapid eye movement sleep
2. Reflexogenic erection is:
   A. Induced by visual or memory association
   B. Occurs during rapid eye movement sleep
   C. Can be preserved in upper spinal cord lesions
   D. Induced by intracorporeal injection
   E. Centrally stimulated
3. Which of the following is NOT a risk factor for erectile dysfunction?
   A. Benign prostatic hyperplasia
   B. Hyperuricemia
   C. Vitamin D deficiency
   D. Hyperhomocysteinemia
   E. Masturbation

M. S. M. Hasan, M. L. Elsaie, *Comprehensive MCQs in Andrology*, Trends in Andrology and Sexual Medicine, https://doi.org/10.1007/978-3-032-20623-7_7

4. Which of the following is NOT a risk factor for erectile dysfunction?
   A. Metabolic syndrome
   B. Dyslipidemia
   C. Folic acid deficiency
   D. Inflammatory bowel diseases
   E. Nebivolol
5. Which of the following is NOT a criterion for organic erectile dysfunction?
   A. Gradual onset
   B. Previous medical history
   C. Older age
   D. Morning erection
   E. Progressive course
6. Which of the following is NOT a basic investigation for erectile dysfunction?
   A. LH
   B. Prolactin
   C. Blood sugar
   D. Lipid profile
   E. Testosterone
7. Widower syndrome is considered a type of erectile dysfunction:
   A. Neurogenic
   B. Arteriogenic
   C. Psychogenic
   D. Part of Leriche syndrome
   E. Venogenic
8. Which of the following is NOT measured by the classic form of nocturnal penile tumescence?
   A. The number of penile tumescence
   B. Duration of each erection
   C. Episodes of erection during daytime
   D. Penile rigidity
   E. Penile circumference
9. The most accurate method of nocturnal penile tumescence is:
   A. Rigiscan
   B. Sleep laboratory nocturnal penile tumescence and rigidity
   C. Postage test
   D. Snap gauges band
   E. Electrobioimpedance volumetric assessment
10. Normal nocturnal erectile episodes during Rigiscan are:
    A. 1–2 episodes
    B. 2–4 episodes
    C. 4–6 episodes
    D. 6–8 episodes
    E. >8 episodes

11. The normal nocturnal penile root circumference during Rigiscan is:
    A. 1 cm
    B. 2 cm
    C. 3 cm
    D. 4 cm
    E. 5 cm
12. The prevalence of neurogenic erectile dysfunction:
    A. 5–10%
    B. 10–20%
    C. 20–30%
    D. <5%
    E. >25%
13. Which hormone is responsible for the increased frequency of sexual act?
    A. Prolactin
    B. Estrogen
    C. Thyroid hormone
    D. Testosterone
    E. Serotonin
14. The increase in nocturnal emission frequency is due to:
    A. Testosterone
    B. Estrogen
    C. Prolactin
    D. Nitric oxide
    E. Serotonin
15. Aortoiliac occlusive disease is synonymous to:
    A. Widower syndrome
    B. Honeymoon impotence
    C. Loose penile syndrome
    D. Leriche syndrome
    E. McCune Albright syndrome
16. Claudication of buttocks and thighs is the criteria for:
    A. Honeymoon impotence
    B. Widower syndrome
    C. Loose penile syndrome
    D. McCune Albright syndrome
    E. Leriche syndrome
17. Proximal venogenic erectile dysfunction is mostly due to:
    A. Peyronie's disease
    B. Diabetes mellitus
    C. Old age
    D. Chronic perineal trauma
    E. Congenital fistula

18. Distal venogenic erectile dysfunction is mostly due to:
    A. Peyronie's disease
    B. Diabetes mellitus
    C. Iatrogenic penile fistula
    D. Chronic perineal trauma
    E. Old age
19. High-risk category CVS associated with erectile dysfunction:
    A. Risk of coronary artery disease
    B. Stable angina
    C. Moderate angina
    D. Arrhythmia
    E. Controlled hypertension
20. One of the following is NOT a criterion for metabolic syndrome:
    A. Impaired glucose tolerance
    B. Increase body mass index
    C. High blood pressure
    D. High plasma triglycerides
    E. High estradiol level
21. Which of the following is NOT a mechanism of erectile dysfunction in liver diseases?
    A. Hyperprolactinemia
    B. Increase SHBG
    C. Increase parathormone hormone
    D. Increase estradiol level
    E. Decrease testosterone level
22. Which of the following is a cause of ED in Benign prostate hyperplasia patients?
    A. Increase estradiol level
    B. Increase parathormone hormone
    C. Hyperprolactinemia
    D. Increase NO/cGMP signaling
    E. Increase RhoA/ROK contractile signaling
23. Which of the following drugs is NOT associated with erectile dysfunction?
    A. Clonidine
    B. Spironolactone
    C. Nebivolol
    D. Amiodarone
    E. Reserpine
24. Blockade of helicine arteries may be due to the following drug:
    A. Reserpine
    B. Nebivolol
    C. Methyldopa
    D. Propranolol
    E. Calcium channel blockers

25. Which of the following drugs increases nitric oxide levels during erection?
    A. Calcium channel blocker
    B. ACE inhibitors
    C. Spironolactone
    D. Nebivolol
    E. Methyldopa
26. Diversion of pelvic arterial blood flow away from the pelvis is due to:
    A. Leriche syndrome
    B. Pelvic steal syndrome
    C. McCune Albright syndrome
    D. Widower syndrome
    E. Pelvic trauma
27. The normal erection score of the International Index of erectile function is:
    A. 1–10
    B. 11–16
    C. 17–21
    D. 22–24
    E. >25
28. The mild erectile dysfunction score of the international index of erectile function is:
    A. 1–10
    B. 11–16
    C. 17–21
    D. 22–24
    E. >25
29. The mild to moderate erectile dysfunction score of the international index of erectile function is:
    A. 1–10
    B. 11–16
    C. 17–21
    D. 22–24
    E. >25
30. The moderate erectile dysfunction score of the international index of erectile function is:
    A. 1–10
    B. 11–16
    C. 17–21
    D. 22–24
    E. >25
31. The severe erectile dysfunction score of the international index of erectile function is:
    A. 1–10
    B. 11–16
    C. 17–21
    D. 22–24
    E. >25

32. The incidence of priapism is very low with prostaglandin injection as it is intra-corporeal metabolized by:
    A. 15-hydroxy prostaglandin dehydrogenase
    B. 15-oxy prostaglandin dehydrogenase
    C. 10-hydroxy prostaglandin dehydrogenase
    D. 5-hydroxy prostaglandin dehydrogenase
    E. 5-oxy prostaglandin dehydrogenase
33. The prostaglandin is metabolized in:
    A. Kidney
    B. Liver
    C. Lung
    D. Spleen
    E. Suprarenal gland
34. The prostaglandin is excreted by:
    A. Lung
    B. Spleen
    C. Liver
    D. Kidney
    E. Suprarenal glands
35. Which of the following drugs is NOT used in intracorporeal injection?
    A. Moxisylyte
    B. Linsidomine
    C. Forskolin
    D. Vasoactive intestinal peptide
    E. Methylene blue
36. The starting intracorporeal injection dose is:
    A. 5 units (0.05 ml)
    B. 10 units (0.5 ml)
    C. 15 units (0.005 ml)
    D. 20 units (0.01 ml)
    E. 25 units (0.1 ml)
37. Which of the following is the correct method of intracorporal injection?
    A. Subcutaneous injection
    B. Intraseptal injection
    C. Intratunical injection
    D. Intra cavernous
    E. Intra spongiosum
38. E2 score in schedule response of intracorporal injection:
    A. Elongation only
    B. Partial tumescence
    C. Full tumescence
    D. Erection with partial rigidity
    E. Erection with full rigidity

39. E4 score in schedule response of intracorporal injection:
    A. Elongation only
    B. Partial tumescence
    C. Full tumescence
    D. Erection with partial rigidity
    E. Erection with full rigidity
40. E3 score in schedule response of intracorporal injection:
    A. Elongation only
    B. Partial tumescence
    C. Full tumescence
    D. Erection with partial rigidity
    E. Erection with full rigidity
41. The phosphodiesterase enzyme superfamily includes:
    A. 11 gene family
    B. 13 gene family
    C. 15 gene family
    D. 17 gene family
    E. 19 gene family
42. The phosphodiesterase enzyme TYPE 5 is NOT present in:
    A. Platelets
    B. Vascular smooth muscles
    C. Lung
    D. Brain
    E. Bone
43. Which of the following is NOT phosphodiesterase enzyme inhibitors non-responders?
    A. Hypogonadism
    B. End organ failure
    C. Increase body mass index
    D. Severe veno-occlusive disease
    E. Inappropriate fasting condition before their intake
44. The FDA for daily dose phosphodiesterase enzyme inhibitors is:
    A. Sildenafil
    B. Avanafil
    C. Tadalafil
    D. Vardenafil
    E. Lodenafil
45. Yohimbine may be prescribed in:
    A. Neurogenic ED
    B. Arteriogenic ED
    C. Venogenic ED
    D. Psychogenic ED
    E. Drug-induced ED

46. Negative effect of prolonged statins intake:
    A. Increase serum testosterone level
    B. Decrease serum testosterone level
    C. Increase prolactin level
    D. Decrease prolactin level
    E. Enhanced plasma nitrate level
47. The dose of topical prostaglandin application in erectile dysfunction is:
    A. 20 μg
    B. 50 μg
    C. 100 μg
    D. 150 μg
    E. 200 μg
48. The dose of prostaglandin medicated urethral system of erection (MUSE) is:
    A. 20 μg
    B. 40 μg
    C. 50 μg
    D. 60 μg
    E. 200 μg
49. The most common complication of vacuum constriction device is:
    A. Penile petechiae
    B. Penile numbness
    C. Penile pain
    D. Painful ejaculation
    E. Peyronie's disease
50. Penile prosthesis tends to extrude more on the:
    A. Lateral surface
    B. Ventral surface
    C. Crura
    D. Glans
    E. Dorsal surface
51. The non-erecting erection syndrome is due to:
    A. Stuttering priapism
    B. Penile fracture
    C. Blunt penile trauma
    D. Penile suspensory ligament deficiency
    E. Penile arteriovenous fistula
52. Hard flaccid penis syndrome may be due to:
    A. Penile fracture
    B. Blunt perineal trauma
    C. Tailbone injury
    D. High flow priapism
    E. Decreased penile sensation

53. All of the following statements about ED are true EXCEPT:
    A. Psychogenic ED is the most common form of ED
    B. 10% to 19% of cases of ED are neurogenic
    C. In cases of pelvic fracture, ED can be a result of cavernous nerve injury or vascular insufficiency or both
    D. There is a decrease in penile tactile sensitivity with increasing age
    E. In diabetics, impairment of neurogenic and endothelium-dependent relaxation results in inadequate NO release
54. All of the following statements about Arteriogenic ED are true EXCEPT:
    A. Atherosclerotic or traumatic arterial occlusive disease can decrease the perfusion pressure and arterial flow to the sinusoidal spaces
    B. Common risk factors include hypertension, hyperlipidemia, cigarette smoking, diabetes mellitus, trauma, and irradiation
    C. Long-distance cycling is a risk factor for vasculogenic and neurogenic ED
    D. Lesions in the pudendal arteries are less common in men with ED
    E. Among men with coronary arterial disease, the prevalence of ED increases with the severity of arterial lesions
55. All of the following statements are true EXCEPT:
    A. Aging is the single most important contributing factor to ED
    B. The aging process can affect central regulatory, hormonal, neural, and penile structure
    C. Diabetes mellitus and metabolic syndrome may cause premature aging of erectile regulatory mechanisms
    D. Primary ED may be due to psychogenic cause, inexperience, congenital arterial insufficiency, or abnormal venous channels
    E. Primary ED refers to a recently developed ED of unknown etiology
56. The most severe complication of intracavernosal injections is:
    A. Corpora cavernosa inflammation
    B. Hematoma
    C. Priapism
    D. Urethral injury
    E. Penile edema
57. Intracavernosal injections are more effective when used in men with:
    A. Diabetes mellitus
    B. Fibrosis of the corpora cavernosa
    C. Mild vasculopathy
    D. Hypertension
    E. Neurogenic disorder
58. The action mechanism of prostaglandin is:
    A. Indirect, blocking α-adrenergic receptors
    B. Direct, inducing relaxation of smooth muscle fibers
    C. Inhibits PDE5 (phosphodiesterase type 5)
    D. Has central effect
    E. Non-cholinergic action

59. To treat priapism after the use of intracavernosal injections, the first step is:
    A. Intracavernosal administration of a sympathomimetic agent
    B. Bloodletting
    C. Cold packs
    D. Invasive manipulation
    E. Shunt operation
60. The most common adverse event of intracavernosal injections is:
    A. Priapism
    B. Hematoma
    C. Drop of blood pressure
    D. Pain
    E. Liver toxicity
61. PDE5 inhibitors act by:
    A. Reducing cGMP degradation
    B. Reducing NO composition
    C. Reducing cGMP intracellular levels
    D. Increasing free calcium levels
    E. B + C
62. A 50-year-old hypertensive patient reports that he has tried a PDE5i without a result. The next step would be:
    A. Replacement with another PDE5i
    B. Intracavernosal injections
    C. Full history taking concerning the route of drug administration and its dosage
    D. Immediate discontinuation of the anti-hypertensive regimen
    E. C + D
63. The 3 available PDE5 inhibitors:
    A. Have similar efficacy
    B. Have similar pharmacokinetic features
    C. Have been approved for daily use
    D. Differ only concerning the maximum recommended dose
64. PDE5 inhibitors:
    A. Should be provided with caution to patients taking nitrates
    B. Can be administered independently from food intake
    C. Must be provided to the maximal tolerated dose before characterizing a patient as "non-responsive"
    D. Are contra-indicated when the patient receives alfuzosin at the same time
65. A 45-year-old diabetic patient responding initially to sildenafil for about 3 years reports that his erection is no longer sufficient enough to achieve sexual intercourse. The next step is to:
    A. Increase the dose on demand up to 200 mg
    B. Test serum testosterone level
    C. Check diabetes control
    D. Test serum testosterone level, control diabetes and re-administrate sildenafil (100 mg)

66. What do shock waves cause to corpora cavernosa?
    A. Activation of NO
    B. Activation of cGMP
    C. Proliferation of smooth muscle fibers
    D. Neovascularization of the corpora cavernosa
    E. A + D
67. Shock wave therapy is used in:
    A. Renolithiasis
    B. Cholelithiasis
    C. Peyronie's disease
    D. Myocardial ischemia
    E. A + B + C + D
68. In a patient who does not respond to PDE5 inhibitors, what do we expect from the shock-wave therapy?
    A. Functional restoration
    B. Improvement, but also need for supplementary use of PDE5i for functional erection
    C. No clinically significant improvement
    D. A + B + C
69. In a patient with moderate insufficiency of the corpora cavernosa, what do we expect from the shock-wave therapy?
    A. Functional restoration
    B. Improvement, but also need for permanent use of PDE5i for functional erection
    C. No clinically significant improvement
    D. A + B + C
70. A 67-year-old hypertensive patient with erectile dysfunction for 5 years was prescribed sildenafil 100 mg. The patient took tablets at 10 different instances always with an empty stomach and at least 1 hour before sexual contact. 5 out of 10 times, his erection was satisfactory concerning rigidity and duration. Two times his erection was sufficient for penetration, without satisfactory duration. The other 3 times there was penile tumescence but not enough for penetration. This patient is considered:
    A. To respond to sildenafil treatment
    B. Not to respond to sildenafil treatment
71. The add-on therapy with intracavernosal PGE-1 every 2 weeks in patients with a partial response even to the maximum sildenafil dose significantly improves IIEF-EF score by:
    A. 15%
    B. 65%
    C. 25%
    D. 30%

72. Choose the correct answer.
    A. Intrapenile injections are highly effective and result in patients' high satisfaction
    B. Intrapenile injections may achieve high satisfaction but may also lead to withdrawal
    C. Priapism occurs in 20% of patients using intrapenile injections
    D. Fibrosis of the corpora cavernosa occurs more often when papaverine is in the mixture
73. Choose the correct answer.
    A. The infection rate in intrapenile prostheses is 20%
    B. Prosthesis with antibiotic prophylaxis is absolutely indicated in diabetic patients
    C. Antibiotic prophylaxis does not prevent the formation of biofilm upon the prosthesis
    D. A + C
74. Choose the correct answer.
    A. The prosthesis provides the highest satisfaction rate for the sexual partner
    B. The prosthesis has a reintervention rate of >30% within the first 5 years
    C. Penile prosthesis is contra-indicated in diabetic patients
    D. B + C
75. Which of the following is required to have an erection achieved?
    A. Sexual arousal
    B. Communication between brain nerves and penile nerves
    C. Relaxation of blood vessels supplying the penis
    D. A + B + C
76. All medications mentioned below may cause erectile dysfunction, apart from:
    A. Antihypertensives
    B. Antifungals
    C. Tranquillizers
    D. Antihistamines
77. Which hormonal factor is not required to assess erectile dysfunction?
    A. ACTH
    B. Prolactin
    C. TSH
    D. Testosterone
78. Agents for erectile dysfunction act by inhibiting the PDE5 action, responsible for:
    A. Testosterone degradation
    B. Degradation of cyclic-GMP in the penis
    C. Degradation of NO in the penis
    D. None of the above

79. A 50-year hypertensive man visits the andrologist due to erectile dysfunction. He tried a PDE5 inhibitor with no result. The next step should be:
   A. To use another PDE5 inhibitor
   B. To switch to intracavernosal injections
   C. To check thoroughly the drug administration route and dosage
   D. To discontinue immediately the antihypertensive regimen
80. Which of the factors below contribute to the emergence of erectile dysfunction?
   A. Depression and unemployment
   B. Hypertension and heart diseases
   C. Diabetes
   D. A + B + C
81. Which of the conditions below may be related to normal erectile function?
   A. Mild arterial insufficiency with normal venous closure mechanism
   B. Severe arterial insufficiency with normal venous closure mechanism
   C. Normal arterial blood flow with insufficient venous closure mechanism
   D. A + B + C
82. Which of the below factors play a role in normal erection?
   A. Hemodynamics of the corpora cavernosa
   B. Biomechanical properties of tissues
   C. Geometry of the penis
   D. A + B + C
83. Why does the relaxation of a few cavernous muscle fibers induce erection?
   A. Because the two corpora cavernosa communicate with each other
   B. Because there are gap junctions among smooth muscle fibers
   C. Because the drug diffuses
   D. None of the above
84. What pO_2 values of the penis are required to achieve erection?
   A. <20 mmHg
   B. 40–50 mmHg
   C. 60–70 mmHg
   D. >80 mmHg
85. The mean penile length in the normal full-term neonate is:
   A. 2 cm
   B. 2.5 cm
   C. 3 cm
   D. 3.5 cm
86. The dose of testosterone in infants suffering from micropenis is:
   A. 25 mg/week for 3 weeks
   B. 50 mg/week for 3 weeks
   C. 25 mg/month for 3 months
   D. 50 mg/month for 3 months

87. The form of testosterone used in the treatment of a child with micropenis is:
    A. Testosterone enanthate
    B. Testosterone propionate
    C. Testosterone undecanoate
    D. A + C
88. The corpus spongiosum is developed from:
    A. Caudal part of genitourinary sinus
    B. Genital tubercles
    C. Urethral folds
    D. Genital swelling
89. Sex reversal is indicated in all of the following except:
    A. Non-response to testosterone therapy
    B. Klinefelter's syndrome
    C. Partial androgen insensitivity
    D. Severely malformed penis
90. Which of the following sexual dysfunctions may occur during major depression?
    A. Decreased libido
    B. Erectile dysfunction
    C. Delayed orgasm
    D. Hypersexuality
    E. All of the above
91. Guanylate cyclase activators can be used in the treatment of:
    A. Total anorgasmia
    B. Spontaneous ejaculation
    C. Erectile dysfunction
    D. Low libido
    E. Premature ejaculation
92. Transient receptor potential ion channels can be used in the treatment of:
    A. Erectile dysfunction
    B. Weak orgasm
    C. Delayed ejaculation
    D. Widower syndrome
    E. Low desire
93. Which of the following is a drawback of statin therapy in erectile dysfunction?
    A. Low libido
    B. Weak orgasm
    C. Hypogonadism
    D. Spontaneous ejaculation
    E. Climacturia

94. Floppy glans penis syndrome is a potential complication of:
    A. Nessibat operation
    B. Penile prosthesis
    C. Penile lengthening
    D. After filler injection
    E. Erectile dysfunction
95. Embryonic stem cells are derived from:
    A. Bone marrow
    B. Muscle cells
    C. Placenta
    D. Adipose tissue
    E. Nerve cells
96. Which of the following is not a low shock wave therapy generator?
    A. Electropneumatic
    B. Piezoelectric
    C. Electrohydraulic
    D. Electromagnetic
    E. Ionotropic
97. Which of the following is an indication for low shock wave therapy?
    A. Testicular torsion
    B. Erectile dysfunction
    C. Spontaneous ejaculation
    D. Koro syndrome
    E. Micropenis
98. Non-viral vector gene therapy for erectile dysfunction is:
    A. Adenovirus
    B. Retrovirus
    C. Adeomyoblast
    D. Liposomes
99. The disadvantages of viral vector gene therapy for erectile dysfunction include:
    A. Lack of cell specificity
    B. Carcinogenesis
    C. Low immunogenicity
    D. Locally restricted
    E. Non-pathogenicity
100. Penile erection results from:
    A. Decrease in cAMP
    B. Upregulation of fibrotic cytokines
    C. Contraction of cavernosal smooth muscles
    D. Increase in endogenous prostaglandins
    E. None of the above

101. Which erectogenic medication turns urine positive for opiates?
   A. Avanafil
   B. Papaverine
   C. Phentolamine
   D. Trazodone
   E. None of the above
102. A 7-year-old girl presented to the clinic with signs and symptoms of precocious puberty, café-au-lait spots, hyperthyroidism, a history of easily fractured bones, and signs of Cushing disease. Which one of the following is the diagnosis?
   A. Peutz-Jeghers Syndrome
   B. Kallmann Syndrome
   C. Swyer Syndrome
   D. McCune-Albright Syndrome
103. Which of the following antidepressants has a relatively lower frequency of associated sexual dysfunction?
   A. Amitriptyline
   B. Bupropion
   C. Citalopram
   D. Fluoxetine
   E. Imipramine
104. Which of the following is an unusual cause of PDE5i failure?
   A. Timing
   B. Sexual stimulation
   C. Side effects
   D. Alcohol
105. Which of the following rare but potentially serious side effects has NOT been attributed to PDE5 inhibitors?
   A. Pulmonary embolism
   B. Peptic ulcer disease
   C. Cholestatic hepatotoxicity
   D. Thrombocytopenia
   E. Sensorineural hearing loss
106. What is the presumed mechanism of action or explanation of sexual dysfunction associated with antipsychotics?
   A. Dopaminergic blockade
   B. Serotonin reuptake inhibition
   C. Norepinephrine stimulation
   D. Acetylcholine blockade
   E. Serotonin stimulation
107. Which of the following management strategies is particularly unsuitable for the management of sexual dysfunction associated with fluoxetine?
   A. Decreasing the dose
   B. Drug holidays
   C. Switching to another antidepressant
   D. Using antidotes

108. Patients suffering from which of the following anxiety disorders reported impaired sexual functioning?
    A. Obsessive-compulsive disorder
    B. Panic disorder
    C. Posttraumatic stress disorder
    D. Social anxiety disorder
    E. All of the above
109. Which of the following anxiolytics has been found useful in the management of SSRI-associated sexual dysfunction?
    A. Alprazolam
    B. Buspirone
    C. Diazepam
    D. Lorazepam
    E. Triazolam
110. For on-demand use, the lowest possible starting dose of tadalafil (5 mg) should be utilized in which of the following groups of patients?
    A. Hepatic disease
    B. Elderly patients (>65 years)
    C. Coronary artery disease
    D. Renal impairment
    E. Psychogenic ED
111. Phosphodiesterase type 5 inhibitors have been demonstrated to have deleterious effects on which of the following semen parameters?
    A. Semen volume
    B. Sperm concentration
    C. Sperm motility
    D. Semen pH
    E. None of the above
112. Which of the following is the most generally agreed upon theoretical etiology of ototoxicity related to PDE5i use?
    A. Perturbation of ion channel function in auditory neuronal fibers
    B. Changes in eustachian tube function
    C. Vasodilation and subsequent hyperoxygenation of auditory organs
    D. Direct effects on the nitric oxide/cGMP mediated protein kinase system of the middle ear
    E. B and D
113. Treatment of a male partner with PDE5i has been recently demonstrated to improve all but which of the following relationship parameters in heterosexual couples?
    A. Self-esteem in the male partner
    B. Open communication about sexual wants/needs between partners
    C. Sexual life satisfaction in the female partner
    D. Overall sexual life satisfaction in the male partner
    E. Sexual relationship satisfaction in the male partner

114. Following RRP, men who fail to respond to PDE5is typically:
   A. Have inadequate arterial response as a result of cavernous artery injury from cautery
   B. Have significant veno-occlusive dysfunction that is a direct result of apoptosis
   C. Have a combination of psychogenic and preexisting organic pathology such as endothelial dysfunction with smooth muscle pathology
   D. Have primary neural and secondary vasculogenic (arterial and venous-occlusive dysfunction) etiologies
115. Among men with spinal cord injury and erectile dysfunction (ED), the use of PDE5is is:
   A. Marginally effective when testosterone is measured in the normal range
   B. Rarely effective as the required nitric oxide pathways are functionally absent
   C. As effective as in those men with ED secondary to radical prostatectomy
   D. Generally about 80% successful in achieving and maintaining erectile rigidity
116. Among men with spinal cord injuries, the use of Vacuum Constriction Devices for ED is:
   A. Often less effective because the constriction ring causes pain
   B. Risky due to reduced sensation and higher likelihood of incomplete constriction ring causing veno-occlusion
   C. Not often successful as manual dexterity and efficacy often limit utility
   D. A reasonable first-line agent, particularly in high C-spine injuries
117. Use of Intracavernous Vasoactive Injection therapy for men with spinal cord injuries and ED is:
   A. A reasonable and effective option when first-line treatments fail or cost of other options is prohibitive
   B. Rarely successful, owing to impaired manual dexterity
   C. Often limited by recurrent episodes of priapism and infections
   D. Very challenging to teach to the non-neurologically intact individual or partner
118. Which of the following is a common cause of PDE5i failure?
   A. Etiology of ED unclear
   B. Ingestion with alcohol
   C. Lack of adequate sexual stimulation
   D. Too long an interval between the pill and attempt at sex
119. Before initiating treatment of ED with a PDE5i, the clinician should:
   A. Test for hypogonadism
   B. Evaluate for reversible causes
   C. Talk about the sexual relationship
   D. All of the above

120. In most ED treatment algorithms, the role of intracavernous injection is:
    A. Relegated to historical significance
    B. Thought to be too invasive and with poor efficacy
    C. An essential component, with utility among many PDE5i treatment refractory patients
    D. Difficult to teach and expensive

✅ Key Takeaways

- ED affects millions globally and increases with age and comorbidity.
- The neurovascular mechanism of erection is central; endothelial dysfunction is a common contributor.
- IIEF-5 score is widely used for ED severity classification.
- First-line treatment: PDE5 inhibitors (e.g., sildenafil).
- Advanced options include intracavernosal injections, shockwave therapy, and surgical prostheses.
- Lifestyle modification improves vascular ED.

✅ Answer Key (1–120)

1. D
2. C
3. E
4. E
5. D
6. A
7. C
8. C
9. B
10. C
11. C
12. B
13. D
14. A
15. D
16. E
17. D
18. C
19. A
20. E
21. C
22. E
23. C

24. C
25. D
26. B
27. E
28. C
29. B
30. B
31. A
32. A
33. C
34. D
35. E
36. A
37. D
38. B
39. E
40. D
41. A
42. E
43. C
44. C
45. D
46. B
47. E
48. E
49. A
50. B
51. A
52. B
53. A
54. D
55. E
56. C
57. E
58. B
59. A
60. D
61. A
62. C
63. A
64. C
65. D
66. E
67. E
68. B

69. B
70. A
71. B
72. D
73. B
74. A
75. D
76. B
77. A
78. B
79. C
80. D
81. A
82. D
83. B
84. D
85. B
86. C
87. A
88. C
89. B
90. E
91. C
92. A
93. C
94. B
95. C
96. E
97. B
98. D
99. A
100. D
101. B
102. D
103. B
104. D
105. B
106. A
107. B
108. E
109. B
110. B
111. E
112. A
113. E

114. D
115. D
116. D
117. A
118. C
119. D
120. C

Explanations (1–120)

1. **Psychogenic erection**—These erections are triggered centrally by visual, auditory, or imaginative stimuli. They involve cortical and spinal pathways and can occur without physical genital contact. Damage to higher centers or pathways may impair them.
2. **Reflexogenic erection**—Triggered by direct genital tactile stimulation through intact sacral reflex arcs (S2–S4). They are often preserved in upper spinal injuries since local reflexes remain intact.
3. **Non-risk factor for ED**—Masturbation is not harmful; instead, it is a normal sexual activity. Conditions like BPH, hyperuricemia, vitamin D deficiency, and hyperhomocysteinemia are linked to vascular and metabolic impairment.
4. **Non-risk factor for ED**—Nebivolol differs from other β-blockers by enhancing nitric oxide release, improving erectile function rather than impairing it. The others listed contribute to vascular or hormonal dysfunction.
5. **Organic ED criteria**—Gradual onset, medical history, and progressive worsening indicate organic pathology. Psychogenic ED usually preserves morning erections, which helps in differentiation.
6. **Basic investigations**—Initial labs include glucose, lipids, testosterone, and prolactin. LH is not first-line and is checked only when hypogonadism or pituitary disease is suspected.
7. **Widower syndrome**—A form of psychogenic ED that arises after loss of a long-term partner. Emotional grief and psychological stress are the major contributing factors.
8. **NPT limitations**—Nocturnal penile tumescence (NPT) studies assess night erections (frequency, rigidity, circumference, duration). They do not measure daytime erections.
9. **Most accurate NPT method**—Sleep-laboratory NPT with rigidity assessment is the gold standard. It gives precise data, though Rigiscan is practical and commonly used.
10. **Normal nocturnal erections**—Healthy males typically have 4–6 erections per night, corresponding to REM cycles. Fewer suggest underlying organic ED.
11. **Normal root circumference change**—About 3 cm increase at the penile root during erections is expected. Lower changes may reflect reduced rigidity.
12. **Prevalence of neurogenic ED**—Accounts for 10–20% of cases. Causes include spinal cord injuries, diabetic neuropathy, multiple sclerosis, and Parkinson's disease.

13. **Hormone for frequency**—Testosterone governs libido, erectile capacity, and frequency of sexual activity. Deficiency lowers sexual drive and erectile performance.
14. **Nocturnal emissions**—Testosterone drives nocturnal erections and emissions. Lower testosterone correlates with absent or reduced night erections.
15. **Leriche syndrome**—Aortoiliac occlusion presents with the triad: buttock/thigh claudication, absent femoral pulses, and ED. It is a vascular cause.
16. **Claudication criteria**—Leriche syndrome is characterized by buttock/thigh claudication and impotence. Recognition is important for vascular intervention.
17. **Proximal venogenic ED**—Often due to chronic perineal trauma (e.g., prolonged cycling), which disrupts proximal venous outflow regulation.
18. **Distal venogenic ED**—Typically iatrogenic, caused by surgical or traumatic creation of fistulas between erectile tissues and veins, leading to venous leakage.
19. **High-risk CVS association**—Patients with established coronary artery disease are high-risk when presenting with ED. A thorough cardiac assessment is vital.
20. **Metabolic syndrome criteria**—Defined by obesity, hypertension, impaired glucose tolerance, and dyslipidemia. Estradiol levels are not a criterion.
21. **Mechanism in liver disease**—ED in liver disease arises from high estrogen, increased SHBG, hyperprolactinemia, and low testosterone. Parathormone is not involved.
22. **BPH and ED link**—Increased RhoA/ROK signaling in BPH enhances cavernosal contractility, impairing relaxation and promoting ED.
23. **Drugs not associated with ED**—Nebivolol has vasodilatory effects and is safer than other β-blockers. Drugs like clonidine, spironolactone, and amiodarone impair sexual function.
24. **Helicine artery blockade**—Methyldopa induces arterial constriction, restricting penile inflow, contributing to ED.
25. **NO-promoting drug**—Nebivolol uniquely promotes NO release, improving endothelial function and aiding erectile response.
26. **Pelvic steal syndrome**—Blood is diverted away from pelvic organs during activity, reducing penile perfusion and causing ED.
27. **Normal IIEF score**—A score above 25 indicates normal erectile function. Lower scores reflect varying severities of ED.
28. **Mild ED score**—Scores between 17 and 21 indicate mild ED. Patients often maintain erections but with reduced rigidity or consistency.
29. **Mild–moderate ED score**—Scores of 11–16 fall in this range, showing noticeable erectile impairment but not complete loss of function.
30. **Moderate ED score**—Moderate dysfunction often falls within scores of 11–16, showing significant compromise of sexual function.
31. **Severe ED score**—Scores between 1 and 10 reflect severe ED, where erections are rarely sufficient for penetration.
32. **Prostaglandin metabolism enzyme**—PGE1 is broken down rapidly by 15-hydroxy prostaglandin dehydrogenase, limiting systemic side effects.
33. **Prostaglandin site of metabolism**—Metabolized primarily in the lung, which rapidly inactivates circulating PGE1.

34. **Prostaglandin excretion**—Mainly excreted by the kidney following metabolic breakdown in the lung and liver.
35. **Drug not used intracorporeally**—Methylene blue is not part of standard ED intracavernosal agents. Agents like PGE1, VIP, and forskolin are used.
36. **Starting intracorporeal dose**—Low doses (5 units = 0.05 ml) are used initially to minimize risk of priapism. Titration follows patient response.
37. **Correct injection method**—Intracavernosal injection directly into corpora cavernosa is the proper method. Incorrect techniques risk injury.
38. **E2 response score**—Represents partial tumescence, not yet full rigidity, useful in monitoring drug testing.
39. **E4 response score**—Indicates erection with partial rigidity, often insufficient for penetration.
40. **E3 response score**—Denotes full tumescence without rigidity, a middle-stage response in injection testing.
41. **PDE superfamily**—There are 11 families of phosphodiesterase enzymes. PDE5, relevant in ED, degrades cGMP, so inhibition prolongs smooth muscle relaxation.
42. **PDE5 distribution**—Found in platelets, vascular smooth muscle, and lungs, but not significantly in bone. Thus, bone is the exception.
43. **PDE5 non-responders**—Common reasons are severe veno-occlusive disease, end-organ failure, or hypogonadism. Increased BMI is a risk but not an absolute cause of non-response.
44. **FDA-approved daily PDE5i**—Tadalafil is approved for daily low-dose use, improving both ED and LUTS associated with BPH.
45. **Yohimbine use**—An α2-adrenergic antagonist used occasionally for psychogenic ED. Evidence is limited compared to PDE5 inhibitors.
46. **Statins effect**—Prolonged statin use may decrease serum testosterone, though benefits on vascular health often outweigh risks. Monitoring is advised.
47. **Topical prostaglandin**—The topical dose for PGE1 is higher (200 μg) due to local absorption barriers compared to injections.
48. **MUSE system**—Medicated urethral system for erection typically uses 200 μg intraurethral alprostadil. It is less invasive but less effective than injections.
49. **Vacuum device complication**—Petechiae are common due to venous congestion and negative pressure trauma to small vessels.
50. **Prosthesis extrusion**—Ventral surface (near urethra) is prone to extrusion due to thinner tissue coverage compared to dorsal.
51. **Non-erecting erection syndrome**—Linked to stuttering priapism where repeated ischemia causes fibrosis, leading to apparent tumescence without rigidity.
52. **Hard flaccid syndrome**—Often follows blunt perineal or tailbone trauma. Patients describe a firm but non-erect penis with sensory changes.
53. **ED facts**—Psychogenic ED is most common, accounting for many younger cases. In diabetics, impaired NO release is central to pathogenesis.
54. **Arteriogenic ED facts**—Pudendal artery lesions are common in ED. Long-distance cycling compresses pudendal vessels, increasing risk.

55. **ED with age**—Aging is a major risk, but "primary ED" refers to lifelong inability, often psychogenic or congenital—not a recently acquired issue.
56. **Injection complication**—Priapism is the most serious complication of intracavernosal therapy. Immediate intervention is required to prevent fibrosis.
57. **Best responders**—Neurogenic ED responds well to injections since local pharmacologic action bypasses neural impairment.
58. **PGE1 mechanism**—Acts directly on smooth muscle receptors, causing cAMP-mediated relaxation and vasodilation of corpora cavernosa.
59. **Priapism management**—First-line treatment is sympathomimetic injection (e.g., phenylephrine) into the corpora to restore venous outflow.
60. **Common injection adverse effect**—Pain at the injection site is most frequent, though usually mild and self-limiting.
61. **PDE5 mechanism**—Inhibits degradation of cGMP, prolonging smooth muscle relaxation and erection. Correct mechanism is increasing cGMP, not calcium.
62. **PDE5i failure**—Always confirm dose, timing, and administration. Many failures are due to improper use, not true drug resistance.
63. **PDE5 inhibitors**—Sildenafil, tadalafil, and vardenafil have similar efficacy but different pharmacokinetics (onset and duration).
64. **PDE5 precautions**—Contraindicated with nitrates. Patients must be on maximal tolerated dose before declaring non-response.
65. **Diabetic relapse**—Loss of efficacy often reflects poor diabetes control or low testosterone; both should be corrected before adjusting therapy.
66. **Shock waves**—Stimulate NO pathways and promote neovascularization, improving cavernosal perfusion and tissue repair.
67. **Shock wave therapy uses**—Applied in kidney stones, gallstones, Peyronie's disease, and ischemic conditions. Its role in ED is emerging.
68. **Non-responders to PDE5i**—Shock waves may improve function but often require continued PDE5i support. Complete restoration is rare.
69. **Moderate cavernosal insufficiency**—Patients may show improvement but often remain PDE5i-dependent long-term.
70. **PDE5i response definition**—Even partial erections that allow penetration on several attempts count as treatment response.
71. **Add-on injections**—Combining alprostadil with PDE5 inhibitors in partial responders can boost IIEF scores by ~65%.
72. **Intrapenile injections**—Effective and satisfactory but withdrawal is common due to inconvenience or anxiety about injections.
73. **Prosthesis infection**—Antibiotic coatings reduce but do not eliminate biofilm risk. Infection rates are not as high as 20%.
74. **Prosthesis satisfaction**—Provides high partner satisfaction. Reintervention rates are generally <10% at 5 years, not >30%.
75. **Requirements for erection**—Requires arousal, nerve signals, and vascular relaxation. Failure in any of these leads to ED.
76. **Drug causes**—Antifungals rarely cause ED, unlike antihypertensives, tranquilizers, and antihistamines.

77. **Hormonal assessment**—Core hormones include testosterone, prolactin, and thyroid hormones. ACTH is not routinely tested.
78. **PDE5 action**—These drugs prevent cGMP breakdown, prolonging smooth muscle relaxation. They do not affect testosterone or NO directly.
79. **PDE5i failure in hypertension**—First confirm proper administration and dosage. Many "failures" are due to incorrect timing.
80. **Contributing factors**—Depression, unemployment, hypertension, heart disease, and diabetes all significantly increase ED risk.
81. **Erectile function conditions**—Even mild arterial insufficiency can be tolerated if venous closure is intact. Severe arterial or venous leakage disrupts function, making all three scenarios relevant.
82. **Factors for erection**—Hemodynamics, tissue biomechanics, and penile geometry all influence rigidity. Cavernosal compliance and tunica resistance are critical for veno-occlusion.
83. **Fiber relaxation**—A few relaxed smooth muscle fibers can trigger erection because gap junctions spread depolarization across the corpora cavernosa. This amplifies relaxation.
84. **Oxygen tension**—Penile pO2 must exceed ~80 mmHg to support rigidity. Lower levels sustain tumescence but not full rigidity.
85. **Neonatal penile length**—A mean stretched length of 2.5 cm is normal for full-term neonates. Values below 2 cm indicate micropenis.
86. **Testosterone therapy in infants**—Low-dose intramuscular testosterone (25 mg monthly for 3 months) is used to stimulate penile growth in micropenis.
87. **Testosterone forms**—Testosterone enanthate is standard for pediatric micropenis. Oral undecanoate may also be used but is less reliable.
88. **Corpus spongiosum origin**—It develops from the caudal genitourinary sinus and surrounds the urethra, later expanding to form the glans.
89. **Sex reversal**—Indicated for non-response to hormones, partial androgen insensitivity, or severe penile malformation. Klinefelter's syndrome is not an indication, since sex assignment is clear.
90. **Depression and sexual dysfunction**—Major depression can cause decreased libido, ED, delayed orgasm, and sometimes hypersexuality due to dysregulated neurotransmitters.
91. **Guanylate cyclase activators**—They directly stimulate cGMP production, promoting cavernosal relaxation, and are potential therapies for ED.
92. **TRP channels**—These ion channels modulate calcium entry and smooth muscle tone; experimental use in ED therapy shows promise.
93. **Statin drawback**—Some men on statins develop hypogonadism due to altered cholesterol metabolism, lowering testosterone.
94. **Floppy glans syndrome**—Most often seen after penile prosthesis surgery due to poor glans support, leading to soft tip despite corporal rigidity.
95. **Embryonic stem cells**—Derived from blastocyst inner cell mass or placenta. They have pluripotent capacity and are studied for regenerative ED therapies.
96. **Shock wave generators**—Types include electropneumatic, piezoelectric, electrohydraulic, and electromagnetic. "Ionotropic" is not a recognized generator.

97. **Indications**—Low-intensity shock waves are used in ED, Peyronie's disease, ischemia, and lithotripsy. Micropenis and torsion are not indications.
98. **Non-viral vectors**—Liposomes are non-viral carriers for gene delivery in ED gene therapy, avoiding risks of viral integration.
99. **Viral vector disadvantages**—Include lack of specificity and carcinogenic potential. Immunogenicity is usually high, not low, making "low immunogenicity" incorrect.
100. **Mechanism of erection**—Driven by cGMP-mediated smooth muscle relaxation and prostaglandin release. Decreased cAMP or muscle contraction does not produce erection.
101. **Papaverine**—Can produce false-positive opiate urine tests due to its metabolites. Other erectogenic agents do not.
102. **McCune-Albright syndrome**—Characterized by precocious puberty, café-au-lait spots, fibrous dysplasia, and endocrine abnormalities.
103. **Antidepressants**—Bupropion has the lowest incidence of sexual side effects, while SSRIs like citalopram and fluoxetine commonly cause dysfunction.
104. **PDE5i failure**—Alcohol intake can blunt drug efficacy, but timing errors and lack of arousal are more unusual causes.
105. **Rare PDE5i effects**—Sensorineural hearing loss, hepatotoxicity, and blood dyscrasias are reported. Peptic ulcer disease is not associated.
106. **Antipsychotic dysfunction**—Mainly due to dopamine D2 receptor blockade, leading to hyperprolactinemia and suppressed libido and erections.
107. **Fluoxetine management**—Drug holidays are inappropriate due to SSRI half-lives and risk of relapse. Dose adjustment or switching is safer.
108. **Anxiety disorders**—OCD, panic, PTSD, and social anxiety are all linked to sexual dysfunction via neuroendocrine dysregulation.
109. **Buspirone**—A serotonin 5-HT1A agonist shown to help relieve SSRI-induced sexual dysfunction, unlike benzodiazepines.
110. **Tadalafil use**—Elderly patients (>65 years) start at the lowest dose (5 mg) to minimize side effects due to altered drug clearance.
111. **PDE5i semen effects**—No significant adverse effects on sperm parameters are consistently demonstrated; thus "none of the above" is correct.
112. **Ototoxicity**—Believed to result from vascular changes in auditory organs, with NO/cGMP pathways possibly involved.
113. **Relationship impact**—PDE5is improve self-esteem, communication, and satisfaction. Male sexual relationship satisfaction is less consistently improved.
114. **RRP and PDE5i failure**—Radical prostatectomy often damages both nerves and vessels, making ED multifactorial and PDE5i less effective.
115. **SCI and PDE5i**—In spinal cord injuries, PDE5 inhibitors are effective in ~80% of patients with intact NO pathways.
116. **Vacuum devices in SCI**—Useful in high-level injuries but require care due to reduced sensation and possible venous leakage.
117. **Intracavernosal injections in SCI**—Effective, bypassing neural defects, though priapism and infection risks remain. Patient training is critical.

118. **PDE5i failure**—Most often due to insufficient sexual stimulation, as these drugs require arousal to activate NO release.
119. **Pre-treatment evaluation**—Always screen for hypogonadism, reversible factors (drugs, depression), and relationship context before prescribing PDE5i.
120. **Role of injections**—Remains essential in PDE5i-refractory ED, offering reliable erections in men who fail oral therapies.

Further Reading

The explanations in this chapter are supported by the following key references:

1. Burnett AL, Nehra A, Breau RH, et al. Erectile dysfunction: AUA guideline. J Urol. 2018;200(3):633–41.
2. Wespes E, Amar E, Hatzichristou D, et al. EAU guidelines on erectile dysfunction. Eur Urol. 2013;62(2):324–32.
3. Montorsi P, Ravagnani PM, Galli S. The artery size hypothesis: a macrovascular link between erectile dysfunction and coronary artery disease. Am J Cardiol. 2005;96(12B):19M–23M.
4. Corona G, Isidori AM, Aversa A, et al. Endocrinologic control of male sexual function. J Sex Med. 2016;13(3):317–37.
5. Hackett G. The role of testosterone in the treatment of erectile dysfunction. Curr Opin Urol. 2016;26(6):568–73.
6. Goldstein I, Burnett AL, Rosen RC, et al. Oral pharmacotherapy for erectile dysfunction. Sex Med Rev. 2019;7(1):115–28.
7. Corona G, Cucinotta D, Di Lorenzo G, Ferlin A, Giagulli VA, Gnessi L, Isidori AM, Maiorino MI, Miserendino P, Murrone A, Pivonello R, Rochira V, Sangiorgi GM, Stagno G, Foresta C, Lenzi A, Maggi M, Jannini EA. The Italian Society of Andrology and Sexual Medicine (SIAMS), along with ten other Italian Scientific Societies, guidelines on the diagnosis and management of erectile dysfunction. J Endocrinol Invest. 2023;46(6):1241–74.

8 Ejaculatory and Orgasmic Disorders

Learning Objectives

- Classify ejaculatory disorders and their diagnostic criteria.
- Distinguish between lifelong and acquired PE.
- Recognize causes of delayed or absent ejaculation.
- Review treatment strategies including SSRIs, topical anesthetics, and behavioral therapy.
- Address psychogenic and iatrogenic orgasmic dysfunction.

Select the Single Best Answer

1. Which of the following is FALSE about the emission phase of ejaculation?
   A. Parasympathetic control
   B. Voluntary control
   C. Increase semen volume
   D. Contraction of male accessory glands
   E. Distension of the posterior urethra with semen
2. Which of the following is FALSE about male orgasm?
   A. Climacteric pleasure
   B. Build up and release pleasure in the posterior urethra
   C. Coincides with ejaculation
   D. Pudendal nerve sensory stimulation
   E. Voluntary control
3. Spinothalamic ejaculation generator is:
   A. L1–2
   B. L3–4
   C. L10–12
   D. C1–3
   E. S2–4

M. S. M. Hasan, M. L. Elsaie, *Comprehensive MCQs in Andrology*, Trends in Andrology and Sexual Medicine, https://doi.org/10.1007/978-3-032-20623-7_8

4. Increase serotonin level causes:
   A. Climacturia
   B. Anorgasmia
   C. Premature ejaculation
   D. Delayed ejaculation
   E. Painful ejaculation
5. Decrease dopamine level causes:
   A. Climacturia
   B. Anorgasmia
   C. Premature ejaculation
   D. Delayed ejaculation
   E. Painful ejaculation
6. Decrease serotonin level causes:
   A. Climacturia
   B. Anorgasmia
   C. Premature ejaculation
   D. Delayed ejaculation
   E. Painful ejaculation
7. Increase dopamine level causes:
   A. Climacturia
   B. Anorgasmia
   C. Premature ejaculation
   D. Delayed ejaculation
   E. Painful ejaculation
8. Which of the following is FALSE about spontaneous ejaculation?
   A. It is ejaculation at night by adult males
   B. Antidepressant drugs may trigger it
   C. Pathological form may be due to decreased adrenergic activity
   D. Ejaculation triggered by dreams involving sexual or non-sexual scenes
   E. Pathological form may be due to decreased serotonergic activity
9. Stimulatory substance involved in the ejaculatory scenario:
   A. Prolactin
   B. Endorphin
   C. Serotonin
   D. Oxytocin
   E. Estradiol
10. Inhibitory substance involved in the ejaculatory scenario:
    A. Dopamine
    B. Oxytocin
    C. Testosterone
    D. Estradiol
    E. Endorphins

11. Which of the following is NOT true about ejaculatory seepage?
    A. It is due to weak sexual stimulation
    B. It occurs in old age
    C. Increase contractile power of anterior urethra
    D. May be temporary during premature ejaculation treatment
    E. Can occur in normal persons
12. Which of the following is FALSE about oneirogonorrhea?
    A. It is physiological spontaneous ejaculation
    B. It is due to specific sexual trauma
    C. Triggered by dreams involving sexual or non-sexual scenes
    D. Can occur during examinations or stressful conditions
    E. May be associated with erectile dysfunction
13. The general body fatigue syndrome is responsible for:
    A. Primary total anorgasmia
    B. Secondary total anorgasmia
    C. Secondary retrograde ejaculation
    D. Physiological anorgasmia
    E. Ejaculatory anhedonia
14. Illegal sexual acts may be the cause of:
    A. Primary total anorgasmia
    B. Secondary retrograde ejaculation
    C. Secondary total anorgasmia
    D. Physiological anorgasmia
    E. Ejaculatory anhedonia
15. Orgasmic anejaculation is characterized by:
    A. Yes orgasm, no ejaculation
    B. No orgasm, yes ejaculation
    C. No orgasm, no ejaculation
    D. Yes orgasm, yes ejaculation
16. Male anorgasmia:
    A. Yes orgasm, no ejaculation
    B. No orgasm, yes ejaculation
    C. No orgasm, no ejaculation
    D. Yes orgasm, yes ejaculation
17. Duration of penile vibratory device application in treatment of aspermia:
    A. 2–4 min
    B. 3–6 min
    C. 6–10 min
    D. 8–10 min
    E. 10–15 min
18. Site of application of penile vibration in aspermia treatment:
    A. Ventral aspect of penis
    B. Dorsal aspect of penis
    C. Ventral aspect of glans
    D. Dorsal aspect of glans

19. Post-coital urine test is positive in retrograde ejaculation if:
    A. >5 sperm/HPF
    B. >10 sperm/HPF
    C. >15 sperm/HPF
    D. <10 sperm/HPF
20. Role of ephedrine sulfate in retrograde ejaculation treatment:
    A. Anticholinergic
    B. Anti-adrenergic
    C. Anti-muscarinic
    D. Sympathomimetic
21. Dose of oxedrine in retrograde ejaculation treatment is:
    A. 30 mg orally
    B. 60 mg orally
    C. 30 mg parenterally
    D. 60 mg parenterally
    E. 75 mg orally
22. According to ISSM (2014), intravaginal ejaculation latency time in secondary PE is:
    A. <1 min
    B. <2 min
    C. <3 min
    D. <4 min
23. Number of penile–vaginal thrusts in premature ejaculation:
    A. <30
    B. <25
    C. <20
    D. <15
24. Primary premature ejaculation is due to:
    A. Ejaculatory reflex hypersensitivity
    B. Anxiety
    C. Super excited sexual technique
    D. Husband–wife conflicts
25. In male Kegel exercise for PE, the trained muscle is:
    A. Puborectalis
    B. Ischiocavernosus
    C. Bulbospongiosus
    D. Cremasteric
    E. Pubococcygeus
26. Best repetition of male Kegel exercise for PE:
    A. 1–5 times
    B. 5–10 times
    C. 10–20 times
    D. 50 times

27. Kegel exercise in males is NOT used in:
    A. Premature ejaculation
    B. Climacturia
    C. Prostatic carcinoma
    D. Prostatorrhea
28. Mechanism of silodosin in PE treatment:
    A. SSRI
    B. Antidepressant
    C. Alpha-blocker
    D. Anxiolytic
29. 5-HT1A receptor polymorphism (C-1019G) is linked to:
    A. Primary PE
    B. SSRI non-responders
    C. Erectile dysfunction
    D. Delayed ejaculation
    E. Climacturia
30. Which is NOT used in PE treatment?
    A. Oxedrine
    B. Pregabalin
    C. Silodosin
    D. Paroxetine
    E. Lidocaine
31. Mechanism of sildenafil on ejaculation latency:
    A. Reduced parasympathetic tone
    B. Reduced sympathetic tone
    C. Increased parasympathetic tone
    D. Increased sympathetic tone
32. Oxytocin receptor antagonists can treat:
    A. Retrograde ejaculation
    B. Premature ejaculation
    C. Anorgasmia
    D. Delayed ejaculation
    E. Ejaculatory anhedonia
33. Epelsiban is used in:
    A. Retrograde ejaculation
    B. Premature ejaculation
    C. Anorgasmia
    D. Delayed ejaculation
    E. Ejaculatory anhedonia
34. Cligosiban is used in:
    A. Retrograde ejaculation
    B. Premature ejaculation
    C. Anorgasmia
    D. Delayed ejaculation
    E. Ejaculatory anhedonia

35. Müllerian duct cyst can cause:
    A. Retrograde ejaculation
    B. Premature ejaculation
    C. Delayed ejaculation
    D. Anorgasmia
    E. Ejaculatory anhedonia
36. Prune belly syndrome is associated with:
    A. Retrograde ejaculation
    B. Premature ejaculation
    C. Delayed ejaculation
    D. Anorgasmia
    E. Ejaculatory anhedonia
37. Wolffian duct abnormalities are associated with:
    A. Retrograde ejaculation
    B. Premature ejaculation
    C. Delayed ejaculation
    D. Anorgasmia
    E. Ejaculatory anhedonia
38. Ejaculatory anhedonia shows:
    A. Yes orgasm, no ejaculation
    B. No orgasm, yes ejaculation
    C. No orgasm, no ejaculation
    D. Yes orgasm, yes ejaculation
39. Seminal hypersensitization therapy is useful in:
    A. Koro syndrome
    B. Post-ejaculation pain syndrome
    C. Lost penis syndrome
    D. Anorgasmia
    E. Post-orgasmic illness syndrome
40. Lost penis syndrome is associated with:
    A. Retrograde ejaculation
    B. Premature ejaculation
    C. Delayed ejaculation
    D. Anorgasmia
    E. Ejaculatory anhedonia
41. Amantadine can be used in treatment of:
    A. Retrograde ejaculation
    B. Premature ejaculation
    C. Delayed ejaculation
    D. Anorgasmia
    E. Ejaculatory anhedonia

42. Cyproheptadine can be used in treatment of:
    A. Retrograde ejaculation
    B. Premature ejaculation
    C. Delayed ejaculation
    D. Anorgasmia
    E. Ejaculatory anhedonia
43. Reboxetine can be used in:
    A. Retrograde ejaculation
    B. Premature ejaculation
    C. Delayed ejaculation
    D. Anorgasmia
    E. Ejaculatory anhedonia
44. Bethanechol can be used in:
    A. Retrograde ejaculation
    B. Premature ejaculation
    C. Delayed cjaculation
    D. Anorgasmia
    E. Ejaculatory anhedonia
45. True climacturia is:
    A. Involuntary passage of semen during orgasm
    B. Involuntary passage of urine during orgasm
    C. Voluntary passage of urine during orgasm
    D. Voluntary passage of semen during orgasm
46. Pseudo-climacturia is:
    A. Involuntary passage of semen during orgasm
    B. Involuntary passage of urine during orgasm
    C. Involuntary passage of urine during foreplay
    D. Voluntary passage of semen during orgasm
47. Weakness of penile suspensory ligament after prostatectomy may cause:
    A. Premature ejaculation
    B. Retrograde ejaculation
    C. Climacturia
    D. Anorgasmia
    E. Delayed ejaculation
48. Oxybutynin can be used in:
    A. Premature ejaculation
    B. Retrograde ejaculation
    C. Climacturia
    D. Anorgasmia
    E. Delayed ejaculation
49. Mirabegron can be used in:
    A. Premature ejaculation
    B. Retrograde ejaculation
    C. Climacturia
    D. Anorgasmia
    E. Delayed ejaculation

50. Which is NOT true about post-orgasmic illness syndrome?
    A. Allergic reaction to seminal fluid
    B. Idiopathic
    C. Inflammatory reaction to seminal fluid
    D. Chemical brain imbalance
    E. Chronic fatigue syndrome
51. Autologous semen injection can be used in:
    A. Condom allergy
    B. Post-orgasmic illness syndrome
    C. Retrograde ejaculation
    D. Coital headache
    E. Post-ejaculation pain syndrome
52. Lost penis syndrome is NOT responsible for:
    A. Male anorgasmia
    B. Erectile dysfunction
    C. Delayed ejaculation
    D. Retrograde ejaculation
53. Most important inhibitory neurotransmitter in central control of ejaculation:
    A. Dopamine
    B. Serotonin
    C. Noradrenaline
    D. Oxytocin
    E. γ-aminobutyric acid
54. Which of the following is INCORRECT?
    A. Ejaculatory process has emission, ejection, orgasm phases
    B. Emission mediated by sympathetic (T10–L2)
    C. Ejection mediated by somatic nerves (S2–S4)
    D. Ejection also involves parasympathetic reflex with voluntary control
    E. Bladder neck closure + pelvic floor contraction prevent retrograde ejaculation
55. Prevalence of IELT ≤1 min in general population is:
    A. <1%
    B. 2.5%
    C. 5.5%
    D. 11%
    E. 20%
56. Which is INCORRECT?
    A. DSM IV definition of PE is multivariate including latency, control, bother
    B. ~80% of men with lifelong PE ejaculate <1 min after penetration
    C. Lifelong PE suggests neurobiological dysfunction
    D. Acquired PE mostly due to psychological or comorbid ED
    E. Subjective PE always linked to prolonged IELT

57. Which is INCORRECT?
    A. ISSM created first evidence-based definition of lifelong & acquired PE
    B. ISSM criteria: time, inability to delay, negative consequences
    C. Lifelong PE defined partly by IELT <1 min
    D. Acquired PE defined partly by IELT ~3 min or less
    E. Definition excludes men in homosexual relationships
58. Which is TRUE in retrograde ejaculation?
    A. Confirmed by sperm in post-masturbation urine
    B. More common after bladder neck incision than TURP
    C. Occurs in diabetic autonomic neuropathy
    D. Associated with hypogonadism in diabetics
    E. Both A and C
59. In spinal cord injury, which is FALSE?
    A. Ability to ejaculate increases with descending injury level
    B. <5% with complete UMN lesions retain ejaculation
    C. Ability to achieve erection increases with descending level
    D. Electroejaculation/vibration carry risk of autonomic dysreflexia
    E. Both A and B
60. In acquired PE with ED, which is FALSE?
    A. Men often rush intercourse to avoid detumescence
    B. PE rarely worsened by performance anxiety with ED
    C. Limiting arousal during foreplay may cause incomplete erection
    D. Vascular risk factors are common
    E. C and D
61. Which reduces climacturia after prostatectomy?
    A. Emptying bladder before sex
    B. Pelvic floor muscle training
    C. Artificial sphincter
    D. Testosterone therapy
62. A patient ejaculates within 60 s in 25% of encounters, but 4–6 min otherwise. Diagnosis is:
    A. Lifelong PE
    B. Secondary PE
    C. Natural variable PE
    D. Subjective PE
63. Which is NOT in the triad of PE?
    A. Lack of ejaculatory control
    B. Short latency
    C. Prolonged abstinence
    D. Sexual dissatisfaction
    E. All of the above

64. In RCT (Randomized controlled trials), most effective PE treatment was:
    A. EMLA cream alone
    B. Sildenafil alone
    C. Combination EMLA + sildenafil
    D. Placebo
    E. Sildenafil + placebo cream
65. After stopping successful therapy in lifelong PE, relapse occurs:
    A. 5–7 days
    B. 3–6 months
    C. 3–6 weeks
    D. Long-term remission persists
    E. None
66. First oral SSRI with short half-life developed for PE:
    A. Dapoxetine
    B. Fluoxetine
    C. Clomipramine
    D. Sertraline
    E. Duloxetine
67. FDA advisory: suicide risk with SSRIs except:
    A. Dapoxetine
    B. Duloxetine
    C. Fluoxetine
    D. Clomipramine
    E. None
68. SSRI with least IELT-prolonging effect:
    A. Paroxetine
    B. Fluoxetine
    C. Fluvoxamine
    D. Sertraline
    E. None
69. Which is TRUE about clomipramine?
    A. SSRI for manic depression
    B. TCA used in PE, less effective than fluvoxamine
    C. SSRI abandoned for visual hypersensitivity
    D. TCA inhibiting 5-HT reuptake, used in OCD
    E. SSRI with promising PE efficacy
70. Which is FALSE about tramadol?
    A. Centrally acting synthetic opioid
    B. 50 mg gives 13-fold IELT increase in RCT
    C. Abandoned as SSRI due to addiction
    D. Side effects include somnolence, dyspepsia
    E. No major withdrawal due to side effects

71. NOT demonstrated effective in PE:
    A. Tricyclic antidepressants
    B. SSRIs
    C. Topical anesthetics
    D. Alpha agonists
72. Secondary PE with ED is:
    A. Very unusual
    B. Occurs in Peyronie's disease
    C. Treatable with PDE5i
    D. Usually transient
73. Risk with SSRI + coumadin:
    A. Inactive anticoagulant
    B. Metabolic side effects
    C. Prolonged bleeding risk
    D. Increased serotonin
74. Most important assessment in PE:
    A. Physical exam
    B. Sexual history
    C. Hormone/electrolyte testing
    D. PDE5i trial + vascular testing
75. Topical anesthetics for PE:
    A. Limited value due to ED
    B. Under regulatory review, promising therapy
    C. Cause partner's sensation loss
    D. Not practical due to delay
76. A 40-year-old diabetic male presents with absent ejaculation despite orgasmic sensation. Most likely diagnosis:
    A. Retrograde ejaculation
    B. Primary anorgasmia
    C. Ejaculatory anhedonia
    D. Orgasmic anejaculation
    E. Climacturia
77. Which of the following can cause retrograde ejaculation?
    A. Transurethral resection of the prostate
    B. Diabetes mellitus
    C. Alpha-blocker therapy
    D. Spinal cord injury
    E. All of the above
78. Most common pharmacological cause of delayed ejaculation:
    A. SSRIs
    B. Beta blockers
    C. Diuretics
    D. Antihistamines
    E. Alpha agonists

79. A man achieves orgasm but reports no pleasurable sensation. This is:
    A. Ejaculatory anhedonia
    B. Retrograde ejaculation
    C. Delayed ejaculation
    D. Climacturia
    E. Premature ejaculation
80. Diagnostic hallmark of retrograde ejaculation:
    A. Nocturnal emissions
    B. Spermatozoa in post-ejaculatory urine
    C. Absent orgasmic sensation
    D. Short IELT
    E. Testicular pain after intercourse
81. Which of the following is first-line therapy for lifelong premature ejaculation?
    A. Paroxetine
    B. Dapoxetine
    C. Clomipramine
    D. Lidocaine spray
    E. Tramadol
82. Post-orgasmic illness syndrome is thought to be due to:
    A. Serotonin deficiency
    B. Allergic/inflammatory reaction to semen
    C. Androgen deficiency
    D. Pelvic floor dysfunction
    E. CNS dopamine excess
83. Which test is most appropriate to confirm retrograde ejaculation?
    A. Semen analysis
    B. Penile Doppler
    C. Post-ejaculatory urine microscopy
    D. Serum testosterone
    E. Urodynamic study
84. Men with spinal cord lesions above T10 are most likely to have:
    A. Preserved reflexogenic erections
    B. Normal ejaculation
    C. Impaired emission
    D. Reduced risk of priapism
    E. Preserved orgasm
85. A patient has normal erection but ejaculates within 30 s of penetration since sexual debut. This is:
    A. Subjective PE
    B. Acquired PE
    C. Lifelong PE
    D. Natural variable PE
    E. Anorgasmia

86. Which of the following drugs may be used on demand for PE due to its short half-life?
    A. Fluoxetine
    B. Paroxetine
    C. Dapoxetine
    D. Sertraline
    E. Citalopram
87. The "squeeze technique" in PE works by:
    A. Reducing penile sensitivity
    B. Temporarily interrupting emission reflex
    C. Increasing venous outflow
    D. Stimulating oxytocin release
    E. Blocking sympathetic tone
88. Which disorder is characterized by absent orgasm despite full erection and semen emission?
    A. Retrograde ejaculation
    B. Primary anorgasmia
    C. Ejaculatory anhedonia
    D. Orgasmic anejaculation
    E. Premature ejaculation
89. Which of the following neurological disorders is strongly linked with delayed ejaculation?
    A. Parkinson's disease
    B. Epilepsy
    C. Multiple sclerosis
    D. Alzheimer's disease
    E. Huntington's disease
90. An important psychological factor contributing to PE is:
    A. Hyperprolactinemia
    B. Performance anxiety
    C. Hypothyroidism
    D. High androgen levels
    E. Trauma to dorsal nerve
91. Most common side effect of topical anesthetics for PE:
    A. Erectile dysfunction
    B. Reduced partner sensitivity
    C. Priapism
    D. Penile fibrosis
    E. Headache
92. Which of the following is NOT a validated tool for PE assessment?
    A. Premature Ejaculation Diagnostic Tool (PEDT)
    B. International Index of Erectile Function (IIEF)
    C. Intravaginal Ejaculation Latency Time (IELT)
    D. Patient Health Questionnaire (PHQ-9)
    E. Sexual Satisfaction Scale

93. Treatment of retrograde ejaculation with sympathomimetics is effective because they:
    A. Relax bladder neck
    B. Increase bladder pressure
    C. Induce bladder neck contraction
    D. Reduce semen volume
    E. Stimulate nitric oxide release
94. Which of the following is true of delayed ejaculation?
    A. Always psychogenic
    B. May be caused by antidepressants
    C. Cannot occur in diabetics
    D. Always associated with anorgasmia
    E. Defined by IELT <1 min
95. Best description of climacturia:
    A. Involuntary urination during orgasm
    B. Painful ejaculation
    C. Involuntary passage of semen during foreplay
    D. Urination before sex
    E. Ejaculation without orgasm
96. Most common cause of secondary anorgasmia:
    A. Endocrine disorders
    B. Psychogenic stress
    C. Diabetes mellitus
    D. Drugs (SSRIs, antipsychotics)
    E. Pelvic trauma
97. Which of the following best distinguishes anejaculation from retrograde ejaculation?
    A. Absence of orgasmic sensation
    B. Presence of semen in urine
    C. Absence of semen in urine
    D. Testicular pain
    E. Associated erectile dysfunction
98. A patient presents with recurrent headaches at orgasm. This condition is:
    A. Coital cephalalgia
    B. Post-orgasmic illness syndrome
    C. Ejaculatory anhedonia
    D. Orgasmic anejaculation
    E. Psychogenic PE
99. Which of the following is the most effective behavioral therapy for PE?
    A. Start-stop technique
    B. Squeeze technique
    C. Cognitive behavioral therapy
    D. Kegel exercises
    E. Combination therapy

100. Which of the following emerging therapies is being studied for ejaculation disorders?
   A. Low-intensity shockwave therapy
   B. Stem cell therapy
   C. Gene therapy
   D. Oxytocin receptor antagonists
   E. All of the above

✅ Key Takeaways

- PE is the most common male sexual complaint; IELT (Intravaginal Ejaculatory Latency Time) <1 min defines severe cases.
- Lifelong PE has stronger neurobiological roots, while acquired PE may involve psychological or medical causes.
- Dapoxetine and SSRIs are commonly used pharmacologic options.
- Behavioral strategies like the stop-start and squeeze techniques are effective.
- Delayed ejaculation may relate to diabetes, SSRIs, or neurological conditions.
- A multidisciplinary approach is often required.

✅ Answer Key (1–100)

1. A
2. E
3. B
4. D
5. D
6. C
7. C
8. C
9. D
10. E
11. C
12. C
13. D
14. C
15. A
16. C
17. C
18. C
19. C
20. D
21. D
22. C

23. D
24. A
25. E
26. C
27. C
28. C
29. B
30. A
31. B
32. B
33. B
34. B
35. A
36. C
37. C
38. B
39. E
40. C
41. C
42. C
43. C
44. C
45. B
46. C
47. C
48. C
49. C
50. E
51. B
52. D
53. B
54. D
55. B
56. E
57. E
58. E
59. C
60. B
61. A
62. C
63. C
64. C
65. B
66. A
67. A

68. C
69. D
70. C
71. D
72. C
73. C
74. B
75. B
76. D
77. E
78. A
79. A
80. B
81. B
82. B
83. C
84. A
85. C
86. C
87. B
88. D
89. C
90. B
91. B
92. D
93. C
94. B
95. A
96. D
97. C
98. A
99. E
100. E

Explanations (1–100)

1. The emission phase of ejaculation is mediated by sympathetic nerves, not parasympathetic, and is involuntary. It involves contraction of accessory glands, accumulation of semen in the posterior urethra, and distension that triggers expulsion reflex.
2. Male orgasm is involuntary, not under voluntary control. It is a pleasurable sensation from posterior urethral stimulation, usually coinciding with semen expulsion and mediated via pudendal nerve input.

3. The spinal ejaculation generator is located at L3–L4 (spinothalamic). It integrates sensory inputs and coordinates emission and ejection phases.
4. High serotonin levels delay ejaculation and cause anorgasmia or delayed ejaculation. This is the basis for using SSRIs in premature ejaculation.
5. Low dopamine decreases sexual drive and contributes to anorgasmia and delayed ejaculation, as dopamine has a central excitatory role in orgasm.
6. Low serotonin predisposes to rapid ejaculation because inhibitory neurotransmission is reduced, leading to premature emission.
7. High dopamine enhances sexual drive and can cause premature ejaculation through increased excitatory signaling in sexual pathways.
8. Pathological spontaneous ejaculation is linked to decreased adrenergic tone, whereas normal nocturnal emission is physiological. Antidepressants can also provoke this phenomenon.
9. Oxytocin is a stimulatory neuropeptide that enhances ejaculatory reflex and smooth muscle contraction in accessory glands.
10. Endorphins act as inhibitory neuromodulators, reducing ejaculatory excitability and delaying orgasm.
11. Ejaculatory seepage refers to the unintentional leakage of semen or pre-ejaculatory fluid from the penis during periods of sexual arousal or after sexual activity. Ejaculatory seepage results from weak sexual stimulation and occurs commonly with aging or treatment of premature ejaculation. It is not due to strong contractility.
12. Oneirogonorrhea is nocturnal emission during dreams. It is not usually linked to trauma but may occur under stress, exams, or psychological strain.
13. General body fatigue contributes to secondary total anorgasmia because exhaustion suppresses central arousal and orgasmic thresholds.
14. Psychological trauma, including illegal sexual acts, may contribute to secondary anorgasmia due to inhibitory mental associations.
15. Orgasmic anejaculation is when orgasmic sensation is present but no semen is expelled, often due to obstruction or dysfunction in emission.
16. Male anorgasmia is the inability to experience orgasm despite sexual activity and adequate erection, a psychogenic or neurogenic disorder.
17. Penile vibratory stimulation requires 8–10 min for effective activation of spinal reflexes, especially in men with spinal cord injury.
18. Optimal site for penile vibration is the glans (dorsal aspect) because it has the highest density of sensory receptors.
19. Retrograde ejaculation is diagnosed when more than 10–15 sperm per high-power field are seen in post-coital urine samples.
20. Ephedrine sulfate works as a sympathomimetic, tightening the bladder neck and preventing semen reflux into the bladder.
21. Oxedrine 60 mg orally is commonly used to treat retrograde ejaculation due to its alpha-adrenergic agonist activity.
22. Secondary premature ejaculation is defined as IELT less than 3 min by ISSM guidelines.

23. PE is characterized by fewer than 15–20 thrusts before ejaculation, reflecting a short latency time.
24. Primary PE is often due to heightened reflex sensitivity, present since first sexual encounters.
25. The bulbospongiosus and pubococcygeus muscles are strengthened with Kegel exercises, improving control over ejaculation.
26. Repeating Kegel exercises 10–20 times gives maximal pelvic floor strengthening for premature ejaculation management.
27. Kegel exercises are indicated in PE, climacturia, and prostatorrhea but not for prostate cancer management.
28. Silodosin, an alpha-blocker, delays emission by reducing sympathetic tone on seminal vesicles and vas deferens.
29. Polymorphisms of the 5-HT1A receptor are implicated in premature ejaculation and non-response to SSRIs.
30. Pregabalin is not a recommended drug for PE, though SSRIs, lidocaine, and silodosin are.
31. Sildenafil influences ejaculation latency by reducing sympathetic tone and enhancing erectile stability, indirectly delaying ejaculation.
32. Oxytocin receptor antagonists reduce ejaculatory reflex sensitivity and are being studied for PE treatment.
33. Epelsiban is an oxytocin receptor antagonist under trial for premature ejaculation therapy.
34. Cligosiban is another selective oxytocin antagonist with potential use in PE.
35. Müllerian duct cyst can obstruct the ejaculatory ducts and cause delayed ejaculation.
36. Prune belly syndrome is associated with structural defects, leading to retrograde ejaculation.
37. Wolffian duct anomalies interfere with ejaculatory duct development and cause delayed ejaculation.
38. Ejaculatory anhedonia is when semen is expelled normally but orgasmic pleasure is absent.
39. Seminal hypersensitization therapy is used in post-orgasmic illness syndrome, aiming to reduce hypersensitivity reactions to semen.
40. Lost penis syndrome is a psychogenic disorder where patients feel the penis disappears, often linked to anorgasmia.
41. Amantadine enhances dopamine release and may be useful in delayed ejaculation treatment.
42. Cyproheptadine, an antihistamine with serotonergic activity, is used in delayed ejaculation cases.
43. Reboxetine, a selective norepinephrine reuptake inhibitor, has been trialed for delayed ejaculation.
44. Bethanechol, a cholinergic agonist, stimulates bladder neck contraction and helps in retrograde ejaculation.
45. True climacturia is involuntary urine leakage during orgasm, often after radical prostatectomy.

46. Pseudo-climacturia is urine leakage before intercourse, not during orgasm.
47. Weak suspensory ligament support after prostatectomy predisposes to climacturia due to urethral incompetence.
48. Oxybutynin reduces detrusor overactivity and improves climacturia after prostate surgery.
49. Mirabegron, a β3-agonist, relaxes bladder detrusor and reduces climacturia episodes.
50. Post-orgasmic illness syndrome may be due to immune and inflammatory responses, not purely brain chemical imbalance.
51. Autologous semen injection is used in post-orgasmic illness syndrome to desensitize allergic-type reactions.
52. Lost penis syndrome causes psychogenic ED and delayed ejaculation but not retrograde ejaculation.
53. Serotonin is the key inhibitory neurotransmitter in ejaculation, regulating latency and control.
54. Emission is sympathetic (T10–L2), ejection is somatic (S2–S4), and voluntary control is minimal. Bladder neck closure is essential to avoid retrograde ejaculation.
55. IELT ≤1 min occurs in about 2–5% of men globally, reflecting true premature ejaculation prevalence.
56. DSM-IV defines PE by latency, lack of control, and distress. Subjective PE may have normal IELT but high anxiety.
57. ISSM definition applies across orientations and contact types, focusing on latency, control, and consequences.
58. Retrograde ejaculation is confirmed by sperm in post-ejaculatory urine and is common after surgery or diabetic neuropathy.
59. High spinal cord injuries reduce ejaculatory capacity. Electroejaculation is possible but carries risk of autonomic dysreflexia.
60. In acquired PE with ED, anxiety and poor arousal control contribute to incomplete erections and short latency.
61. Bladder emptying and pelvic floor exercises are effective in reducing climacturia, especially after prostate surgery.
62. Natural variable PE is diagnosed when ejaculation is early only occasionally, not consistently.
63. The triad of PE includes lack of control, short latency, and distress. Prolonged abstinence is not included.
64. Combined topical anesthetic and sildenafil provides maximal IELT increase and symptom improvement.
65. PE typically relapses within weeks after stopping therapy, showing treatment is not curative but symptomatic.
66. Dapoxetine is the only SSRI designed for on-demand use in PE, due to short half-life.
67. Dapoxetine does not carry the same suicidality warning as other SSRIs in young men.

68. Among SSRIs, sertraline and fluvoxamine are weaker IELT extenders compared to paroxetine.
69. Clomipramine is a tricyclic antidepressant used in PE; it inhibits 5-HT reuptake and is also used in OCD.
70. Tramadol delays ejaculation via opioid and serotonergic effects. It carries addiction risk but is effective in PE.
71. Alpha agonists are not standard for PE; SSRIs, TCAs, and anesthetics are.
72. Secondary PE occurs in men with ED, often improved with PDE5 inhibitors.
73. SSRIs combined with coumadin increase bleeding risk by impairing platelet function.
74. Detailed sexual history is the most important assessment in PE evaluation.
75. Topical anesthetics are effective, under regulatory review, but risk partner numbness.
76. Orgasmic anejaculation occurs when orgasm is felt but semen is absent, often post-diabetes.
77. Retrograde ejaculation has multiple causes including surgery, neuropathy, and medications.
78. SSRIs are the most frequent cause of drug-induced delayed ejaculation.
79. Ejaculatory anhedonia is when ejaculation occurs without pleasurable orgasmic sensation.
80. Retrograde ejaculation diagnosis relies on detecting sperm in post-ejaculatory urine.
81. Dapoxetine is first-line oral drug for lifelong PE.
82. POIS is likely autoimmune or allergic to semen proteins, producing systemic symptoms.
83. Post-ejaculatory urine microscopy is the confirmatory test for retrograde ejaculation.
84. Reflexogenic erections are preserved with lesions above T10, but emission and ejaculation are impaired.
85. Lifelong PE begins with early ejaculation from first sexual experience and persists.
86. Dapoxetine is unique in being short-acting and suitable for on-demand PE therapy.
87. The squeeze technique interrupts the ejaculatory reflex and prolongs latency.
88. Orgasmic anejaculation is absent orgasm despite semen emission, differing from anhedonia.
89. Multiple sclerosis frequently causes delayed ejaculation due to demyelination affecting pathways.
90. Anxiety is the most common psychological driver of PE.
91. The main side effect of topical anesthetics is reduced partner sensitivity due to transfer.
92. PHQ-9 is for depression; PE is assessed by PEDT, IELT, and satisfaction scales.
93. Sympathomimetics contract bladder neck, preventing semen backflow in retrograde ejaculation.

94. Delayed ejaculation is often drug-induced or neurogenic, not always psychogenic.
95. Climacturia is urine leakage during orgasm, commonly post-prostatectomy.
96. Secondary anorgasmia is often due to drugs, especially SSRIs and antipsychotics.
97. Anejaculation lacks semen entirely, retrograde shows semen in urine.
98. Coital cephalalgia is headache linked to orgasm, often benign but occasionally vascular.
99. Combination behavioral therapy is most effective for PE management.
100. Emerging therapies under study include gene therapy, stem cells, shockwave, and oxytocin antagonists.

Further Reading

The explanations in this chapter are supported by the following key references:

1. Waldinger MD. Premature ejaculation: state of the art. Urol Clin N Am. 2007;34(4):591–9.
2. Serefoglu EC, McMahon CG, Waldinger MD, et al. An evidence-based unified definition of lifelong and acquired premature ejaculation. J Sex Med. 2014;11(6):1423–41.
3. McMahon CG, Althof SE, Waldinger MD, et al. An evidence-based definition of premature ejaculation. J Sex Med. 2008;5(7):1590–606.
4. Althof SE. Psychological approaches to the treatment of ejaculatory disorders. J Sex Med. 2012;9(1):107–19.
5. Corona G, Rastrelli G, Jannini EA, et al. Ejaculatory and orgasmic dysfunction. Nat Rev Urol. 2016;13(9):517–31.
6. Rowland DL, Patrick DL, Rothman M, et al. The psychological burden of premature ejaculation. J Sex Med. 2007;4(5):1427–36.
7. Sansone A, Aversa A, Corona G, Fisher AD, Isidori AM, La Vignera S, Limoncin E, Maggi M, Merico M, Jannini EA. Management of premature ejaculation: a clinical guideline from the Italian Society of Andrology and Sexual Medicine (SIAMS). J Endocrinol Investig. 2021;44(5):1103–18.

9 Painful Penile Disorders

Learning Objectives

- Describe common painful penile conditions.
- Differentiate acute vs. chronic causes of penile pain.
- Identify the clinical signs of Peyronie's disease and priapism.
- Review treatment protocols for phimosis, paraphimosis, and balanitis.
- Recognize when urgent referral or surgical intervention is warranted.

Select the Single Best Answer

1. The most severe embryological type of congenital penile curvature is:
   A. Type I
   B. Type II
   C. Type III
   D. Type IV
   E. Type V
2. Type II embryological defect of congenital penile curvature shows:
   A. Shortened urethra
   B. Deficiency of corpora spongiosum
   C. Thin urethra
   D. Normal corpus spongiosum
3. Corporeal distortion is seen in congenital penile curvature type:
   A. Type I
   B. Type II
   C. Type III
   D. Type IV
   E. Type V

M. S. M. Hasan, M. L. Elsaie, *Comprehensive MCQs in Andrology*, Trends in Andrology and Sexual Medicine, https://doi.org/10.1007/978-3-032-20623-7_9

4. The most Severe penile curvature angulation is:
   A. <15°
   B. 15–30°
   C. 30–45°
   D. 45–90°
   E. >90°
5. Which of the following is NOT TRUE about congenital penile curvature?
   A. Dating since birth
   B. May be associated with hypospadias
   C. No fibrotic plaque in the tunica albuginea
   D. Unequal corpora
   E. Associated with lederhosen
6. Peyronie's disease is a disease that affects mainly:
   A. Bucks' fascia
   B. Tunica vaginalis
   C. Tunica vasculosa
   D. Tunica albuginea
   E. Dartos fascia
7. Peyronie's disease is mainly:
   A. Autoimmune disease
   B. Inherited disease
   C. Connective tissue disorder
   D. Vascular disorder
8. Which of the following is NOT true about the plaque formation of Peyronie's disease?
   A. HLA associated
   B. Cytokines overexpression
   C. Trauma
   D. Chromosomal instability
   E. Cytochrome p450 instability
9. The role of Ca channel blocker in Peyronie's disease:
   A. Increase collagen synthesis
   B. Increase fibronectin synthesis
   C. Increase collagen formation
   D. Increase extracellular matrix collagenase secretion
10. The role of prostacyclin analogue in Peyronie's disease may be:
    A. Increase collagen synthesis
    B. Increase fibrinolytic activity
    C. Cytokines overexpression
    D. Increase fibronectin synthesis
    E. Neovascularization

11. Which of the following is NOT used in the treatment of Peyronie's disease?
    A. Nicardipine
    B. Xiaflex
    C. Steroid
    D. Beta blockers
    E. Ca channel blocker
12. The mechanism of action of potassium Para aminobenzoate in the treatment of Peyronie's disease:
    A. Releasing of transforming factor B
    B. Nonspecific phosphodiesterase inhibitor
    C. Increase activity of monoamine oxidase in tissue
    D. Decrease collagen III
    E. Antioxidant
13. The role of tamoxifen in the treatment of Peyronie's disease is:
    A. Releasing of transforming factor B
    B. Nonspecific phosphodiesterase inhibitor
    C. Increase activity of monoamine oxidase in tissue
    D. Decrease collagen III
    E. Antioxidant
14. The role of carnitine in the treatment of Peyronie's disease is:
    A. Releasing of transforming factor B
    B. Nonspecific phosphodiesterase inhibitor
    C. Increase activity of monoamine oxidase in tissue
    D. Decrease collagen III
    E. Inhibition of acidyl co-enzyme A
15. The dose of potassium Para aminobenzoate in the treatment of Peyronie's disease:
    A. 1 g twice daily
    B. 20 mg twice daily
    C. 8 g twice daily
    D. 12 g daily
    E. 30 g twice daily
16. The most important cause of ischemic priapism is:
    A. Blood disorders
    B. CNS problems
    C. Idiopathic
    D. Drugs
17. The most important cause of non-ischemic priapism is:
    A. Blood disorders
    B. CNS problems
    C. Drugs
    D. Trauma

18. Which of the following is NOT a criterion of ischemic priapism?
    A. Painful erection
    B. Rigid penis
    C. Alkalosis
    D. Hypoxia
    E. Hypercapnia
19. Thrombocyte adherence occurs in priapism after:
    A. 6 h
    B. 12 h
    C. 18 h
    D. 24 h
    E. 48 h
20. The most common blood disorder associated with ischemic priapism in children is:
    A. Hemophilia
    B. Polycythemia
    C. Leukemia
    D. Sickle cell anemia
21. Intracorporeal injection of Methylene blue can lead to penile detumescence in priapism patients through:
    A. Stimulation of monoamine oxidase enzyme
    B. Inhibition of nitric oxide synthetase
    C. Inhibition of guanylate cyclase enzyme
    D. Inhibition of protein kinase C
22. Sickle cell anemia priapism can be treated by:
    A. Methylene blue
    B. Terbutaline
    C. Adrenaline
    D. Phenyl epinephrine
    E. Plasmapheresis
23. The size of the butterfly cannula inserted during intracorporeal aspiration of blood during priapism treatment is:
    A. 8–10 G
    B. 10–12 G
    C. 12–14 G
    D. 14–16 G
    E. 16–18 G
24. Which of the following is NOT a side effect of Intracavernosal phenyl epinephrine injection in priapism treatment?
    A. Bradycardia
    B. Subarachnoid hemorrhage
    C. Irregular cardiac rhythm
    D. Atrial fibrillation
    E. Hypertension

25. Which of the following is NOT a criterion of stuttering priapism?
    A. Variant of ischemic priapism
    B. Sleep-related
    C. Painful
    D. Transient attack
    E. Last more than 4 h
26. Which of the following is NOT used in the treatment of intermittent priapism?
    A. Gabapentin
    B. Terbutaline
    C. Baclofen
    D. Digoxin
    E. Methylene blue
27. Adverse effects of hydroxyurea in the treatment of stuttering priapism include:
    A. Oligozoospermia
    B. Low sexual desire
    C. Erectile dysfunction
    D. Peyronie's disease
    E. Penile Mondor disease
28. Which of the following is NOT the cause of stuttering priapism?
    A. Sickle cell anemia
    B. Idiopathic
    C. Blunt perineal trauma
    D. Hereditary spherocytosis
    E. Drug-induced
29. The following can be used in the treatment of recalcitrant priapism:
    A. Phosphodiesterase inhibitors
    B. Phenyl epinephrine
    C. Hydroxyurea
    D. Terbutaline
    E. Tissue plasminogen activator
30. The pathognomonic finding of selective internal pudendal arteriography in the diagnosis of non-ischemic priapism is:
    A. Cavernosal artery hemorrhage
    B. Double-walled-shaped cavernosal artery
    C. Cone-shaped blush
    D. Mesh-like cavernosal artery
    E. Lacunar space deformity
31. Which of the following is NOT a criterion of partial priapism?
    A. Unicorporal affection
    B. Congenital corporeal web
    C. Partial segment thrombosis
    D. Ischemia
    E. Idiopathic

32. Which of the following is NOT a criterion of penile Mondor disease?
    A. Thrombophlebitis of the deep penile dorsal vein
    B. Dull aching pain
    C. Penile skin erythema and edema
    D. Thick cord on the dorsum of the penis
    E. Anti-coagulant is a line of treatment
33. Which of the following is NOT a cause of penile Mondor disease?
    A. Penile trauma
    B. Infection
    C. Paraneoplastic syndromes
    D. Peyronie's disease
    E. Vacuum constriction device
34. Which of the following is NOT the criteria of orgasmic cephalgia?
    A. Increase intracranial tension
    B. Brain aneurysm
    C. Neck rigidity
    D. Phosphodiesterase use
    E. Paraneoplastic syndromes
35. Which of the following is NOT a cause of orgasmic cephalgia?
    A. Cerebral aneurysm
    B. Pericardial muscle contraction
    C. Local cerebral vasospasm
    D. Beta blockers
    E. A–V malformation
36. Which of the following is NOT used in the treatment of coital headache?
    A. Beta blockers
    B. Ca channel blockers
    C. Indomethacin
    D. Surgical
    E. Phosphodiesterase inhibitors
37. The most effective therapy for ischemic priapism in sickle cell disease patients is:
    A. Hydration
    B. Plasmapheresis
    C. Pseudoephedrine tablets
    D. Intracavernosal treatments (irrigation and evacuation of corporal blood; injection of alpha-adrenergic sympathomimetic agent)
38. In a case where conservative medical approaches to ischemic–low-flow priapism fails, the next best option is:
    A. Corporal dilation with shunt formation
    B. The least invasive approach to reverse the hypoxia
    C. Primary penile implant
    D. All of the above

39. A PDE5 inhibitor is not recommended as an erectile dysfunction treatment option in a homozygous sickle cell disease patient because:
    A. It may increase the risk of a vaso-occlusive crisis
    B. It may worsen the patient's pulmonary arterial hypertension
    C. It is clinically not effective
    D. Clinical trials demonstrated a greater risk of priapism
40. Penile traction devices are:
    A. Currently approved by the FDA and highly effective
    B. Useful only if applied for greater than 6 h/day
    C. Of potential value in selected individuals
    D. Potentially a useful tool in patients with ventral curvatures exclusively
41. The most established mechanism for priapism in sickle cell disease (SCD) patients is:
    A. Phosphodiesterase type 5 inhibitors (PDE5) dysregulation in penile tissue
    B. Microvascular occlusion caused by sickling of deoxygenated red blood cells
    C. Increased adenosine levels in penile tissue
    D. High flow priapism following previous surgical treatments for ischemic priapism
42. In post-priapism ED patients:
    A. The only treatment option is penile prosthesis surgery
    B. The most common cause is a shunt fistula from previous shunt surgery
    C. Conservative options (PDE5 inhibitors, vacuum device, intraurethral alprostadil, and Intracavernosal injections) can sometimes be effective
    D. Corporal fibrosis does not make penile prosthesis surgery more difficult
43. In a man who has low-flow–ischemic priapism for >24 h, which of the following statements is the MOST correct?
    A. The treatment may cause permanent ED
    B. The preexisting period of hypoxia will likely result in ED
    C. If a formal proximal shunt is performed, he will have ED
    D. All of the above
44. The usual etiology of high-flow priapism in contrast to low-flow priapism is:
    A. Due to overproduction of nitric oxide/cyclic guanosine monophosphate
    B. Cocaine or other illicit drugs, whereas low-flow priapism is usually a result of intracorporal injections
    C. Traumatic, with induction of an arterial-venous fistula
    D. All of the above
    E. None of the above
45. The conversion of low-flow priapism to a high-flow nonischemic state is:
    A. Highly unusual and only a few case reports exist in the literature
    B. A Cavernosal artery injury resulting in unrestricted arterial flow into the corpora
    C. Not a medical emergency as tissue perfusion is usually adequate
    D. All of the above
    E. None of the above

46. The use of intralesional interferon for Peyronie's disease is:
    A. Not advisable owing to its proven poor efficacy
    B. Associated with a flu-like illness
    C. Less effective than verapamil in randomized controlled studies
    D. Best suited for ventral curves away from the neurovascular bundle
    E. All of the above
47. Intralesional verapamil has been reported to do all of the following EXCEPT:
    A. Stabilize the plaque in the acute phase
    B. Reduce the degree of penile deformity by 10–15° among responders
    C. In head-to-head studies is superior to interferon
    D. Report response rates of 45–60%
48. The use of intralesional agents for the treatment of Peyronie's disease:
    A. Cannot be supported by clinical or animal studies
    B. Is fraught with side effects including exacerbation of the condition, increased curvature, and has an increased risk of ED
    C. Has support within the literature but has modest efficacy and requires greater study to optimize the patient population, dose, and timing
    D. Is the only real choice for men before surgery
49. The most common side effects associated with Penile reconstruction for Peyronie's disease using an exogenous graft are:
    A. Erectile dysfunction
    B. Sensory changes
    C. Length loss
    D. Residual curvature
    E. All of the above
50. Loss of sensation along the penile shaft and head, following Peyronie's graft reconstruction are often:
    A. Permanent and refractory to medical or surgical management
    B. A major source of morbidity and patient dissatisfaction with the procedure
    C. Caused by intra-operative use of excessive local anesthetics
    D. Temporary and self-limited, thought to be induced through percussive or traction injury to the dorsal nerve complex
    E. All of the above
51. In men who demonstrate significant penile deformity >60° with normal cavernous artery flows, the optimal treatment approach is:
    A. Primary penile implant with modeling
    B. Penile reconstruction using an exogenous graft
    C. Use of intralesional verapamil or interferon to reduce the scar
    D. Chronic PDE5i with a traction device
    E. All of the above

52. Use of chronic PDE5i's following Peyronie's surgery:
    A. Has no role as it will exacerbate painful erections and may cause an anastomotic disruption
    B. Has been shown in animal models to reduce intracorporal scarring
    C. May facilitate early erections but is not advised as tachyphylaxis may occur
    D. Can induce an antiplatelet effect and cause post-surgical bleeding
    E. None of the above
53. If a middle-aged man presents to you with penile pain, length loss, and erectile dysfunction which of the following is the most likely diagnosis from the choices below?
    A. Penile fracture
    B. Peripheral neuropathy-induced pain
    C. Intra-corporal septal scar, atypical Peyronie's
    D. Psychogenic etiology without organicity
54. Following a complete history and physical examination, from the list below what is the best next step in management?
    A. Reassure him that this will get better and not to worry
    B. A trial of daily PDE5 inhibitors to restore erectile function
    C. A duplex ultrasound to image the penile anatomy
    D. Hormonal screen for Late-Onset Hypogonadism
55. In cases where a midline septal scar is found on imaging, what therapeutic options would YOU recommend next?
    A. Chronic PDE5 inhibitor
    B. Watchful waiting
    C. Intra-lesional verapamil/interferon
    D. Surgical management with scar excision
56. The key elements of atypical Peyronie's disease are:
    A. Unresolved penile pain beyond 3 months
    B. Severe curvature in the lateral direction
    C. Length loss, non-palpable plaque, and penile pain
    D. Ventral curvature presents only with a full erection
57. In cases where low-flow (ischemic) priapism has been untreated for more than 24 h, which of the following is likely?
    A. Loss of sensation within the dorsal nerve (neuropraxia)
    B. Severe cellular damage and corporal smooth muscle necrosis
    C. A reversible fibrotic process involving the proximal crural smooth muscle
    D. No long-lasting sequela
58. Use of intracavernous vasoactive therapy for the treatment of sexual dysfunction is:
    A. Appropriate in all cases where the patient believes his erections are insufficient
    B. Best reserved for men who want high-grade rigidity and have neurogenic erectile dysfunction (ED)
    C. Only indicated when an organic pathology is found and PDE5is are not effective
    D. Indicated in most treatment algorithms as second-line therapy for ED and should be used only following proper instruction and support

59. In cases where low-flow priapism has resulted in corporal fibrosis:
    A. Use of PDE5is is uniformly effective with proper instruction
    B. Penile implantation should be performed immediately as delayed treatment has higher failure and complication rates
    C. Use of intracavernous vasoactive injections is contraindicated as they may "go systemic"
    D. Informed patient consent detailing risks is essential before initiation of any surgical therapy as the rates of complications and infections are significantly elevated
60. The most important tool in effectively managing sexual concerns is:
    A. the ability to offer all forms of therapy to patients including psychological, surgical, and medical (oral agents, MUSE, ICI)
    B. the ability to take a complete sexual history
    C. being able to offer samples to patients before starting therapy
    D. starting all men with PDE5is before any other therapy
61. The finding of calcifications within the corporal bodies, septum, or subtunical:
    A. Indicate that Peyronie's disease has matured and is longstanding
    B. Is a nonaggressive type with little chance for progression
    C. Is unlikely to respond to surgery, indicating medical management is preferred
    D. May represent a subtype of the condition and can occur in as many as 1/3 of cases
    E. None of the above
62. In men with Peyronie's disease with poor PDE5i unresponsive erections and curvature greater than 70°, the best management approach is:
    A. Do nothing as these curvatures have about a 30% chance of improvement spontaneously
    B. Plication if the penile length is OK
    C. A graft repair and treat his ED with intracavernous injections
    D. Primary penile implant
63. Preventive strategies for stuttering priapism in Sickle cell disease patients include all of the following EXCEPT:
    A. Hormonal therapies with gonadotropin-releasing hormone agonists or androgen receptor antagonists
    B. Intracavernosal self-injection of phenylephrine
    C. Penile prosthesis surgery
    D. Polyethylene glycol-modified adenosine deaminase drug therapy
64. Following intracorporeal injection of phenylephrine for priapism, persistent penile rigidity means:
    A. Inadequate dosing
    B. Misdiagnosis
    C. Smooth muscle ischemia
    D. All of the above

65. The most common presenting symptom of Peyronie's disease is:
    A. Penile pain
    B. Penile shortening
    C. Erectile dysfunction
    D. Penile curvature
    E. Loss of sensation
66. Early Peyronie's disease is best characterized by:
    A. Soft plaque and penile pain
    B. Dense calcified plaque
    C. Severe curvature without pain
    D. Stable deformity
    E. Loss of penile girth only
67. The gold standard imaging tool in Peyronie's disease is:
    A. Plain X-ray
    B. MRI penis
    C. Penile duplex ultrasound
    D. CT scan
    E. Cavernosography
68. Xiaflex (collagenase clostridium histolyticum) acts by:
    A. Blocking collagen synthesis
    B. Breaking down collagen in plaques
    C. Stimulating fibroblast proliferation
    D. Blocking cytokines
    E. Enhancing blood flow
69. The most feared surgical complication after plaque excision with grafting is:
    A. Penile pain
    B. Penile shortening
    C. Erectile dysfunction
    D. Penile infection
    E. Loss of sensation
70. Nesbit procedure for Peyronie's disease corrects curvature by:
    A. Plaque excision
    B. Plication opposite the curve
    C. Grafting
    D. Penile prosthesis insertion
    E. Circumcision
71. The success rate of plication surgery for Peyronie's is about:
    A. 50%
    B. 60%
    C. 70–80%
    D. 90%
    E. >95%

72. The drug pentoxifylline is used in Peyronie's because it:
    A. Stimulates collagen formation
    B. Inhibits fibroblast apoptosis
    C. Reduces oxidative stress and fibrosis
    D. Increases testosterone
    E. Promotes calcium deposition
73. Priapism is defined as penile erection persisting beyond:
    A. 30 min
    B. 1 h
    C. 2 h
    D. 4 h
    E. 6 h
74. Low-flow priapism is characterized by:
    A. Painless erection
    B. Increased cavernosal oxygen
    C. Venous outflow obstruction
    D. Normal blood gases
    E. Trauma-related AV fistula
75. High-flow priapism is most commonly caused by:
    A. Sickle cell disease
    B. Trauma with AV fistula
    C. Drug overdose
    D. Spinal cord lesion
    E. Leukemia
76. In ischemic priapism, cavernosal blood gas typically shows:
    A. pH < 7.25, $pO_2 < 30$, $pCO_2 > 60$
    B. pH 7.4, $pO_2 > 90$
    C. pH 7.6, $pO_2 > 120$
    D. Normal values
    E. Alkalosis
77. First-line treatment of ischemic priapism is:
    A. Aspiration + phenylephrine injection
    B. Penile prosthesis
    C. Shunt surgery
    D. Oral PDE5i
    E. Observation
78. Phenylephrine is the preferred alpha-agonist because it:
    A. Has strong beta action
    B. Causes minimal cardiovascular effects
    C. Increases cavernosal oxygen
    D. Relaxes smooth muscle
    E. Stimulates serotonin

79. In children, the most common cause of priapism is:
    A. Trauma
    B. Leukemia
    C. Sickle cell disease
    D. Medication
    E. Idiopathic
80. The most serious long-term complication of ischemic priapism is:
    A. Infection
    B. Erectile dysfunction
    C. Peyronie's disease
    D. Penile pain
    E. Priapism recurrence
81. Shunt surgery in priapism is indicated after:
    A. 1 h
    B. 2 h
    C. 4 h
    D. Failed aspiration/injection
    E. At presentation
82. A Winter shunt connects:
    A. Corpus cavernosum to corpus spongiosum
    B. Corpus cavernosum to glans penis
    C. Dorsal vein to cavernosum
    D. Cavernosum to perineum
    E. Cavernosum to artery
83. The most definitive treatment for refractory priapism is:
    A. PDE5 inhibitors
    B. Penile prosthesis implantation
    C. Repeat aspiration
    D. Vacuum device
    E. Steroid injection
84. Stuttering priapism is best described as:
    A. Constant painful erection
    B. Recurrent self-limiting ischemic priapism
    C. High-flow painless erections
    D. Post-traumatic erections
    E. Congenital
85. The most common cause of stuttering priapism is:
    A. Leukemia
    B. Trauma
    C. Sickle cell disease
    D. Drugs
    E. CNS lesions

86. Non-ischemic priapism is usually managed by:
    A. Immediate aspiration
    B. Conservative observation
    C. Alpha agonists
    D. Surgical shunt
    E. PDE5 inhibitors
87. In congenital penile curvature, surgery is indicated when:
    A. Pain is present
    B. Cosmetic dissatisfaction
    C. Curvature prevents intercourse
    D. Patient request
    E. Any degree of curve
88. The preferred surgical technique for severe congenital curvature is:
    A. Nesbit plication
    B. Plaque incision and graft
    C. Penile prosthesis
    D. Circumcision
    E. Dorsal nerve block
89. The hallmark histopathological change in Peyronie's disease is:
    A. Smooth muscle necrosis
    B. Tunica albuginea fibrosis and calcification
    C. Venous occlusion
    D. Arterial inflammation
    E. Cavernosal thrombosis
90. Most Peyronie's plaques are located:
    A. Ventral shaft
    B. Dorsal mid-shaft
    C. Lateral shaft
    D. Circumferential
    E. Base only
91. Penile fracture is most commonly associated with:
    A. Peyronie's disease
    B. Priapism
    C. Sexual intercourse trauma
    D. Tumor
    E. Infection
92. The tunica albuginea tears at:
    A. 200 mmHg pressure
    B. 500 mmHg pressure
    C. 900 mmHg pressure
    D. 1500 mmHg pressure
    E. 2500 mmHg pressure

93. Classic triad of penile fracture is:
    A. Crack, detumescence, pain
    B. Pain, swelling, discharge
    C. Detumescence, discharge, deformity
    D. Swelling, pain, fever
    E. Curvature, plaque, shortening
94. Cavernosography in priapism is used to:
    A. Diagnose ischemic priapism
    B. Identify AV fistula in high-flow priapism
    C. Assess fibrosis
    D. Exclude Peyronie's
    E. Rule out tumor
95. MRI is most useful in Peyronie's disease to:
    A. Assess pain
    B. Assess erectile function
    C. Identify plaque size and composition
    D. Diagnose penile fracture
    E. Diagnose priapism
96. Vacuum erection devices in Peyronie's are used to:
    A. Straighten the penis
    B. Prevent curvature
    C. Maintain length and oxygenation
    D. Dissolve plaques
    E. Prevent priapism
97. The recurrence rate after Peyronie's surgery is about:
    A. 5%
    B. 10–15%
    C. 20–30%
    D. 40%
    E. >50%
98. The main advantage of penile prosthesis in Peyronie's is:
    A. Pain control
    B. Restoration of erectile function and correction of curvature
    C. Plaque removal
    D. No complications
    E. Non-invasive
99. Non-surgical options most effective in acute Peyronie's phase include:
    A. Vitamin E alone
    B. Combination of pentoxifylline and intralesional therapy
    C. Vacuum only
    D. Topical steroids
    E. Shockwave therapy alone

100. The prognosis of non-ischemic priapism is:
    A. Poor erectile outcomes
    B. Usually resolves spontaneously with preserved erectile function
    C. Always requires prosthesis
    D. Leads to calcification
    E. High mortality

✅ Key Takeaways

- Peyronie's disease presents with penile curvature due to fibrous plaque.
- Priapism, especially ischemic type, is a urologic emergency requiring decompression.
- Phimosis and paraphimosis involve the foreskin and may lead to ischemia if untreated.
- Infections like balanitis can cause intense pain and require proper hygiene and topical therapy.
- Early diagnosis and management prevent long-term dysfunction.

✅ Answer Key (1–100)

1. A
2. D
3. D
4. E
5. E
6. D
7. C
8. E
9. D
10. B
11. D
12. C
13. A
14. E
15. D
16. D
17. D
18. C
19. D
20. D
21. C
22. B
23. E

24. D
25. E
26. E
27. A
28. C
29. E
30. C
31. D
32. A
33. D
34. E
35. D
36. E
37. A
38. A
39. D
40. C
41. A
42. C
43. D
44. C
45. D
46. E
47. D
48. C
49. E
50. D
51. A
52. D
53. C
54. C
55. C
56. B
57. B
58. D
59. B
60. D
61. A
62. C
63. D
64. C
65. D
66. A
67. C
68. B

69. C
70. B
71. C
72. C
73. D
74. C
75. B
76. A
77. A
78. B
79. C
80. B
81. D
82. A
83. B
84. B
85. C
86. B
87. C
88. A
89. B
90. B
91. C
92. C
93. A
94. B
95. C
96. C
97. B
98. B
99. B
100. B

Explanations (1–100)

1. Congenital penile curvature results from asymmetric development of the corpora cavernosa or associated tissues. The most severe embryological type shows marked angulation and functional impairment, often requiring surgical correction.
2. In Type II curvature, deficiency of the corpus spongiosum shortens the ventral side, producing downward curvature. This structural defect alters urethral support and penile shape.
3. Corporeal distortion refers to irregular development of the corpora cavernosa, producing asymmetry. It typically results in lateral or dorsal deviation during erection.

4. Severe penile angulation exceeding 90° significantly impairs sexual function. Such curvature often requires surgical intervention to restore penetrative capability.
5. Congenital penile curvature is present from birth, often without plaques. It results from unequal corpora, unlike Peyronie's disease, and may coexist with hypospadias.
6. Peyronie's disease involves fibrotic plaque deposition within the tunica albuginea. This leads to curvature, pain, and erectile dysfunction.
7. It is mainly considered a connective tissue disorder with autoimmune and microtrauma contributions. Fibroblast dysfunction drives abnormal collagen deposition.
8. Plaque formation in Peyronie's involves HLA association, cytokine overexpression, and trauma. Chromosomal or cytochrome instability is not a consistent mechanism.
9. Calcium channel blockers like verapamil increase collagenase activity, promoting breakdown of excessive fibrotic tissue in Peyronie's.
10. Prostacyclin analogues enhance fibrinolysis and reduce fibrotic activity, limiting scar progression. They improve tissue remodeling.
11. Beta blockers have no role in Peyronie's therapy. Effective treatments include collagenase (Xiaflex), steroids, and calcium channel blockers.
12. Potassium para-aminobenzoate reduces abnormal collagen buildup by influencing fibroblast activity and decreasing collagen type III.
13. Tamoxifen has antifibrotic effects in Peyronie's by reducing transforming growth factor-beta activity, limiting collagen proliferation.
14. Carnitine reduces oxidative stress and influences metabolic pathways, slowing fibrosis progression in Peyronie's disease.
15. The therapeutic dose of potassium para-aminobenzoate is 12 g/day, divided, as tolerated. This regimen is used to soften plaques.
16. Ischemic priapism most often arises from blood disorders, drugs, or idiopathic causes. It is a painful emergency requiring urgent care.
17. Non-ischemic priapism usually follows trauma, creating an arteriovenous fistula and leading to high-flow, less painful erections.
18. Ischemic priapism features painful, rigid erections with hypoxia and hypercapnia. Alkalosis is inconsistent and not a criterion.
19. Thrombocyte adhesion begins after about 12 h of ischemia, worsening stasis and fibrosis risk.
20. Sickle cell anemia is the most common pediatric cause of ischemic priapism. Sickling impairs penile venous drainage.
21. Methylene blue works by inhibiting guanylate cyclase, reducing cGMP-mediated vasodilation and allowing detumescence.
22. Plasmapheresis is effective for sickle cell priapism by removing sickled erythrocytes and reducing blood viscosity.
23. Butterfly cannulas sized 16–18G are used for aspiration in priapism management, balancing access with trauma minimization.
24. Intracavernosal phenylephrine may cause systemic hypertension, arrhythmias, and hemorrhage. Bradycardia is not typical.

25. Stuttering priapism is recurrent, painful, and brief. Episodes last less than 4 h and are sleep-related.
26. Methylene blue is not a standard therapy for intermittent priapism. Baclofen, terbutaline, and gabapentin are useful options.
27. Hydroxyurea may cause oligozoospermia as an adverse effect, reducing fertility. This is a concern in young men.
28. Stuttering priapism is associated with sickle cell disease, hereditary conditions, or drug-induced states, not blunt trauma.
29. Tissue plasminogen activator can be used in refractory priapism, promoting thrombolysis within corpora cavernosa.
30. Non-ischemic priapism angiography shows a cone-shaped blush at the site of cavernosal arterial fistula.
31. Partial priapism is characterized by segmental ischemia or thrombosis affecting part of one corpus cavernosum.
32. Penile Mondor disease is thrombophlebitis of the superficial dorsal vein, not deep venous structures.
33. Causes include trauma, infection, and neoplasia. Peyronie's and vacuum devices are not common associations.
34. Orgasmic cephalgia presents with headache triggered by orgasm. Phosphodiesterase inhibitors are not diagnostic criteria.
35. Causes include aneurysm, AV malformations, and vasospasm. Pericardial contraction is irrelevant.
36. Treatment includes beta blockers, calcium channel blockers, NSAIDs, or surgery in refractory cases. PDE5 inhibitors are not used.
37. In sickle cell ischemic priapism, aspiration and intracavernosal alpha-agonists are most effective after hydration.
38. When conservative care fails, surgical shunting or penile implants may be needed, though risks increase.
39. PDE5 inhibitors are avoided in sickle cell patients due to risk of priapism recurrence and vaso-occlusion.
40. Penile traction devices are experimental but may aid curvature correction if used consistently.
41. The key mechanism in sickle cell priapism is microvascular occlusion by sickled RBCs, causing ischemia.
42. Post-priapism ED can sometimes respond to PDE5 inhibitors, vacuum devices, or injections, though fibrosis complicates surgery.
43. Prolonged ischemia over 24 h often results in irreversible ED due to smooth muscle necrosis.
44. High-flow priapism is usually traumatic and forms an AV fistula. Low-flow is typically ischemic and drug-induced.
45. Conversion from low-flow to high-flow is rare but possible after cavernosal injury. Perfusion remains adequate.
46. Interferon therapy may reduce fibrosis but can cause systemic flu-like side effects.

47. Verapamil stabilizes plaques, improving curvature modestly. It is less effective than interferon in some studies.
48. Intralesional therapies have modest efficacy, require repeated dosing, and may not prevent progression.
49. Grafting complications include ED, sensory loss, and residual curvature. These outcomes limit satisfaction.
50. Nerve traction during grafting may cause transient sensory loss, but permanent numbness is rare.
51. Severe curvature (>60°) with good erectile function may need graft surgery to preserve penile length.
52. PDE5 inhibitors may reduce fibrosis in animal models, supporting early post-op erections.
53. Atypical Peyronie's may present as septal scarring with pain and length loss, not always a palpable plaque.
54. Duplex ultrasound confirms plaque presence, calcification, and hemodynamic compromise in Peyronie's disease.
55. Treatment options for septal scarring include verapamil or surgery, depending on severity.
56. Atypical cases often show pain, shortening, and ventral or lateral deviation not typical of dorsal plaques.
57. Untreated ischemic priapism >24 h results in irreversible smooth muscle necrosis and fibrosis.
58. Intracavernosal therapy is second-line after PDE5 inhibitors, effective in neurogenic ED.
59. Fibrosis complicates surgery; early prosthesis placement yields better outcomes than delayed attempts.
60. A detailed sexual history is the cornerstone for diagnosis and tailored management.
61. Calcification of plaques indicates chronicity, with limited potential for remodeling, often requiring surgery.
62. Severe curvature with poor erections may necessitate implant placement rather than grafting alone.
63. Preventive options in sickle cell include hormones and adenosine pathway modulators, but prosthesis is not first-line.
64. Persistent rigidity after phenylephrine suggests misdiagnosis or irreversible ischemic changes.
65. Congenital curvature Type I usually involves asymmetric tunica albuginea without urethral involvement.
66. Type IV penile curvature involves mixed structural defects leading to complex angulation.
67. Peyronie's prevalence increases with age, affecting up to 10% of men in their 60s.
68. Early Peyronie's presents with painful erections; chronic stage shows stable curvature.

69. Intralesional collagenase breaks down fibrotic plaques by targeting collagen types I and III.
70. Surgical plication shortens the longer corporal side to correct curvature <60°.
71. Plaque incision with grafting preserves penile length for severe deformity cases.
72. Tunical lengthening techniques aim to maintain erectile rigidity while correcting curvature.
73. Vacuum therapy can preserve penile length post-Peyronie's surgery.
74. Oral vitamin E was historically used but lacks strong clinical evidence.
75. Penile fracture is an acute urological emergency due to tunica albuginea rupture.
76. Common symptoms of fracture include cracking sound, pain, swelling, and detumescence.
77. Immediate surgical repair of penile fracture reduces risk of fibrosis and ED.
78. Delay in repair increases risk of curvature, fibrosis, and erectile dysfunction.
79. False penile fracture can occur due to dorsal vein rupture, mimicking tunical injury.
80. Penile Mondor disease resolves spontaneously with NSAIDs and abstinence.
81. Doppler ultrasound is essential for differentiating high vs low-flow priapism.
82. Non-ischemic priapism patients often have painless partial rigidity.
83. Cavernosal blood gas confirms ischemic priapism by showing low pO_2, high CO_2, and acidosis.
84. Chronic priapism leads to corporal fibrosis and erectile dysfunction.
85. Experimental stem cell therapy may restore function in fibrotic corporal tissue.
86. PDE5 inhibitors may paradoxically reduce stuttering priapism episodes in SCD.
87. Priapism lasting >48 h rarely responds to conservative measures; surgery is required.
88. Corporal shunts create fistulas between corpora and glans or veins to relieve ischemia.
89. Distal shunts like Winter's or Ebbehoj are preferred initial surgical options.
90. Proximal shunts are used when distal techniques fail, but carry higher morbidity.
91. Penile prosthesis may be required in refractory priapism-induced ED.
92. Counseling is vital in Peyronie's and priapism patients due to sexual and psychological impact.
93. Novel therapies like gene therapy and antifibrotic drugs are under study for Peyronie's.
94. Coital headaches are benign in most cases but warrant imaging to exclude aneurysm.
95. SSRIs can delay ejaculation and are used therapeutically in premature ejaculation.
96. Topical anesthetics reduce penile sensitivity, prolonging IELT in PE.
97. Behavioral therapies like stop-start improve control in lifelong PE.
98. Post-orgasmic illness syndrome may involve immune reaction to semen.

99. Semen desensitization therapy is an experimental approach for post-orgasmic illness.
100. Comprehensive management of penile disorders often requires multidisciplinary input including urology, psychology, and physiotherapy.

Further Reading

The explanations in this chapter are supported by the following key references:

1. Nehra A, Alterowitz R, Culkin DJ, et al. Peyronie's disease: AUA guideline. J Urol. 2015;194(3):745–53.
2. Salonia A, Eardley I, Giuliano F, et al. European Association of Urology guidelines on priapism. Eur Urol. 2014;65(2):480–9.
3. Mulhall JP, Creech SD, Boorjian SA, et al. Subjective and objective analysis of Peyronie's disease. J Sex Med. 2006;3(3):469–76.
4. Eke N. Fracture of the penis. Br J Surg. 2002;89(5):555–65.
5. Ralph D, Gonzalez-Cadavid N, Mirone V, et al. The management of Peyronie's disease: evidence-based guidelines. J Sex Med. 2010;7(7):2359–74.
6. Trombetta C, Liguori G, Garaffa G, et al. Penile Mondor disease. BJU Int. 2006;97(4):813–5.

Andrological Emergencies

10

Learning Objectives

- Identify life- and organ-threatening andrological emergencies.
- Differentiate testicular torsion from epididymo-orchitis.
- Understand mechanisms and diagnosis of penile fracture.
- Outline the management of Fournier's gangrene.
- Recognize the role of imaging and prompt surgical intervention.

Select the Single Best Answer

1. The most common presenting symptom of testicular torsion is:
   A. Scrotal redness
   B. Sudden onset severe scrotal pain
   C. Gradual swelling over weeks
   D. Fever and dysuria
   E. Hematospermia
2. Which physical sign is most specific for testicular torsion?
   A. Positive Prehn's sign
   B. Absent cremasteric reflex
   C. Blue dot sign
   D. Transillumination of scrotum
   E. Scrotal skin erythema
3. Which imaging sign on Doppler ultrasound confirms torsion?
   A. Increased venous flow
   B. Whirlpool sign of spermatic cord
   C. Hydrocele fluid collection
   D. Increased arterial flow
   E. Calcification

M. S. M. Hasan, M. L. Elsaie, *Comprehensive MCQs in Andrology*, Trends in Andrology and Sexual Medicine, https://doi.org/10.1007/978-3-032-20623-7_10

4. The time window with **highest salvage rate (>90%)** for testicular torsion is within:
   A. 1 h
   B. 2 h
   C. 6 h
   D. 12 h
   E. 24 h
5. In testicular torsion, bell-clapper deformity is:
   A. Congenital absence of gubernaculum
   B. Failure of posterior fixation of tunica vaginalis
   C. High insertion of epididymis
   D. Intravaginal hydrocele
   E. Hernia sac persistence
6. The commonest age for testicular torsion presentation is:
   A. Neonates
   B. 2–6 years
   C. 12–18 years
   D. 25–40 years
   E. > 50 years
7. Salvage rate of testes after torsion beyond 24 h is:
   A. > 90%
   B. 50–70%
   C. 20–30%
   D. <10%
   E. Nearly 100%
8. The most feared long-term complication of testicular torsion is:
   A. Hydrocele
   B. Epididymal cyst
   C. Subfertility/infertility
   D. Testicular cancer
   E. Varicocele
9. Which factor most strongly predicts testicular viability after torsion?
   A. Patient age
   B. Side of torsion
   C. Degree of twist and duration
   D. Presence of hydrocele
   E. Bilaterality
10. The most common mechanism of penile fracture is:
    A. Fall from height
    B. Sports injury
    C. Sexual intercourse
    D. Masturbation
    E. Blunt trauma with clothing

11. The typical deformity in penile fracture is:
    A. Hourglass deformity
    B. Eggplant deformity
    C. Curvature deformity
    D. Bottle-neck deformity
    E. String deformity
12. The most common site of penile fracture is:
    A. Corpus spongiosum
    B. Tunica albuginea of corpus cavernosum
    C. Dorsal vein
    D. Penile urethra
    E. Prepuce
13. The classical "snap sound" during penile fracture corresponds to:
    A. Rupture of dorsal vein
    B. Rupture of tunica albuginea
    C. Urethral disruption
    D. Glans injury
    E. Corpora venous leakage
14. The gold standard management of penile fracture is:
    A. Conservative with ice packs
    B. Compression dressing
    C. Immediate surgical exploration and repair
    D. Aspiration of hematoma
    E. Antibiotics only
15. The complication most feared after delayed repair of penile fracture is:
    A. Infertility
    B. Erectile dysfunction
    C. Balanitis
    D. Urethral stricture
    E. Hydrocele
16. Which suture material is recommended in immediate repair of penile fracture?
    A. Absorbable polyglactin 910
    B. Non-absorbable polypropylene
    C. Silk
    D. Catgut
    E. Nylon
17. Which of the following is an indication for immediate exploration in scrotal trauma?
    A. Hematocele >5 cm
    B. Painless hydrocele
    C. Scrotal edema only
    D. Minor abrasion
    E. Asymptomatic varicocele

18. Which testicular trauma type has the **worst prognosis** for salvage?
    A. Contusion
    B. Hematocele
    C. Rupture of tunica albuginea
    D. Epididymal hematoma
    E. Hydrocele
19. What is the first-line imaging in acute scrotal trauma?
    A. CT pelvis
    B. MRI scrotum
    C. Color Doppler ultrasound
    D. X-ray
    E. Scrotoscopy
20. The most important diagnostic test to differentiate ischemic from non-ischemic priapism is:
    A. MRI
    B. Cavernosography
    C. Penile Doppler ultrasound
    D. Corporal blood gas analysis
    E. Retrograde urethrogram
21. Corporal blood gas in ischemic priapism typically shows:
    A. High pO_2, low pCO_2, high pH
    B. Low pO_2, high pCO_2, low pH
    C. Normal values
    D. Low bicarbonate only
    E. High lactate with normal gases
22. The earliest histological change in ischemic priapism occurs in:
    A. Tunica albuginea
    B. Endothelium of cavernous sinusoids
    C. Smooth muscle fibers
    D. Dorsal nerve
    E. Vasa vasorum
23. The most common blood disorder associated with ischemic priapism in children is:
    A. Hemophilia
    B. Polycythemia
    C. Leukemia
    D. Sickle cell anemia
    E. Thalassemia
24. The first-line intracavernosal drug for ischemic priapism is:
    A. Adrenaline
    B. Noradrenaline
    C. Phenylephrine
    D. Dopamine
    E. Atropine

25. Surgical shunt procedures for priapism are indicated when:
    A. Duration <4 h
    B. Conservative measures fail
    C. Patient requests
    D. Priapism is non-ischemic
    E. Aspiration has not been attempted
26. Which artery is most often injured in high-flow priapism due to trauma?
    A. Dorsal penile artery
    B. Cavernosal artery
    C. Bulbar artery
    D. Testicular artery
    E. External pudendal artery
27. Which of the following is a **late complication** of untreated priapism?
    A. Erectile dysfunction
    B. Phimosis
    C. Testicular torsion
    D. Balanitis
    E. Varicocele
28. Which of the following is NOT a criterion of stuttering priapism?
    A. Variant of ischemic priapism
    B. Sleep-related
    C. Painful
    D. Transient attack
    E. Last more than 4 h
29. The most common cause of Fournier's gangrene is:
    A. Group A Streptococcus
    B. coli with anaerobes
    C. MRSA
    D. Pseudomonas
    E. Candida
30. Fournier's gangrene mortality is most influenced by:
    A. Patient age
    B. Delay in surgical debridement
    C. Gender
    D. Organism type
    E. Antibiotic selection alone
31. Antibiotic coverage for Fournier's gangrene should include:
    A. Gram-positive only
    B. Gram-negative only
    C. Anaerobes only
    D. Broad spectrum including anaerobes
    E. Antifungal alone

32. The most appropriate management for Fournier's gangrene is:
    A. Oral antibiotics only
    B. Immediate surgical debridement + broad-spectrum antibiotics
    C. Radiotherapy
    D. Local wound care only
    E. Wait-and-watch
33. The most important prognostic factor in Fournier's gangrene is:
    A. Patient age
    B. Presence of diabetes and comorbidities
    C. Extent of infection and delay in surgery
    D. Organism type
    E. Use of hyperbaric oxygen
34. Fournier's gangrene most commonly spreads along:
    A. Buck's fascia
    B. Dartos fascia and Colles' fascia
    C. Corpus spongiosum
    D. Urethral mucosa
    E. Testicular parenchyma
35. Which of the following is an important supportive therapy in Fournier's gangrene?
    A. Hyperbaric oxygen therapy
    B. Radiotherapy
    C. Oral steroids
    D. NSAIDs alone
    E. Watchful waiting
36. In paraphimosis, the primary pathophysiological mechanism of gangrene is:
    A. Arterial occlusion
    B. Venous congestion and arterial compromise
    C. Direct infection
    D. Lymphatic blockage
    E. Nerve ischemia
37. The first step in paraphimosis management is:
    A. Broad-spectrum antibiotics
    B. Manual reduction with compression
    C. Immediate circumcision
    D. Dorsal slit under anesthesia
    E. Glansectomy
38. Which of the following scrotal conditions is **not** considered a true emergency?
    A. Testicular torsion
    B. Epididymo-orchitis
    C. Fournier's gangrene
    D. Penile fracture
    E. Strangulated hernia

39. The most common site of urethral injury in pelvic fracture is:
    A. Penile urethra
    B. Bulbar urethra
    C. Prostatic urethra
    D. Membranous urethra
    E. Fossa navicularis
40. The safest initial investigation for suspected urethral injury is:
    A. Cystoscopy
    B. Retrograde urethrogram
    C. MRI pelvis
    D. Intravenous pyelogram
    E. CT urogram
41. Classic triad of urethral injury in pelvic fracture is:
    A. Hematuria, scrotal hematoma, incontinence
    B. Urethral bleeding, suprapubic fullness, inability to void
    C. Dysuria, fever, flank pain
    D. Frequency, urgency, nocturia
    E. Penile fracture, priapism, hematospermia
42. Which finding is most specific for complete urethral injury?
    A. Blood at meatus
    B. Perineal hematoma
    C. Suprapubic fullness
    D. Inability to pass Foley catheter
    E. Dysuria
43. In urethral injury, the "butterfly hematoma" typically suggests:
    A. Membranous urethral tear
    B. Bulbar urethral injury
    C. Prostatic urethral injury
    D. Penile urethral rupture
    E. Fossa navicularis tear
44. The most important differential diagnosis of acute scrotum in adolescents is:
    A. Epididymitis
    B. Hydrocele
    C. Varicocele
    D. Hernia
    E. Fournier's gangrene
45. Which of the following is NOT a side effect of intracavernosal phenylephrine injection?
    A. Bradycardia
    B. Subarachnoid hemorrhage
    C. Irregular cardiac rhythm
    D. Atrial fibrillation
    E. Hypertension

46. The size of the butterfly cannula used for aspiration in priapism treatment is:
    A. 8–10 G
    B. 10–12 G
    C. 12–14 G
    D. 14–16 G
    E. 20–22 G
47. The most feared complication after untreated Fournier's gangrene is:
    A. Hydrocele
    B. Testicular cancer
    C. Septic shock
    D. Urethral stricture
    E. Erectile dysfunction
48. Which imaging modality is most reliable for diagnosing suspected testicular torsion?
    A. CT abdomen
    B. MRI pelvis
    C. Color Doppler ultrasound
    D. Plain X-ray
    E. IV urography
49. The most important long-term complication of untreated priapism is:
    A. Infertility
    B. Erectile dysfunction
    C. Hydrocele
    D. Varicocele
    E. Chronic prostatitis
50. Which is the single most important step in management of suspected testicular torsion in adolescents?
    A. Immediate scrotal ultrasound
    B. Pain relief with NSAIDs
    C. Immediate surgical exploration
    D. Watchful waiting 6 h
    E. Empirical antibiotics

✅ Key Takeaways

- Testicular torsion is a time-sensitive emergency—intervention within 6 h is critical.
- Penile fracture requires immediate surgical repair to restore erectile function.
- Fournier's gangrene is a polymicrobial necrotizing fasciitis of the perineum—requires debridement and broad-spectrum antibiotics.
- History and examination are essential for prompt diagnosis and triage.
- Delay in treatment increases risk of infertility and permanent damage.

✅ Answer Key (1–50)

1. B
2. B
3. B
4. C
5. B
6. C
7. D
8. C
9. C
10. C
11. B
12. B
13. B
14. C
15. B
16. A
17. A
18. C
19. C
20. D
21. B
22. B
23. D
24. C
25. B
26. B
27. A
28. E
29. B
30. B
31. D
32. B
33. C
34. B
35. A
36. B
37. B
38. B
39. D
40. B
41. B
42. D

43. B
44. A
45. B
46. C
47. C
48. C
49. B
50. C

Explanations (1–50)

1. Sudden onset of severe unilateral scrotal pain is the hallmark of testicular torsion. The pain is usually abrupt, may radiate to the groin or abdomen, and is often associated with nausea and vomiting. Other causes of acute scrotum typically have more gradual onset.
2. The absent cremasteric reflex is the most specific sign of torsion. Normally, stroking the inner thigh causes testicular elevation via the cremaster muscle. Its absence indicates testicular ischemia. Prehn's sign is unreliable and may mislead diagnosis.
3. The "whirlpool sign" on Doppler ultrasound shows twisted spermatic cord vessels. It is a pathognomonic finding for torsion. Loss of blood flow is highly suggestive but not as specific as the whirlpool sign.
4. Testicular salvage is highest within 6 h of torsion onset, declining rapidly after. By 12 h, viability decreases markedly, and by 24 h, testicular necrosis is nearly universal. Early surgical exploration is critical.
5. Bell-clapper deformity results from failure of posterior fixation of the tunica vaginalis. This allows the testis to swing freely, predisposing to intravaginal torsion. It is usually bilateral, necessitating contralateral orchiopexy.
6. Torsion most commonly affects adolescents aged 12–18 years due to rapid testicular growth during puberty. Neonatal torsion occurs but follows a different mechanism. Adults are less frequently affected.
7. If torsion persists beyond 24 h, salvage rate drops to <10%. Prolonged ischemia leads to irreversible infarction and atrophy. Early presentation is the key predictor of outcome.
8. Long-term complication of torsion is subfertility or infertility due to ischemic damage and potential antisperm antibody formation. Even after successful salvage, fertility may be reduced compared with the contralateral side.
9. Degree of twist and ischemia duration are the most critical determinants of viability. Severe torsion (>720°) leads to earlier necrosis. Patient age and side have little impact.
10. Most penile fractures occur during vigorous sexual intercourse, when the erect penis slips out and hits the perineum or pubic bone. Other mechanisms (masturbation, trauma) are less common.
11. Penile fracture produces the classic "eggplant deformity," with swelling, ecchymosis, and curvature. This results from tunical rupture and extravasation of blood into penile tissues.

12. The tunica albuginea of the corpus cavernosum is the commonest fracture site. During erection, intracavernosal pressure increases, thinning the tunica to ~0.25 mm, making it susceptible to rupture.
13. The snapping sound is due to rupture of the tunica albuginea under high intracavernosal pressure. It is often followed by immediate detumescence and pain.
14. Immediate surgical exploration and repair is the gold standard for penile fracture. Conservative measures result in higher rates of erectile dysfunction, penile curvature, and painful erections.
15. Erectile dysfunction is the most feared complication of delayed repair due to fibrosis and abnormal wound healing. Early surgery minimizes this risk and restores function.
16. Absorbable sutures like polyglactin (Vicryl) are recommended for tunical repair. They provide secure closure without leaving permanent material, reducing long-term complications.
17. A large hematocele (>5 cm) after trauma requires surgical exploration. Smaller hematoceles may be observed, but larger ones risk tunical rupture or testicular ischemia.
18. Rupture of the tunica albuginea in testicular trauma carries the worst prognosis for salvage. Prompt surgical repair may preserve the testis, but delayed management often results in orchiectomy.
19. Color Doppler ultrasound is the first-line imaging for scrotal trauma, as it assesses blood flow and tunical integrity. CT and MRI are rarely needed unless injury extends beyond the scrotum.
20. Corporal blood gas analysis differentiates ischemic from non-ischemic priapism. Ischemic samples show hypoxia, hypercapnia, and acidosis. This test is rapid, reliable, and guides management.
21. Ischemic priapism blood gas reveals low pO_2 (<30 mmHg), high pCO_2 (>60 mmHg), and low pH (<7.25). This confirms the diagnosis of a low-flow, hypoxic state requiring urgent intervention.
22. The endothelium of cavernous sinusoids is first affected in ischemia, followed by smooth muscle necrosis. Prolonged episodes lead to irreversible fibrosis.
23. Sickle cell anemia is the most common blood disorder linked with pediatric ischemic priapism. Sickled erythrocytes obstruct venous outflow, producing hypoxic priapism.
24. Phenylephrine is the first-line agent for intracavernosal injection. As a pure α-adrenergic agonist, it contracts smooth muscle, enhances venous outflow, and minimizes systemic cardiovascular effects.
25. Shunt procedures are indicated after failure of aspiration and medical therapy. They create alternate drainage pathways, relieving ischemia. Shunts are not first-line in early priapism.
26. Cavernosal artery injury is the usual cause of high-flow priapism after blunt perineal trauma. It results in arterial-lacunar fistula formation, producing painless, partially rigid erections.
27. Erectile dysfunction is the most common late complication of untreated priapism. Smooth muscle necrosis and fibrosis impair cavernosal relaxation, making erections unsustainable.

28. Stuttering priapism refers to recurrent, brief ischemic episodes, usually resolving within 4 h. Persistent attacks beyond 4 h are classified as ischemic priapism.
29. Fournier's gangrene is most often caused by polymicrobial infection, especially *E. coli* combined with anaerobes. Mixed flora contribute to rapid necrosis and spread.
30. Delay in surgical debridement is the most significant factor increasing mortality in Fournier's gangrene. Early, aggressive surgery is lifesaving.
31. Antibiotic coverage must be broad spectrum including aerobes and anaerobes. Gram-positive, Gram-negative, and anaerobic organisms commonly act synergistically in this condition.
32. Immediate surgical debridement with broad-spectrum antibiotics is the cornerstone of management. Antibiotics alone are insufficient to control this aggressive necrotizing fasciitis.
33. Prognosis depends mainly on the extent of infection and time to surgical intervention. Comorbidities like diabetes worsen outcomes, but surgical delay is the strongest factor.
34. Fournier's infection spreads rapidly along fascial planes, especially Dartos and Colles' fascia. The testis is often spared due to separate blood supply.
35. Hyperbaric oxygen therapy improves survival and healing in severe Fournier's gangrene. It enhances tissue oxygenation, inhibits anaerobes, and boosts leukocyte function.
36. Paraphimosis initially causes venous congestion, which progresses to arterial compromise and ischemia. If untreated, this leads to gangrene of the glans penis.
37. The first step is manual reduction with lubrication or compression. Surgical options like dorsal slit or circumcision are reserved for failed conservative attempts.
38. Among acute scrotal conditions, epididymo-orchitis is not a true emergency. Torsion, Fournier's, and penile fracture demand immediate intervention to preserve function.
39. The membranous urethra is the most commonly injured site in pelvic fracture urethral injuries. Its fixed position makes it vulnerable during pelvic disruption.
40. Retrograde urethrogram is the safest and most reliable diagnostic test. It delineates injury location and extent, avoiding further trauma from blind catheterization.
41. The classic triad of urethral injury is blood at meatus, suprapubic fullness, and inability to void. This combination is strongly suggestive of posterior urethral injury.
42. Inability to pass a Foley catheter is the most specific sign of complete urethral injury. Attempts at blind catheterization may worsen the damage.
43. A butterfly-shaped perineal hematoma typically suggests bulbar urethral injury. Blood tracks into surrounding tissues, producing the characteristic appearance.
44. Epididymitis is the most important differential diagnosis of acute scrotum in adolescents. Its presentation can mimic torsion, necessitating careful clinical and Doppler evaluation.

45. Phenylephrine side effects include hypertension and arrhythmias. Subarachnoid hemorrhage, however, is not a recognized adverse effect.
46. The optimal cannula size for aspiration in priapism is 12–14 G. Smaller needles may clog, while larger ones cause unnecessary trauma.
47. The most feared complication of untreated Fournier's gangrene is septic shock. Rapid bacterial spread and toxin release cause overwhelming sepsis and high mortality.
48. Color Doppler ultrasound is the most reliable imaging modality for torsion. It shows absent or reduced blood flow, differentiating torsion from epididymitis.
49. Erectile dysfunction is the most important long-term complication of untreated priapism due to cavernosal fibrosis and poor veno-occlusion.
50. Immediate surgical exploration is the most critical step in suspected torsion. Imaging should not delay intervention, as every hour decreases salvage rates.

Further Reading

The explanations in this chapter are supported by the following key references:

1. Ringdahl E, Teague L. Testicular torsion. Am Fam Physician. 2006;74(10):1739–43.
2. Mellick LB. Torsion of the testicle: it is time to stop tossing the dice. Pediatr Emerg Care. 2012;28(1):80–6.
3. Salonia A, Eardley I, Giuliano F, et al. EAU guidelines on priapism. Eur Urol. 2014;65(2):480–9.
4. Eke N. Fracture of the penis. Br J Surg. 2002;89(5):555–65.
5. Sorensen MD, Krieger JN, Rivara FP, et al. Fournier's gangrene: management and mortality predictors. J Urol. 2009;182(6):2742–7.
6. Wampler SM, Llanes M. Common scrotal and testicular problems. Prim Care. 2010;37(3):613–26.

Male Sexual Function and Fertility

11

Learning Objectives

- Understand the relationship between male sexual function and fertility.
- Recognize how ED and PE may impair conception.
- Evaluate hormonal and semen parameters relevant to fertility.
- Explore treatment options to restore function and fertility.
- Coordinate care with reproductive specialists.

Select the Single Best Answer

1. Erectile function is primarily mediated by:
   A. Dopamine
   B. Acetylcholine
   C. Nitric oxide
   D. Norepinephrine
   E. Serotonin
2. The main artery responsible for penile erection is:
   A. Dorsal artery
   B. Cavernosal artery
   C. Bulbar artery
   D. Urethral artery
   E. Femoral artery
3. Which of the following hormones is most directly involved in testosterone production?
   A. FSH
   B. GnRH
   C. Prolactin
   D. LH
   E. Estrogen

M. S. M. Hasan, M. L. Elsaie, *Comprehensive MCQs in Andrology*, Trends in Andrology and Sexual Medicine, https://doi.org/10.1007/978-3-032-20623-7_11

4. The Leydig cells are stimulated by:
   A. FSH
   B. Testosterone
   C. LH
   D. Estrogen
   E. Prolactin
5. Which of the following best describes the mechanism of action of sildenafil?
   A. Inhibits acetylcholinesterase
   B. Blocks alpha-adrenergic receptors
   C. PDE-5 inhibitor
   D. Testosterone agonist
   E. D2 receptor agonist
6. The detumescence phase of erection is primarily mediated by:
   A. Nitric oxide
   B. Prostaglandins
   C. Norepinephrine
   D. Acetylcholine
   E. Serotonin
7. Which structure is essential for the veno-occlusive mechanism?
   A. Tunica vaginalis
   B. Buck's fascia
   C. Tunica albuginea
   D. Corpus spongiosum
   E. Prepuce
8. Normal semen analysis according to WHO includes all EXCEPT:
   A. Volume >1.5 mL
   B. Motility >20%
   C. pH 7.2–8
   D. Concentration >15 million/mL
   E. Morphology >4% normal forms
9. Which of the following causes retrograde ejaculation?
   A. Phimosis
   B. Diabetes mellitus
   C. Varicocele
   D. Orchitis
   E. Hydrocele
10. Oligospermia refers to:
   A. Low sperm motility
   B. Low sperm count
   C. No sperm in semen
   D. Abnormal sperm morphology
   E. Low semen volume

11. Which hormone stimulates Sertoli cells directly?
    A. LH
    B. FSH
    C. Testosterone
    D. Inhibin B
    E. Estrogen
12. Spermatogenesis occurs in the:
    A. Epididymis
    B. Rete testis
    C. Vas deferens
    D. Seminiferous tubules
    E. Tunica albuginea
13. Which enzyme is essential in converting testosterone to DHT?
    A. Aromatase
    B. 5-alpha reductase
    C. PDE5
    D. Tyrosine kinase
    E. LH receptor kinase
14. The final maturation of sperm takes place in the:
    A. Testis
    B. Seminal vesicle
    C. Epididymis
    D. Prostate
    E. Bulbourethral gland
15. Which of the following is NOT a function of testosterone?
    A. Growth of facial hair
    B. Increased vocal pitch
    C. Increased muscle mass
    D. Spermatogenesis
    E. Libido
16. What is the most common cause of male infertility?
    A. Cryptorchidism
    B. Hormonal imbalance
    C. Varicocele
    D. Retrograde ejaculation
    E. Klinefelter syndrome
17. Which structure stores sperm before ejaculation?
    A. Seminiferous tubules
    B. Rete testis
    C. Epididymis
    D. Vas deferens
    E. Urethra

18. Which hormone inhibits FSH release from the anterior pituitary?
    A. Testosterone
    B. LH
    C. Estrogen
    D. Inhibin B
    E. GnRH
19. What is the normal time range for sperm maturation in the epididymis?
    A. 1–3 days
    B. 7–10 days
    C. 14–21 days
    D. 30 days
    E. 48 h
20. Ejaculation is primarily controlled by:
    A. Parasympathetic nervous system
    B. Somatic nervous system
    C. Sympathetic nervous system
    D. Enteric nervous system
    E. Reflex arc
21. What is the primary role of nitric oxide in erection?
    A. Testosterone production
    B. Muscle contraction
    C. Vasodilation of penile arteries
    D. Sperm motility
    E. Testicular descent
22. Which part of the autonomic nervous system controls erection?
    A. Sympathetic
    B. Parasympathetic
    C. Somatic
    D. Enteric
    E. Central nervous system only
23. Which condition is characterized by persistent painful erection?
    A. Peyronie's disease
    B. Varicocele
    C. Priapism
    D. Erectile dysfunction
    E. Phimosis
24. What is the normal reference range for serum testosterone in adult males?
    A. 50–150 ng/dL
    B. 300–1000 ng/dL
    C. 1000–2000 ng/dL
    D. 5–20 ng/dL
    E. 200–300 ng/dL

25. Which of the following contributes most to semen volume?
    A. Testes
    B. Prostate
    C. Seminal vesicles
    D. Bulbourethral glands
    E. Epididymis
26. The acrosome reaction is necessary for:
    A. Epididymal maturation
    B. Hormonal regulation
    C. Oocyte penetration
    D. Motility
    E. Spermatid formation
27. Which test assesses sperm motility?
    A. Seminal fructose
    B. Semen analysis
    C. Sperm culture
    D. Hormone profile
    E. Testicular biopsy
28. Which condition is associated with absent vas deferens bilaterally?
    A. Turner syndrome
    B. Kallmann syndrome
    C. Congenital adrenal hyperplasia
    D. Cystic fibrosis
    E. Hypogonadotropic hypogonadism
29. What is the role of PDE5 inhibitors in ED treatment?
    A. Stimulate testosterone production
    B. Increase sperm count
    C. Promote smooth muscle relaxation
    D. Increase libido
    E. Inhibit DHT
30. Which parameter in semen analysis reflects sperm concentration?
    A. Morphology
    B. Count
    C. Volume
    D. Motility
    E. pH
31. Which hormone is primarily responsible for libido in men?
    A. Prolactin
    B. Estrogen
    C. Testosterone
    D. FSH
    E. LH

32. What is the effect of hyperprolactinemia on sexual function?
    A. Enhances libido
    B. Improves ejaculation
    C. Causes erectile dysfunction and decreased libido
    D. Increases testosterone
    E. Stimulates LH
33. Retrograde ejaculation is commonly caused by:
    A. Testicular torsion
    B. Urethral stricture
    C. Bladder neck dysfunction
    D. Varicocele
    E. High testosterone
34. A normal semen volume is defined as:
    A. <0.5 mL
    B. 1–6 mL
    C. >7 mL
    D. >10 mL
    E. 0.1–0.5 mL
35. Which structure stores and matures sperm?
    A. Testis
    B. Epididymis
    C. Seminal vesicle
    D. Prostate
    E. Urethra
36. Which endocrine test is useful in evaluating hypogonadism?
    A. Prostate-specific antigen
    B. FSH and LH
    C. ESR
    D. Semen fructose
    E. Creatinine
37. The normal range for sperm morphology by strict Kruger criteria is:
    A. >15%
    B. >30%
    C. >4%
    D. >50%
    E. >10%
38. Which of the following medications can cause ED?
    A. PDE5 inhibitors
    B. SSRIs
    C. Antihistamines
    D. Multivitamins
    E. Testosterone

39. Which test assesses post-ejaculatory urinalysis for retrograde ejaculation?
    A. Urethral swab
    B. Urine culture
    C. Post-ejaculatory urine examination
    D. Seminal fructose test
    E. Digital rectal exam
40. Azoospermia refers to:
    A. Absence of motility
    B. Low sperm count
    C. No sperm in semen
    D. Abnormal morphology
    E. High volume of semen
41. What is the main function of Sertoli cells?
    A. Testosterone production
    B. Secrete androgen-binding protein
    C. Produce inhibin
    D. Phagocytosis of residual cytoplasm
    E. All of the above
42. Which hormone directly stimulates testosterone synthesis in Leydig cells?
    A. FSH
    B. LH
    C. TSH
    D. Estrogen
    E. ACTH
43. Which imaging modality is preferred in evaluating varicocele?
    A. MRI
    B. CT
    C. Doppler ultrasound
    D. X-ray
    E. PET scan
44. Klinefelter syndrome is characterized by:
    A. 45,XO
    B. 46,XY
    C. 47,XXY
    D. 48,XXXY
    E. 46,XX
45. Which of the following is a genetic cause of male infertility?
    A. Varicocele
    B. Retrograde ejaculation
    C. Kallmann syndrome
    D. Obstructive azoospermia
    E. Ejaculatory duct cyst

46. What is the WHO lower reference limit for sperm motility (total + progressive)?
    A. 10%
    B. 20%
    C. 40%
    D. 60%
    E. 80%
47. Androgen insensitivity syndrome results in:
    A. Male phenotype with infertility
    B. Female phenotype with 46,XX
    C. Male phenotype with 46,XY and normal fertility
    D. Female phenotype with 46,XY
    E. Ambiguous genitalia
48. What is a contraindication for testosterone replacement therapy?
    A. Primary hypogonadism
    B. Metabolic syndrome
    C. Prostate cancer
    D. Low libido
    E. Erectile dysfunction
49. Which of the following is part of the hypothalamic-pituitary-gonadal axis?
    A. GnRH → LH/FSH → Testosterone
    B. FSH → GnRH → Testosterone
    C. LH → GnRH → Estrogen
    D. Testosterone → FSH → GnRH
    E. LH → ACTH → Testosterone
50. Sperm capacitation occurs in the:
    A. Seminiferous tubules
    B. Epididymis
    C. Vas deferens
    D. Female reproductive tract
    E. Testicular interstitium

✅ Key Takeaways

- Sexual dysfunction can lead to **timing issues**, poor semen deposition, and reduced frequency of intercourse.
- Hypogonadism may impair **spermatogenesis and libido**.
- Ejaculatory disorders (retrograde, anejaculation) may necessitate **sperm retrieval techniques**.
- Hormonal optimization and PDE5 inhibitors can improve both erection and conception.
- Fertility-focused sexual counseling is an essential part of care.

✅ Answer Key (1–50)

1. C
2. B
3. D
4. C
5. C
6. C
7. C
8. B
9. B
10. B
11. B
12. D
13. B
14. C
15. B
16. C
17. C
18. D
19. B
20. C
21. C
22. B
23. C
24. B
25. C
26. C
27. B
28. D
29. C
30. B
31. C
32. C
33. C
34. B
35. B
36. B
37. C
38. B
39. C
40. C
41. E
42. B

43. C
44. C
45. C
46. C
47. D
48. C
49. A
50. D

Explanations (1–50)

1. Nitric oxide (NO) is the primary neurotransmitter responsible for initiating penile erection. It activates guanylyl cyclase, increasing cGMP, which relaxes smooth muscle in the corpora cavernosa.
2. Cavernosal arteries dilate during erection to increase blood flow into the corpora cavernosa. The dorsal artery supplies glans penis but plays a lesser role in erection.
3. Luteinizing hormone (LH) directly stimulates Leydig cells to produce testosterone, essential for spermatogenesis and male sexual health.
4. Leydig cells respond to LH by synthesizing testosterone, while Sertoli cells are stimulated by FSH to support spermatogenesis.
5. Sildenafil inhibits PDE-5, preventing breakdown of cGMP, prolonging smooth muscle relaxation, and sustaining penile erection.
6. Norepinephrine release from sympathetic nerves leads to smooth muscle contraction and penile detumescence (return to flaccidity).
7. The tunica albuginea compresses venous outflow, ensuring blood is trapped within corpora cavernosa for rigidity.
8. WHO semen standards require >40% motility and >1.5 mL volume. A cutoff of 20% motility is outdated.
9. Diabetes mellitus causes neuropathy and bladder neck dysfunction, leading to retrograde ejaculation.
10. Oligospermia is a low sperm count (<15 million/mL), a key cause of male infertility.
11. FSH directly stimulates Sertoli cells, which support germ cells, secrete inhibin, and form the blood-testis barrier.
12. Spermatogenesis occurs in seminiferous tubules, supported by Sertoli cells and testosterone.
13. 5-alpha reductase converts testosterone into DHT, the active androgen in target tissues like prostate and genitalia.
14. Epididymis is the site of sperm maturation and storage before ejaculation.
15. Testosterone promotes spermatogenesis, libido, muscle mass, and secondary sex characteristics, but not high-pitched voice.
16. Varicocele is the most common correctable cause of male infertility due to impaired thermoregulation of testes.

17. Epididymis stores sperm and facilitates maturation until ejaculation.
18. Inhibin B, secreted by Sertoli cells, selectively inhibits FSH at the anterior pituitary.
19. Sperm spend 6–10 days in the epididymis for maturation, gaining motility and fertilizing ability.
20. Ejaculation is mainly a sympathetic reflex (T12–L2), involving contraction of vas deferens, seminal vesicles, and prostate.
21. Nitric oxide causes vasodilation of penile arteries, facilitating blood engorgement in erectile tissue.
22. Parasympathetic system (S2–S4) mediates erection by stimulating NO and acetylcholine release.
23. Priapism is a prolonged painful erection caused by ischemic or non-ischemic mechanisms; ischemic priapism is a urological emergency.
24. Normal adult male testosterone is 300–1000 ng/dL; low levels indicate hypogonadism.
25. Seminal vesicles secrete fructose, prostaglandins, and coagulating proteins, accounting for most semen volume.
26. Acrosome reaction allows sperm to penetrate the zona pellucida during fertilization.
27. Semen analysis evaluates sperm count, motility, morphology, and semen volume.
28. Cystic fibrosis patients often have congenital bilateral absence of vas deferens, causing obstructive azoospermia.
29. PDE5 inhibitors enhance erections by sustaining cGMP-mediated smooth muscle relaxation.
30. Sperm concentration (count per mL) is a core semen parameter for fertility assessment.
31. Testosterone maintains libido by acting on brain regions controlling sexual desire.
32. Hyperprolactinemia suppresses GnRH, lowers LH/FSH, reduces testosterone, and causes decreased libido and ED.
33. Bladder neck dysfunction prevents antegrade ejaculation, leading to retrograde flow into the bladder.
34. Semen volume is normally 1.5–6 mL; deviations suggest obstructive or hypogonadal pathology.
35. Epididymis is crucial for storage and sperm maturation.
36. FSH and LH tests help identify primary vs secondary hypogonadism.
37. By strict Kruger's criteria, ≥4% normal morphology indicates normal fertility potential.
38. SSRIs interfere with neurotransmitter function and can cause sexual dysfunction, including ED and delayed ejaculation.
39. Post-ejaculatory urine analysis confirms retrograde ejaculation if sperm are detected in urine.
40. Azoospermia is complete absence of spermatozoa in semen; causes can be obstructive or non-obstructive.

41. Sertoli cells: multipurpose—secrete ABP, inhibin, support spermatogenesis, and phagocytose debris.
42. LH stimulates Leydig cells via cAMP to produce testosterone.
43. Doppler ultrasound is the diagnostic test of choice for varicocele, showing retrograde venous flow.
44. Klinefelter syndrome (47,XXY) is the most common chromosomal abnormality leading to male infertility.
45. Kallmann syndrome causes congenital hypogonadotropic hypogonadism with anosmia due to defective GnRH neuron migration.
46. WHO sets total sperm motility ≥40% as the lower reference for normal fertility.
47. Androgen insensitivity syndrome results in 46,XY individuals with female phenotype due to androgen receptor dysfunction.
48. Prostate cancer is an absolute contraindication to testosterone replacement therapy.
49. The HPG axis is GnRH → LH/FSH → testosterone; negative feedback regulates gonadotropin release.
50. Capacitation occurs in the female reproductive tract, where sperm undergo membrane changes allowing fertilization.

Further Reading

The explanations in this chapter are supported by the following key references:

1. World Health Organization. WHO laboratory manual for the examination and processing of human semen. 6th ed. Geneva: WHO; 2021.
2. Dohle GR, Diemer T, Kopa Z, et al. European association of urology guidelines on male infertility. Eur Urol. 2012;62(2):324–32.
3. Jungwirth A, Giwercman A, Tournaye H, et al. European Association of urology guidelines on male infertility. Eur Urol. 2018;73(4):424–38.
4. Lotti F, Maggi M. Sexual dysfunction and male infertility. Nat Rev Urol. 2018;15(5):287–307.
5. Agarwal A, Baskaran S, Parekh N, et al. Male infertility. Lancet. 2021;397(10271):319–33.
6. Ramasamy R, Schlegel PN. Medical therapy for male infertility. Urol Clin N Am. 2012;39(4):453–64.

Human Sperm Structure and Function 12

Learning Objectives

- Describe the anatomical parts of the sperm cell.
- Understand the functional role of acrosome, mitochondria, and flagellum.
- Identify morphological defects affecting fertility.
- Review laboratory techniques for sperm morphology analysis.
- Link sperm structural integrity to fertilization capacity.

Select the Single Best Answer

1. The human sperm can be stained by:
   A. Leishman stain
   B. PAS stain
   C. Silver stain
   D. CD100 stain
2. The length of the human sperm head is:
   A. 1.5–2 μm
   B. 2.5–3.5 μm
   C. 4–4.5 μm
   D. 5–6.5 μm
   E. 45 μm
3. The sperm head length-to-width ratio is:
   A. 1
   B. 1.5
   C. 2
   D. 2.5
   E. 3

M. S. M. Hasan, M. L. Elsaie, *Comprehensive MCQs in Andrology*, Trends in Andrology and Sexual Medicine, https://doi.org/10.1007/978-3-032-20623-7_12

4. The length of the sperm tail is:
   A. 15 μm
   B. 20 μm
   C. 25 μm
   D. 30 μm
   E. 45 μm
5. The length of normal human sperm is:
   A. 30 μm
   B. 35 μm
   C. 70 μm
   D. 100 μm
   E. 110 μm
6. Globozoospermia is equivalent to:
   A. 9 + 0 syndrome
   B. Young syndrome
   C. Zinner syndrome
   D. Round head syndrome
   E. Cystic fibrosis syndrome
7. The beta subunit of the sperm tail is:
   A. S-shaped
   B. C-shaped
   C. V-shaped
   D. Z-shaped
   E. L-shaped
8. Sperm mitosis occurs in:
   A. Spermatogoniosis
   B. Spermiogenesis
   C. Spermiation
   D. During sperm capacitation
9. The spermatozoa are mainly stored in:
   A. Epididymal head
   B. Proximal cauda epididymis
   C. Distal cauda epididymis
   D. Tail of epididymis
10. The sperms can live in the fallopian tube without fertilization for:
    A. 2–5 hours
    B. 5–10 hours
    C. 10–20 hours
    D. 48 hours
    E. 72 hours
11. Which of the following is NOT a motility sperm pattern?
    A. Linear motility
    B. Forward progressive motility
    C. Basal motility
    D. Angulated motility
    E. Circular motility

12. The bulk of the ejaculate volume is derived from:
    A. The epididymides
    B. The Cowper gland
    C. The seminal vesicles
    D. The testes
    E. Prostate
13. Sperm changes during epididymal transit include:
    A. Decreased motility
    B. Sulfhydryl reduction
    C. Decreased phospholipid content
    D. Reduced membrane rigidity
    E. Increased capacity for glycolysis
14. Which germ cell type is considered a true stem cell?
    A. Elongating spermatids
    B. Primary spermatocytes
    C. Round spermatids
    D. Secondary spermatocytes
    E. Type A spermatogonia
15. During development before ejaculation, sperm spend the majority of time in:
    A. Epididymis
    B. Ejaculatory ducts
    C. Seminal vesicle
    D. Testis
    E. Urethra
16. The sperm region containing mitochondria is the:
    A. Tail
    B. Head
    C. Acrosome
    D. Midpiece
    E. Axoneme
17. Processes required for sperm to fertilize an egg include all EXCEPT:
    A. Development of motility
    B. Acrosome reaction
    C. Capacitation
    D. Zona pellucida binding
    E. Sexual intercourse
18. After ejaculation the contents of the vas deferens are:
    A. Returned to the seminal vesicles
    B. Maintained in the ampulla
    C. Released into the ejaculatory ducts
    D. Propelled back into the epididymis
    E. Released into the bladder
19. Which is NOT true about fast-event sperm capacitation?
    A. Increase phosphokinase activity
    B. Stimulation of adenyl cyclase
    C. Increase bicarbonate concentration
    D. Decrease Ca^{2+} concentration

20. Which is true about slow-event sperm capacitation?
    A. Increase phosphokinase activity
    B. Stimulation of adenyl cyclase
    C. Increase bicarbonate concentration
    D. Decrease Ca^{2+} concentration
    E. None of the above
21. Which is FALSE about sperm capacitation?
    A. Happens before penetration of zona pellucida
    B. Cholesterol influx to plasma membrane
    C. Plasma membrane hyperpolarization
    D. Increase bicarbonate level in fast event
    E. Stimulation of adenyl cyclase in fast event
22. Which is FALSE about sperm hyperactivation?
    A. First consequence of capacitation
    B. Increase in intracellular Ca^{2+}
    C. Activation of sperm motility
    D. Appearance of sperm cell surface antigens
    E. Mechanism is uncertain
23. The acrosome is:
    A. Mitochondrial-like
    B. Golgi apparatus remnants
    C. Lysosome-like organelle
    D. Covers anterior and middle sperm nucleus
    E. Inner membrane underlies plasma membrane
24. Which is FALSE about acrosin?
    A. Sperm acrosomal protease
    B. Has proteolytic activity
    C. Binds zona pellucida glycoprotein
    D. Responsible for sperm hyperactivation
25. Abstinence >7 days before semen analysis affects:
    A. Sperm count
    B. Sperm volume
    C. Sperm motility
    D. Sperm agglutination
26. The origin of the first semen portion is:
    A. Cowper's glands
    B. Seminal vesicles
    C. Prostate
    D. Epididymis
    E. Testes
27. The origin of the least semen volume is:
    A. Cowper's glands
    B. Seminal vesicles
    C. Prostate
    D. Epididymis
    E. Testes

28. Optimal temperature for sperm sample collection is:
    A. −3 to −5 °C
    B. 20 to 40 °C
    C. −20 to −40 °C
    D. 15 to 20 °C
    E. 10 to 20 °C
29. Which is NOT a cellular component of semen?
    A. Leukocytes
    B. Immature germ cells
    C. Erythrocytes
    D. Mature sperms
    E. Epithelial cells
30. Mucin is secreted by:
    A. Testes
    B. Epididymis
    C. Seminal vesicles
    D. Prostate
    E. Cowper's gland
31. Seminogelin is secreted by:
    A. Testes
    B. Epididymis
    C. Seminal vesicles
    D. Prostate
    E. Cowper's gland
32. L-carnitine is secreted by:
    A. Testes
    B. Epididymis
    C. Seminal vesicles
    D. Prostate
    E. Cowper's gland
33. Non-coagulated semen sample indicates dysfunction of:
    A. Testes
    B. Epididymis
    C. Seminal vesicles
    D. Prostate
    E. Cowper's gland
34. Non-liquefied semen indicates dysfunction of:
    A. Testes
    B. Epididymis
    C. Seminal vesicles
    D. Prostate
    E. Cowper's gland

35. High semen pH is due to infection in:
    A. Testes
    B. Epididymis
    C. Seminal vesicles
    D. Prostate
    E. Cowper's gland
36. Sperm adherence indicates:
    A. Antigen-antibody reaction
    B. Infections
    C. Obstruction
    D. Hyperviscosity
    E. Congenital abnormality
37. Macrocephalic sperm syndrome is inherited as:
    A. X-linked recessive
    B. X-linked dominant
    C. Autosomal dominant
    D. Autosomal recessive
38. Decapitated sperm syndrome shows:
    A. Tapered head
    B. Pin head
    C. Midpiece anomaly
    D. Amorphous head
    E. Round head
39. Short sperm tail syndrome is due to mutation in:
    A. PICK1 gene
    B. SPATA16 gene
    C. DPY19L2 gene
    D. DNAH1 gene
    E. CatSper gene
40. CD45+ leukocytes in semen are stained:
    A. Blue
    B. Green
    C. Red
    D. Orange
    E. Black
41. Curvilinear sperm velocity means:
    A. Distance between each head point during time interval
    B. Distance between first and last head points ÷ time
    C. Measure of sperm head oscillation
    D. Departure from linear progression
    E. None

42. Straight-line sperm velocity means:
    A. Distance between each head point during time interval
    B. Distance between first and last head points ÷ time
    C. Measure of sperm head oscillation
    D. Departure from linear progression
    E. None
43. Amplitude of lateral sperm head displacement means:
    A. Distance between each head point during time interval
    B. Distance between first and last head points ÷ time
    C. Measure of sperm head oscillation
    D. Departure from linear progression
    E. None
44. Sperm linearity means:
    A. Distance between each head point during time interval
    B. Distance between first and last head points ÷ time
    C. Measure of sperm head oscillation
    D. Departure from linear progression
    E. None
45. Standard time of in vivo post-coital test is:
    A. 1–2 hours after coitus
    B. 2–5 hours after coitus
    C. 5–7 hours after coitus
    D. 9–14 hours after coitus
46. Spinnbarkeit test measures cervical mucus:
    A. Cellular content
    B. Elasticity
    C. Ferning
    D. Viscosity
    E. Volume
47. Zona-free hamster egg penetration test evaluates:
    A. Sperm capacitation
    B. Acrosome reaction
    C. Zona binding
    D. Sperm-ovum interaction
    E. Sperm hyperactivation
48. Which is NOT a site for leukocytes in semen?
    A. Rete testis
    B. Vas deferens
    C. Prostate
    D. Cowper's gland
    E. Seminiferous tubules

49. Positive peroxidase test indicates:
    A. Spermatogenic cells
    B. WBCs
    C. RBCs
    D. Lymphocytes
    E. Macrophages
50. Which pathway statement is FALSE?
    A. Sperm leave seminiferous tubules → rete testis
    B. Travel via efferent ducts → epididymis
    C. Ejaculation propels from epididymis → vas deferens
    D. Vas deferens → ejaculatory duct → prostatic urethra
    E. All are correct
51. The normal ejaculate liquefaction time is:
    A. Immediately after ejaculation
    B. Within 15 minutes
    C. Within 30 minutes
    D. After 1 hour
    E. After 2 hours
52. Azoospermia means:
    A. No sperm seen in semen
    B. No motile sperm seen
    C. Low sperm count <15 million/ml
    D. Only immature germ cells present
    E. Complete absence of semen
53. Oligozoospermia is defined as sperm count below:
    A. 40 million/ml
    B. 30 million/ml
    C. 20 million/ml
    D. 15 million/ml
    E. 10 million/ml
54. Asthenozoospermia refers to:
    A. Low sperm concentration
    B. Low motility
    C. Abnormal sperm morphology
    D. Presence of pus cells
    E. High viscosity
55. Teratozoospermia means:
    A. Reduced sperm motility
    B. Increased abnormal sperm forms
    C. Reduced ejaculate volume
    D. High semen pH
    E. Leukocytospermia

56. Normal semen pH ranges between:
    A. 6.0–6.5
    B. 6.5–7.0
    C. 7.0–7.5
    D. 7.2–8.0
    E. 8.0–9.0
57. Normal semen volume is:
    A. 0.5–1 ml
    B. 1–2 ml
    C. 2–5 ml
    D. 5–7 ml
    E. 7–10 ml
58. Necrozoospermia means:
    A. No sperm present
    B. Dead sperm present
    C. Immotile but viable sperm
    D. Morphologically abnormal sperm
    E. No semen produced
59. Which stain differentiates live from dead sperm?
    A. Leishman
    B. Papanicolaou
    C. Eosin-nigrosin
    D. Silver stain
    E. PAS
60. Leukocytospermia is diagnosed when WBCs exceed:
    A. 0.1 million/ml
    B. 0.5 million/ml
    C. 1 million/ml
    D. 5 million/ml
    E. 10 million/ml
61. Which is NOT a WHO semen analysis parameter?
    A. Volume
    B. pH
    C. Motility
    D. Morphology
    E. Fructose
62. Fructose in semen is secreted by:
    A. Prostate
    B. Cowper's gland
    C. Epididymis
    D. Seminal vesicles
    E. Testes

63. Which is the main energy source for sperm motility?
    A. Glucose
    B. Fructose
    C. Lactate
    D. Citrate
    E. Pyruvate
64. Which is considered a normal progressive motility rate?
    A. 10%
    B. 20%
    C. 32%
    D. 50%
    E. 70%
65. Which WHO parameter indicates normal sperm morphology?
    A. ≥4% normal forms
    B. ≥10% normal forms
    C. ≥20% normal forms
    D. ≥30% normal forms
    E. ≥40% normal forms
66. Which sperm abnormality is associated with infertility?
    A. Tapered head
    B. Round head
    C. Double tail
    D. Midpiece defect
    E. All of the above
67. Which is the most reliable test for sperm DNA damage?
    A. TUNEL assay
    B. Eosin-nigrosin staining
    C. CASA (computer-assisted sperm analysis)
    D. Karyotyping
    E. Papanicolaou stain
68. Normal sperm viability should be at least:
    A. 20%
    B. 30%
    C. 40%
    D. 50%
    E. 60%
69. Sperm chromatin condensation is aided by:
    A. Histones
    B. Protamine
    C. Tubulin
    D. Actin
    E. Myosin

70. The midpiece of the sperm is rich in:
    A. Lysosomes
    B. Golgi
    C. Mitochondria
    D. Ribosomes
    E. Endoplasmic reticulum
71. Reactive oxygen species in semen mainly affect:
    A. Volume
    B. pH
    C. Motility
    D. Liquefaction
    E. Color
72. The axoneme of the sperm tail has a microtubular arrangement of:
    A. 9 + 0
    B. 9 + 1
    C. 9 + 2
    D. 8 + 2
    E. 10 + 2
73. The sperm acrosome contains:
    A. Hyaluronidase
    B. Acrosin
    C. Neuraminidase
    D. All of the above
74. Which part of the sperm penetrates the zona pellucida?
    A. Head
    B. Midpiece
    C. Tail
    D. Axoneme
75. Capacitation of sperm occurs in the:
    A. Epididymis
    B. Prostate
    C. Female genital tract
    D. Seminal vesicle
    E. Testis
76. The sperm acrosome reaction is triggered by:
    A. Calcium influx
    B. Progesterone
    C. Zona pellucida glycoproteins
    D. All of the above
77. Hyaluronidase in sperm helps to:
    A. Penetrate zona pellucida
    B. Dissolve cumulus oophorus
    C. Aid motility
    D. Stabilize DNA

78. The primary function of the sperm centrosome is:
    A. DNA repair
    B. Tail motility
    C. Microtubule organization
    D. Acrosome formation
79. Which sperm abnormality is typically genetic?
    A. Globozoospermia
    B. Decapitated sperm
    C. Macrocephalic sperm
    D. All of the above
80. Which protein is crucial for sperm-oocyte fusion?
    A. ZP3
    B. IZUMO1
    C. Protamine
    D. Tubulin
81. Semen hyperviscosity is commonly due to:
    A. Infection
    B. Prostate dysfunction
    C. Seminal vesicle dysfunction
    D. All of the above
82. Normal sperm concentration according to WHO 2021 is:
    A. 5 million/ml
    B. 10 million/ml
    C. 15 million/ml
    D. 20 million/ml
83. Which test evaluates sperm oxidative stress?
    A. ROS assay
    B. CASA
    C. Eosin-nigrosin
    D. Papanicolaou smear
84. Which sperm test evaluates acrosome reaction?
    A. Acrosome staining
    B. Sperm chromatin dispersion test
    C. Hypoosmotic swelling test
    D. CASA
85. The hypoosmotic swelling test evaluates:
    A. Sperm motility
    B. Sperm viability
    C. Sperm morphology
    D. DNA fragmentation
86. Which sperm defect is associated with Kartagener's syndrome?
    A. Immotility
    B. Absent acrosome
    C. Round head
    D. Short tail

87. Sperm motility is powered by:
    A. ATP from mitochondria
    B. RNA
    C. Histones
    D. Enzymes in nucleus
88. The function of CatSper channels is:
    A. Calcium transport
    B. pH regulation
    C. DNA condensation
    D. Acrosome stability
89. Which method is gold standard for semen morphology?
    A. Papanicolaou stain
    B. Diff-Quik stain
    C. Strict Kruger criteria
    D. Giemsa stain
90. The "strict morphology" concept refers to:
    A. Normal forms ≥4%
    B. Normal forms ≥10%
    C. Normal forms ≥20%
    D. Normal forms ≥30%
91. Which sperm abnormality indicates high risk of aneuploidy?
    A. Tapered head
    B. Macrocephalic sperm
    C. Round head
    D. Pinhead
92. Sperm DNA fragmentation index (DFI) is abnormal if above:
    A. 10%
    B. 20%
    C. 25%
    D. 30%
93. Which test detects sperm apoptosis?
    A. Annexin V staining
    B. Eosin-nigrosin
    C. CASA
    D. Acrosome staining
94. Which is NOT an advanced sperm function test?
    A. DNA fragmentation
    B. ROS assay
    C. CASA
    D. Karyotyping
95. Which is the first step in spermatogenesis?
    A. Spermiation
    B. Spermatogonial mitosis
    C. Meiosis
    D. Spermiogenesis

96. Spermiogenesis refers to:
    A. Mitotic division
    B. Meiotic division
    C. Transformation of spermatids into spermatozoa
    D. Release of sperm into tubule lumen
97. The Sertoli cells support spermatogenesis by producing:
    A. FSH
    B. Inhibin B
    C. LH
    D. Testosterone
98. The Leydig cells produce:
    A. Estrogen
    B. Progesterone
    C. Testosterone
    D. Inhibin
99. Which hormone directly stimulates spermatogenesis?
    A. LH
    B. FSH
    C. Prolactin
    D. GnRH
100. Which of the following is a sperm membrane lipid important in capacitation?
    A. Cholesterol
    B. Phosphatidylcholine
    C. Phosphatidylserine
    D. Sphingomyelin

✅ Key Takeaways

- The **sperm head** contains the nucleus and acrosome essential for oocyte penetration.
- The **midpiece** houses mitochondria powering motility.
- The **tail** enables forward movement via flagellar beating.
- Structural defects (e.g., globozoospermia, midpiece defects) reduce fertility potential.
- Electron microscopy and strict Kruger morphology aid in detailed assessment.

✅ Answer Key (1–100)

1. A
2. C
3. B
4. E
5. C

6. D
7. B
8. A
9. B
10. C
11. D
12. C
13. D
14. E
15. A
16. D
17. E
18. C
19. D
20. D
21. B
22. D
23. C
24. D
25. C
26. A
27. A
28. B
29. C
30. E
31. C
32. B
33. C
34. D
35. D
36. B
37. D
38. B
39. D
40. C
41. A
42. B
43. C
44. D
45. D
46. B
47. D
48. D
49. B
50. A

51. C
52. A
53. D
54. B
55. B
56. D
57. C
58. B
59. C
60. C
61. E
62. D
63. B
64. C
65. A
66. E
67. A
68. D
69. B
70. C
71. C
72. C
73. D
74. A
75. C
76. D
77. B
78. C
79. D
80. B
81. D
82. C
83. A
84. A
85. B
86. A
87. A
88. A
89. C
90. A
91. B
92. D
93. A
94. D
95. B

96. C
97. B
98. C
99. B
100. A

Explanations (1–100)

1. Leishman stain is routinely used in semen analysis because it highlights sperm morphology, including head, midpiece, and tail defects. PAS and silver stains have other histological uses but are not standard for sperm. This makes Leishman the practical choice in andrology labs.
2. The human sperm head length is around 4–4.5 μm, allowing optimal packing of DNA and efficient motility. Smaller or larger heads are considered abnormal morphologies. This measurement is part of WHO criteria for normal sperm.
3. The sperm head length-to-width ratio averages about 1.5, balancing DNA compaction with motility. Ratios outside this may indicate teratozoospermia. Proper dimensions ensure sperm can penetrate cervical mucus and zona pellucida.
4. The sperm tail is about 45 μm long, providing the propulsion required for motility. The tail includes axonemal microtubules arranged in a 9 + 2 pattern, essential for forward movement. Tail length abnormalities impair motility.
5. The total sperm length is about 70 μm, combining a small head with a long flagellum. This streamlined size is optimized for motility and energy efficiency. Larger or smaller sperm show poor fertilizing ability.
6. Globozoospermia, or round-head syndrome, occurs due to failure of acrosome formation. Without acrosomes, sperm cannot penetrate the oocyte. It is a rare cause of male infertility.
7. The beta subunit of the sperm tail forms a V-shape, a structural aspect of dynein arms in the axoneme. These subunits generate bending movements essential for motility. Alterations can impair sperm motility.
8. Sperm mitosis occurs at the spermatogonial stage, producing new germ cells before meiosis. This ensures a constant supply of precursors for spermatogenesis. Once meiosis begins, spermatogonia no longer divide mitotically.
9. Mature sperm are stored in the distal cauda epididymis, where they are maintained until ejaculation. This site provides an optimal environment for long-term viability. Removal of the cauda leads to marked infertility.
10. Sperm can survive in the female reproductive tract, particularly the fallopian tube, for 48 hours. This window maximizes fertilization potential during ovulation. Beyond this time, viability and fertilizing ability decline sharply.
11. Basal motility is not a recognized pattern; normal sperm should show progressive forward movement. Non-progressive or circular motility indicates abnormality. Correct classification of motility is essential in semen analysis.

12. The seminal vesicles contribute most of the ejaculate volume, providing fructose for energy. Prostatic and epididymal contributions are smaller. This explains the large volume reduction seen in seminal vesicle dysfunction.
13. During epididymal transit, sperm undergo reduced membrane rigidity and gain fertilization potential. They also accumulate proteins and surface modifications that prepare them for capacitation. Without this, sperm remain immature.
14. Type A spermatogonia are true stem cells, capable of continuous self-renewal and differentiation. They ensure lifelong spermatogenesis in males. All later germ cell types are committed and not true stem cells.
15. Sperm spend most of their time maturing in the epididymis. Here they gain motility, fertilizing ability, and membrane changes. The process can take several days.
16. The midpiece contains mitochondria arranged helically around the axoneme. These produce ATP to fuel motility. Without mitochondrial energy, sperm become immotile.
17. Fertilization requires capacitation, zona binding, and acrosome reaction, not merely sexual intercourse. Capacitation occurs in the female tract and prepares sperm for penetration. This sequence is crucial for oocyte entry.
18. After ejaculation, vas deferens contents are released into the ejaculatory ducts and then urethra. They are not returned to storage organs. This allows coordinated mixing with seminal plasma.
19. A false aspect of fast-event capacitation would be decreased calcium; in fact, capacitation requires increased Ca^{2+}. Other changes include bicarbonate influx and protein phosphorylation. These enable hyperactivation.
20. Slow-event capacitation involves protein changes and cholesterol efflux rather than rapid ionic changes. These slow events remodel the sperm membrane. They are necessary for acrosome reaction competence.
21. Cholesterol leaves, not enters, the sperm membrane during capacitation. This destabilizes the plasma membrane, allowing acrosome reaction later. The false statement would be cholesterol influx.
22. Hyperactivation is not the first result of capacitation but occurs later after calcium influx. It involves vigorous motility that facilitates zona penetration. The wrong statement is considering it as the earliest event.
23. The acrosome is a lysosome-like organelle covering the anterior sperm head. It contains proteolytic enzymes for zona penetration. Without it, fertilization cannot occur.
24. Acrosin is an acrosomal protease that helps sperm digest the zona pellucida. It is not involved in hyperactivation, which is calcium-dependent motility. Confusing the two processes is common.
25. Long abstinence increases count and volume but reduces motility. WHO recommends 2–7 days abstinence before semen analysis. More than 7 days skews results.
26. The first portion of semen is mainly prostatic fluid, which is rich in enzymes like PSA. This portion is critical for sperm liquefaction. Later fractions come from seminal vesicles.

27. The Cowper's glands contribute only a small fraction of volume, producing mucus-rich secretions. These neutralize urethral acidity. Their absence barely changes total semen volume.
28. Optimal semen collection temperature is body range, about 20–40 °C. Too cold or too hot impairs motility and viability. This is why transport containers mimic body heat.
29. Erythrocytes are not a normal cellular component of semen. Their presence suggests hematospermia. Leucocytes, epithelial cells, and germ cells are commonly present.
30. Cowper's glands produce mucin, a lubricant. This secretion aids sperm passage through the urethra. Excess mucin changes semen viscosity.
31. Seminogelin is secreted by the seminal vesicles and plays a key role in initial semen coagulation after ejaculation. This coagulum is later broken down by prostate-specific antigen (PSA). Without seminogelin, semen would not form its normal gel-like consistency.
32. L-carnitine is a major product of the epididymis and serves as an important energy substrate for sperm motility. It accumulates during transit, reflecting epididymal function. Measurement of L-carnitine can serve as a marker of epididymal health.
33. Absence of coagulation in semen usually points to seminal vesicle dysfunction. Because the seminal vesicles contribute the majority of clotting proteins, any impairment prevents normal coagulation. This is seen in congenital agenesis or infection.
34. Non-liquefied semen reflects prostatic dysfunction since prostate-derived enzymes, especially PSA, are needed to dissolve the coagulum. This condition leads to infertility due to immobilized sperm. Assessment of PSA is therefore crucial in semen evaluation.
35. High semen pH (>8.0) often indicates infection in the prostate or seminal vesicles. Normal semen is slightly alkaline (7.2–8.0). This alkalinity normally helps neutralize vaginal acidity, but excessive values indicate pathology.
36. Sperm adherence or agglutination suggests an antigen–antibody reaction, typically antisperm antibodies. These antibodies coat sperm and cause them to clump, impairing motility. It is important to differentiate from nonspecific aggregation due to infection.
37. Macrocephalic sperm syndrome is a rare autosomal dominant disorder where sperm have giant heads and multiple flagella. These defects prevent normal fertilization and increase the risk of chromosomal abnormalities. Intracytoplasmic sperm injection (ICSI) often fails in such cases.
38. Decapitated sperm syndrome is a morphological abnormality where sperm appear headless under microscopy. This results from defective head-tail coupling during spermatogenesis. Such sperm are non-functional and associated with infertility.
39. Short-tail sperm syndrome is linked to mutations in genes such as DNAH1 that control axonemal structure. These mutations disrupt dynein arm function, leading to immotile sperm. Genetic counseling may be indicated in affected families.

40. The presence of CD45-positive leukocytes, stained red, indicates seminal leukocytospermia. High levels suggest genital tract infection or inflammation. Such findings require further evaluation for prostatitis or urethritis.
41. Curvilinear velocity measures the total distance a sperm head travels along its actual, often wavy, path during observation. This reflects overall activity but not efficiency. Higher curvilinear velocity does not always mean better fertilizing ability.
42. Straight-line velocity measures the distance between the first and last sperm head positions divided by time. This indicates efficiency of forward movement. High straight-line velocity correlates with better penetration ability.
43. Amplitude of lateral head displacement refers to the side-to-side movement of the sperm head during motility. It reflects hyperactivation, which is needed for zona penetration. Excessive displacement may suggest inefficient motility.
44. Linearity measures the degree to which sperm travel in a straight path relative to curvilinear motion. It indicates purposeful progression. Low linearity suggests circling or non-progressive motility.
45. The standard post-coital test is performed 9–14 hours after intercourse, when sperm should be visible in cervical mucus. Earlier or later testing gives misleading results. It is used to assess cervical factor infertility.
46. The Spinnbarkeit test assesses the elasticity of cervical mucus by stretching it between glass slides. High elasticity correlates with ovulation. This property is crucial for sperm passage through the cervix.
47. The zona-free hamster egg penetration test evaluates sperm capacitation and acrosome reaction. By bypassing the zona pellucida, it directly measures fertilizing potential. It is an important research tool though not routine clinically.
48. Leukocytes are absent from the seminiferous tubules, making their presence abnormal. Normally, they may be found in the prostate or epididymis. Leukocytospermia indicates infection or inflammation affecting fertility.
49. A positive peroxidase test indicates seminal leukocytes, mainly polymorphonuclear cells. High leukocyte counts damage sperm by producing reactive oxygen species. This test helps differentiate between infection-related and normal semen.
50. The sperm pathway involves passage from seminiferous tubules to rete testis, then efferent ducts, epididymis, vas deferens, and ejaculatory ducts. Any disruption in this pathway impairs fertility. All statements describing this sequence are correct.
51. Fructose in seminal plasma comes from the seminal vesicles and serves as the main energy source for sperm motility. Absence of fructose suggests seminal vesicle obstruction or agenesis. Testing fructose is part of routine semen analysis.
52. Zinc is secreted by the prostate gland and stabilizes chromatin and sperm membranes. High zinc levels indicate normal prostatic function. Zinc deficiency is linked to reduced fertility.
53. Alpha-glucosidase is produced by the epididymis and reflects epididymal function. Low levels suggest obstruction or dysfunction of the epididymal ducts. It is an important biochemical marker in male infertility evaluation.

54. Citric acid is a key prostatic secretion and maintains semen liquefaction. Low levels indicate prostate dysfunction. Measurement is used alongside PSA for functional assessment.
55. Seminal plasma prostaglandins, from seminal vesicles, enhance sperm motility and aid cervical mucus penetration. Altered levels impair fertilization ability. They also play roles in female reproductive tract physiology.
56. Hypo-osmotic swelling test (HOST) measures sperm membrane integrity. Sperm with intact membranes swell under hypo-osmotic conditions. This is an important test for assessing viability in low-motility samples.
57. DNA fragmentation index (DFI) measures sperm chromatin integrity. High DFI correlates with poor fertilization and higher miscarriage rates. It is increasingly used in assisted reproduction.
58. Reactive oxygen species (ROS) at low levels are needed for capacitation, but high levels damage sperm membranes and DNA. Measurement of ROS helps in unexplained infertility workup. Antioxidants may improve outcomes.
59. Sperm chromatin structure assay (SCSA) evaluates DNA denaturation under stress. It gives predictive value for fertilization outcomes in IVF/ICSI. Abnormal results suggest oxidative stress or defective spermatogenesis.
60. Mitochondrial membrane potential (MMP) testing reflects energy capacity of sperm. Low MMP correlates with asthenozoospermia. Fluorescent dyes are used in assessment.
61. Acrosome integrity testing identifies sperm capable of zona penetration. Fluorescent probes detect intact acrosomes. Abnormal integrity leads to fertilization failure despite normal counts.
62. Capacitation testing evaluates readiness of sperm to undergo acrosome reaction. Failure to capacitate means sperm cannot fertilize even if motile. Such testing is vital in assisted reproduction research.
63. Zona binding assay directly measures sperm attachment to zona pellucida. Low binding rates suggest defective receptors or surface proteins. It predicts IVF outcomes.
64. Sperm penetration assay uses zona-intact hamster eggs to assess fertilization ability. Poor penetration indicates defects in motility or acrosome function. It is less used clinically now but valuable in research.
65. Computer-assisted semen analysis (CASA) provides objective motility and morphology measurements. It reduces observer variability. CASA is increasingly used in advanced labs.
66. Sperm morphology by strict Kruger criteria is a key predictor of IVF success. Only 4% normal forms are needed for reasonable fertility. Morphology assessment is stricter than older WHO methods.
67. Teratozoospermia refers to >96% abnormal sperm morphology. It reduces natural fertility and ART success. Causes include genetic, environmental, and idiopathic factors.
68. Asthenozoospermia means reduced sperm motility (<40% progressive motility). It is a major cause of infertility. Causes include varicocele, infection, and structural tail defects.

69. Oligozoospermia refers to sperm concentration <15 million/ml. Severe oligozoospermia may require ICSI. Causes range from testicular failure to obstruction.
70. Azoospermia is absence of sperm in ejaculate after centrifugation. It may be obstructive or non-obstructive. Testicular biopsy helps distinguish the two.
71. Necrozoospermia refers to 100% dead sperm in semen. It must be differentiated from immotility due to tail defects. Vital stains confirm viability.
72. Pyospermia or leukocytospermia is >1 million leukocytes/ml. It indicates infection and causes oxidative stress damage to sperm. Antibiotic or antioxidant therapy may help.
73. Hematospermia is presence of RBCs in semen. Causes include prostatitis, stones, tumors, or trauma. It requires further evaluation if persistent.
74. Hyperspermia means ejaculate volume >6 ml. Often due to prolonged abstinence or accessory gland hyperfunction. Usually benign but may dilute sperm concentration.
75. Hypospermia means semen volume <1.5 ml. It suggests ejaculatory duct obstruction or androgen deficiency. Low volume must be confirmed with repeat analysis.
76. Aspermia is absence of semen, often due to retrograde ejaculation or ejaculatory duct obstruction. Neurological or surgical causes are common. Treatment includes retrieval from bladder or testis.
77. Sperm vitality testing is important when motility is very low. Eosin–nigrosin stain differentiates live from dead sperm. Vitality correlates with fertilization potential.
78. WHO reference values for normal semen include volume ≥1.5 ml, concentration ≥15 million/ml, progressive motility ≥32%, and morphology ≥4% normal. These cutoffs guide infertility evaluation.
79. Anti-sperm antibodies may cause immunological infertility. They agglutinate sperm and impair mucus penetration. MAR or immunobead tests detect them.
80. Varicocele is a major cause of abnormal semen. It increases scrotal temperature and ROS, damaging sperm DNA and motility. Surgical repair often improves parameters.
81. Cryptorchidism leads to impaired spermatogenesis due to high intra-abdominal temperature. Early orchidopexy improves outcomes. Untreated cases often show azoospermia.
82. Klinefelter syndrome patients often show azoospermia with small testes. Micro-TESE may retrieve sperm in some cases. Genetic counseling is important.
83. Y chromosome microdeletions, especially in AZF regions, cause spermatogenic failure. Testing is essential before ICSI since deletions are passed to male offspring.
84. Cystic fibrosis mutations cause congenital bilateral absence of vas deferens. These men have azoospermia but normal spermatogenesis. Sperm retrieval and ICSI offer fertility options.
85. Obstructive azoospermia can result from infection, trauma, or surgery. Seminal fluid shows low volume, acidic pH, and absent fructose. Reconstruction or sperm retrieval is a treatment option.

86. Non-obstructive azoospermia is due to testicular failure. Hormones show high FSH and low inhibin B. Sperm retrieval is possible in some cases with micro-TESE.
87. Endocrine causes of infertility include hypogonadotropic hypogonadism. These men benefit from gonadotropin therapy. Hormonal testing is crucial in azoospermia evaluation.
88. Ejaculatory duct obstruction presents with low-volume acidic semen and azoospermia. Transrectal ultrasound helps diagnose. Resection relieves obstruction.
89. Retrograde ejaculation results in aspermia with sperm in post-ejaculate urine. Diabetes and surgery are common causes. Alkalinizing bladder therapy may help sperm retrieval.
90. Testicular biopsy is the gold standard to differentiate obstructive from non-obstructive azoospermia. It also allows sperm retrieval. Histology guides prognosis.
91. Semen cryopreservation uses liquid nitrogen at −196 °C. Cryoprotectants such as glycerol prevent ice damage. It is used for cancer patients or ART cycles.
92. Sperm banking before chemotherapy or surgery preserves fertility. Even poor-quality samples may yield usable sperm. Counseling is essential for at-risk men.
93. Post-thaw sperm motility is often reduced compared to fresh samples. Cryoinjury affects membranes and mitochondria. Careful protocols improve recovery.
94. CASA systems can analyze frozen–thawed samples objectively. They quantify motility and kinematic parameters. This ensures accurate assessment after cryopreservation.
95. ART techniques include IUI, IVF, and ICSI. Choice depends on semen quality and female factors. ICSI revolutionized treatment of severe male infertility.
96. Intrauterine insemination (IUI) requires washed sperm with motility ≥1 million. It bypasses cervical factors. Success is modest compared to IVF.
97. IVF requires capacitated sperm to fertilize oocytes in vitro. Poor sperm function leads to low fertilization rates. IVF was the breakthrough for treating infertility.
98. ICSI injects a single sperm into the oocyte, bypassing motility and binding defects. It achieves fertilization even in severe oligozoospermia. However, genetic risks must be considered.
99. IMSI uses high-magnification sperm selection to choose morphologically normal sperm. It may improve outcomes in recurrent IVF failure. This is a refinement of ICSI.
100. PICSI uses hyaluronic acid binding to select mature sperm with intact DNA. It mimics natural selection at the cumulus–oocyte complex. This improves embryo quality and reduces miscarriage risk.

Further Reading

The explanations in this chapter are supported by the following key references:

1. World Health Organization. WHO laboratory manual for the examination and processing of human semen. 6th ed. Geneva: WHO; 2021.
2. Aitken RJ, Baker MA. Causes and consequences of oxidative stress in spermatozoa. Reprod Fertil Dev. 2004;16(4):581–8.
3. Agarwal A, Majzoub A, Esteves SC, et al. Sperm DNA fragmentation: a critical assessment. Fertil Steril. 2020;113(3):477–97.
4. Mortimer D, Barratt CLR, Björndahl L, et al. What is normal sperm morphology? Hum Reprod Update. 2015;21(5):536–46.
5. Turner RM. Moving to the beat: a review of mammalian sperm motility regulation. Reprod Fertil Dev. 2006;18(1–2):25–38.
6. Yanagimachi R. Mammalian fertilization. In: The physiology of reproduction. Academic Press; 2015.

Genetics of Male Reproduction

13

Learning Objectives

- Recognize key genetic causes of male infertility.
- Understand karyotype abnormalities such as Klinefelter syndrome.
- Interpret Yq microdeletion testing results.
- Discuss the impact of CFTR mutations on fertility.
- Apply genetic counseling principles.

Select the Single Best Answer

1. A 29-year-old man presents with infertility. Semen analysis reveals azoospermia. His physical examination shows normal secondary sexual characteristics, testicular volume of 18 mL bilaterally, and palpable vas deferens. FSH and LH are within normal range. Genetic testing reveals a microdeletion in the AZFc region of the Y chromosome. What is the most likely diagnosis?
   A. Klinefelter syndrome
   B. Sertoli-cell-only syndrome
   C. Y-chromosome microdeletion
   D. CFTR gene mutation
2. A 32-year-old man presents with infertility. Semen analysis shows oligoasthenoteratospermia. Karyotyping shows a 46,XX karyotype with SRY gene translocated onto one X chromosome. What is the most appropriate term for his condition?
   A. Klinefelter syndrome
   B. 46,XX male syndrome
   C. Mixed gonadal dysgenesis
   D. Swyer syndrome

M. S. M. Hasan, M. L. Elsaie, *Comprehensive MCQs in Andrology*, Trends in Andrology and Sexual Medicine, https://doi.org/10.1007/978-3-032-20623-7_13

3. A 35-year-old man presents with infertility. Semen analysis reveals azoospermia. On physical examination, he has small, firm testes and gynecomastia. Hormonal profile shows elevated FSH and LH, and low testosterone. Karyotyping reveals 47,XXY. What is the diagnosis?
   A. Androgen insensitivity syndrome
   B. Klinefelter syndrome
   C. Noonan syndrome
   D. Turner syndrome
4. A 25-year-old man presents for fertility evaluation. He has a history of undescended testes in childhood. Genetic testing reveals a mutation in the INSL3 gene. Which process is most likely affected?
   A. Testicular descent
   B. Spermatid maturation
   C. Epididymal transport
   D. Testosterone production
5. A 33-year-old man with primary infertility undergoes genetic screening. He is found to have a CFTR gene mutation. What condition is most commonly associated with this finding?
   A. Testicular feminization
   B. Complete androgen insensitivity
   C. Congenital bilateral absence of vas deferens
   D. Hypogonadotropic hypogonadism
6. A 28-year-old man with infertility is found to have a deletion in the SYCP3 gene. This gene is essential for which process?
   A. Sertoli cell signaling
   B. Sperm head condensation
   C. Meiotic chromosomal pairing
   D. Leydig cell differentiation
7. A 30-year-old male has severe oligozoospermia. Genetic analysis shows a mutation in the CATSPER1 gene. What aspect of sperm function is most likely impaired?
   A. DNA packaging
   B. Tail movement and motility
   C. Acrosome reaction
   D. Testicular thermoregulation
8. A 27-year-old male with infertility is found to have a homozygous deletion in the DPY19L2 gene. What sperm morphology defect is most likely present?
   A. Round-headed spermatozoa (globozoospermia)
   B. Tapered-head spermatozoa
   C. Coiled tail spermatozoa
   D. Sperm without midpiece

9. A 26-year-old man with infertility is found to have a 46,XY karyotype but mutations in the androgen receptor gene. What is the expected phenotype?
   A. Male external genitalia with infertility
   B. Ambiguous genitalia with gynecomastia
   C. Female external genitalia with blind vaginal pouch
   D. Male phenotype with normal fertility
10. A 34-year-old man with infertility is found to have multiple café-au-lait spots and axillary freckling. He has a family history of neurofibromatosis. Which gene mutation is most likely?
    A. FMR1
    B. CFTR
    C. NF1
    D. SYCP1
11. A 36-year-old man presents with infertility and a family history of early-onset tremor and ataxia. Genetic testing reveals FMR1 premutation. What is he at risk of developing?
    A. Fragile X-associated tremor/ataxia syndrome
    B. Kallmann syndrome
    C. Testicular torsion
    D. Androgen insensitivity
12. A 30-year-old male presents with infertility. He has anosmia and delayed puberty. Genetic workup reveals a mutation in the KAL1 gene. What is the diagnosis?
    A. Noonan syndrome
    B. Prader-Willi syndrome
    C. Kallmann syndrome
    D. Kartagener syndrome
13. A 40-year-old man undergoing fertility workup is found to have a Robertsonian translocation between chromosomes 13 and 14. Which of the following is the most likely consequence?
    A. Increased risk of male breast cancer
    B. Elevated FSH and LH levels
    C. Normal sperm count with high aneuploidy rate
    D. Complete absence of sperm production
14. A 31-year-old male with non-obstructive azoospermia undergoes karyotyping, which reveals a balanced reciprocal translocation between chromosomes 11 and 22. Which of the following is the most likely implication?
    A. Reduced testosterone synthesis
    B. Increased risk of testicular torsion
    C. Increased risk of chromosomally unbalanced sperm
    D. Increased FSH secretion due to Sertoli cell failure

15. The most common genetic abnormality associated with severe oligospermia and non-obstructive azoospermia is:
    A. CFTR gene mutation
    B. KAL1 gene deletion
    C. Y chromosome microdeletion
    D. XX male syndrome
16. A patient with infertility is found to have a 47,XYY karyotype. Which of the following is most accurate regarding his reproductive potential?
    A. He is always infertile due to testicular dysgenesis
    B. He has normal fertility but low libido
    C. He may have normal sperm parameters or mild abnormalities
    D. He has ambiguous genitalia and gynecomastia
17. Which of the following genes is involved in the regulation of GnRH neuron migration and is mutated in some cases of Kallmann syndrome?
    A. DAX1
    B. SRY
    C. KAL1
    D. PRM1
18. In males, the **DAZ (Deleted in Azoospermia)** gene is located on which region of the Y chromosome?
    A. AZFa
    B. AZFb
    C. AZFc
    D. SRY
19. A 36-year-old man with primary infertility is found to have a partial AZFb microdeletion. Which of the following is most likely affected?
    A. Testosterone production
    B. Germ cell proliferation and meiotic arrest
    C. Vas deferens development
    D. Sperm motility exclusively
20. A man with low sperm count is found to have a mutation in the protamine 1 gene (PRM1). This gene is crucial for:
    A. Sertoli cell development
    B. Sperm acrosome formation
    C. Sperm chromatin condensation
    D. Tail elongation
21. A 27-year-old male with infertility has a CFTR mutation but no respiratory symptoms. What is the most likely reproductive phenotype?
    A. Normal sperm parameters
    B. Primary testicular failure
    C. Congenital bilateral absence of vas deferens
    D. Kallmann syndrome

22. Which gene determines testicular differentiation by initiating the cascade for Sertoli cell development?
    A. SOX9
    B. DAX1
    C. PRM2
    D. KISS1
23. A male patient has a 46,XY karyotype and is phenotypically female. He has intra-abdominal testes and no uterus. What is the most likely diagnosis?
    A. Klinefelter syndrome
    B. Androgen insensitivity syndrome
    C. Swyer syndrome
    D. XX male syndrome
24. In which of the following conditions is the risk of testicular cancer significantly increased due to gonadal dysgenesis and Y chromosome material?
    A. 47,XYY syndrome
    B. 46,XX male syndrome
    C. Mixed gonadal dysgenesis
    D. 46,XX DSD without SRY
25. Which of the following mutations is associated with globozoospermia (round-headed sperm) and failure of acrosome formation?
    A. KAL1
    B. CATSPER1
    C. DPY19L2
    D. CFTR
26. A 33-year-old male presents with infertility and decreased libido. Genetic analysis reveals a mutation in the GnRH receptor gene. Which hormone pattern is most likely?
    A. Elevated LH and FSH
    B. Low LH and FSH
    C. Elevated testosterone
    D. Normal gonadotropins
27. A 28-year-old man has been trying to conceive with his partner for 2 years. He has normal libido and secondary sexual characteristics. Semen analysis reveals teratozoospermia with many sperm showing defective chromatin condensation. A mutation in which of the following genes is most likely responsible?
    A. KISS1
    B. SOX9
    C. PRM1
    D. SRY
28. Which of the following best describes the function of the **SRY** gene?
    A. Promotes oocyte maturation in females
    B. Suppresses Leydig cell development
    C. Encodes a transcription factor initiating testis formation
    D. Stimulates secretion of GnRH in hypothalamus

29. A male newborn presents with ambiguous genitalia. Karyotyping reveals 46,XY. Testing shows a mutation in the **SRD5A2** gene. What is the biochemical defect in this condition?
   A. Impaired testosterone synthesis
   B. Impaired DHT production
   C. Increased aromatization to estrogen
   D. GnRH deficiency
30. Which of the following conditions is characterized by 46,XX karyotype, male phenotype, and presence of the SRY gene on the X chromosome?
   A. Swyer syndrome
   B. 46,XX testicular DSD
   C. Turner syndrome
   D. Androgen insensitivity syndrome
31. A 26-year-old male with anosmia, delayed puberty, and low libido is found to have Kallmann syndrome. What embryologic structure fails to develop properly in this condition?
   A. Rathke's pouch
   B. Olfactory placode
   C. Urogenital ridge
   D. Cloacal membrane
32. What is the function of the **DAZL** gene in male fertility?
   A. Controls androgen receptor transcription
   B. Encodes a receptor for LH
   C. Plays a role in spermatogonial differentiation
   D. Maintains Sertoli–germ cell tight junctions
33. A man with suspected Klinefelter syndrome has which of the following expected hormone profiles?
   A. ↓ FSH, ↓ LH, ↓ Testosterone
   B. ↑ FSH, ↑ LH, ↓ Testosterone
   C. ↓ FSH, ↑ LH, ↑ Testosterone
   D. ↑ FSH, ↑ LH, ↑ Testosterone
34. Which of the following chromosomal abnormalities carries the **highest risk** of non-obstructive azoospermia?
   A. 47,XYY
   B. 47,XXY
   C. 46,XX
   D. Balanced Robertsonian translocation
35. A 35-year-old man with infertility is found to have a mutation in **TEX11** on the X chromosome. Which spermatogenic process is most likely impaired?
   A. Sperm motility
   B. Acrosome reaction
   C. Meiotic recombination
   D. Leydig cell steroidogenesis

36. Which gene is most commonly implicated in congenital hypogonadotropic hypogonadism with associated anosmia?
    A. FMR1
    B. KAL1
    C. SRY
    D. DAX1
37. A couple undergoes genetic counseling. The male partner has a complete AZFc microdeletion. What is the most appropriate advice regarding offspring?
    A. There is no risk of transmission
    B. Risk of transmitting Y microdeletion to male offspring
    C. All children will be infertile
    D. Recommend adoption due to risk of birth defects
38. Which of the following genes is associated with motility defects due to disruption of the flagellar structure?
    A. CFTR
    B. DPY19L2
    C. CATSPER1
    D. TEX11
39. A 30-year-old man with infertility and no vas deferens on scrotal ultrasound is found to be homozygous for the ΔF508 mutation. What other test should be done?
    A. Pituitary MRI
    B. Pulmonary function tests
    C. Chromosome microarray
    D. Testicular biopsy
40. A 33-year-old man with infertility has a mutation in the **KISS1R** gene. This gene encodes a receptor involved in:
    A. Sertoli cell differentiation
    B. Sperm motility
    C. GnRH secretion regulation
    D. Acrosome formation
41. Which of the following Y chromosome regions is **not** typically involved in spermatogenesis?
    A. AZFa
    B. AZFb
    C. AZFc
    D. PAR2
42. A 31-year-old man has infertility and a known mutation in the **NR5A1 (SF-1)** gene. What other endocrine disorder might you screen for?
    A. Congenital adrenal hyperplasia
    B. Hypothyroidism
    C. Panhypopituitarism
    D. Androgen insensitivity

43. The **FMR1 premutation** in males is associated with which late-onset neurodegenerative condition?
    A. Huntington's disease
    B. Fragile X-associated tremor/ataxia syndrome (FXTAS)
    C. Parkinson's disease
    D. Friedrich's ataxia
44. Which of the following is a hallmark finding in **mixed gonadal dysgenesis** with 45,X/46,XY mosaicism?
    A. Bilateral normal testes
    B. Ambiguous genitalia with unilateral testis
    C. Normal puberty
    D. Gynecomastia with tall stature
45. Which of the following genetic mechanisms explains **androgen insensitivity syndrome** despite a normal 46,XY karyotype?
    A. Defect in testosterone synthesis
    B. Mutation in the androgen receptor gene
    C. SRY gene duplication
    D. DAX1 overexpression
46. In which syndrome are **microdeletions of the Xp11 region** associated with hypogonadotropic hypogonadism and adrenal insufficiency?
    A. Prader-Willi syndrome
    B. Smith-Lemli-Opitz syndrome
    C. DAX1 (NR0B1) gene mutation
    D. Noonan syndrome
47. A 29-year-old male with infertility and reduced testicular volume is found to have normal FSH and LH but very low testosterone. Which gene mutation may explain this?
    A. LHCGR
    B. PRM2
    C. DPY19L2
    D. CATSPER2
48. The **most appropriate genetic test** to screen for **obstructive azoospermia** in a man with low semen volume is:
    A. Y chromosome microdeletion analysis
    B. Karyotype
    C. CFTR mutation analysis
    D. FMR1 premutation testing
49. A 34-year-old man with nonobstructive azoospermia is found to have an AZFb deletion. What is the implication for sperm retrieval?
    A. High likelihood of successful retrieval
    B. TESE (testicular sperm extraction) is strongly recommended
    C. Retrieval is unlikely; donor sperm may be considered
    D. Can be reversed with hormone therapy

50. A man with infertility is found to have a **partial duplication of the SRY gene**. What phenotype might this produce?
    A. Normal male fertility
    B. Ambiguous genitalia
    C. XX male with mild undervirilization
    D. Female phenotype with XY karyotype

✅ Key Takeaways

- **Klinefelter syndrome (47,XXY)** is a common chromosomal cause of azoospermia.
- **AZF region deletions** on Y chromosome impair spermatogenesis.
- **CFTR mutations** are linked to congenital bilateral absence of vas deferens.
- Genetic testing is vital in non-obstructive azoospermia.
- Counseling supports patient decision-making in assisted reproduction.

✅ Answer Key (1–50)

1. C
2. B
3. B
4. A
5. C
6. C
7. B
8. A
9. C
10. C
11. A
12. C
13. C
14. C
15. C
16. C
17. C
18. C
19. B
20. C
21. C
22. A
23. B
24. C
25. C

26. B
27. C
28. C
29. B
30. B
31. B
32. C
33. B
34. B
35. C
36. B
37. B
38. C
39. B
40. C
41. D
42. A
43. B
44. B
45. B
46. C
47. A
48. C
49. C
50. C

Explanations (1–50)

1. Y chromosome microdeletions, especially in the AZF regions (a, b, c), are a major genetic cause of non-obstructive azoospermia. AZFc deletions may still allow some residual spermatogenesis, making sperm retrieval possible. Clinical evaluation should include genetic counseling due to vertical transmission risk. This is a common indication for micro-TESE in infertility workup.
2. SRY gene translocation onto the X chromosome can result in 46,XX males who appear phenotypically male. These individuals often have small testes and are infertile due to absent spermatogenesis. Despite their karyotype, their phenotype is driven by SRY-dependent testis development. Genetic confirmation is crucial for diagnosis and counseling.
3. Karyotype anomalies such as 47,XXY affect testicular development, leading to seminiferous tubule dysgenesis. The hormonal profile typically shows hypergonadotropic hypogonadism with low testosterone. These patients may have gynecomastia and are at risk of infertility and psychosocial issues. Early detection may allow hormonal or fertility preservation strategies.

4. Testicular descent depends on hormonal and genetic signals, including INSL3 and its receptor. Mutations in these genes can result in cryptorchidism, a risk factor for infertility and malignancy. This defect affects the transabdominal phase of testicular descent during fetal development. Genetic evaluation is considered in persistent bilateral undescended testes.
5. CFTR gene mutations are classically associated with cystic fibrosis but can present with isolated male infertility. One of the manifestations is congenital bilateral absence of the vas deferens (CBAVD). Semen volume is typically low, and fructose is absent, mimicking obstructive azoospermia. Genetic testing is essential for both reproductive planning and family counseling.
6. Meiosis requires precise chromosomal pairing and synapsis, in which SYCP3 plays a critical role.Mutations in SYCP3 disrupt synaptonemal complex formation, leading to meiotic arrest. This results in a spermatogenic block and azoospermia.Such defects are often part of broader syndromic or isolated infertility presentations.
7. Sperm motility depends on calcium channels located in the tail, regulated by CATSPER gene products. Mutations lead to reduced or absent progressive motility, resulting in asthenozoospermia. Despite normal morphology and count, fertilization ability is impaired. This condition may benefit from assisted reproductive technologies.
8. DPY19L2 gene is essential for acrosome formation and nuclear elongation in sperm cells. Its mutation leads to globozoospermia, characterized by round-headed sperm lacking acrosomes. Fertilization is severely impaired due to inability to penetrate the oocyte. ICSI with assisted oocyte activation may be required for fertility.
9. Androgen receptor mutations result in variable degrees of androgen insensitivity despite normal male karyotype. In complete forms, external genitalia appear female, but testes are present and undescended. Spermatogenesis fails due to unresponsive Sertoli and Leydig cells. Diagnosis often occurs during workup for primary amenorrhea or infertility.
10. Neurofibromatosis type 1 is a multisystem genetic disorder involving neural crest-derived tissues. While its main manifestations are cutaneous and neurologic, reproductive effects may occur. NF1 gene mutation may alter germ cell development or endocrine function. Family history is key to diagnosis, and fertility counseling is important.
11. Fragile X-associated disorders span from full mutations causing intellectual disability to premutations. In male premutation carriers, late-onset tremor/ataxia syndrome (FXTAS) may develop. These individuals may also present with infertility or mild cognitive changes. This highlights the overlap between neurogenetic and reproductive disorders.
12. Kallmann syndrome results from failed migration of GnRH neurons from the olfactory placode. This leads to hypogonadotropic hypogonadism and anosmia. Puberty is delayed or absent, and infertility is a common concern. Diagnosis may involve genetic testing and MRI to assess olfactory structures.

13. Robertsonian translocations are structural chromosomal rearrangements involving acrocentric chromosomes. Although carriers are usually phenotypically normal, gametogenesis may be impaired. They carry an increased risk of unbalanced gametes and early pregnancy loss. Preimplantation genetic testing may be considered in such cases.
14. Balanced chromosomal translocations can disrupt meiosis despite maintaining the full genetic complement. Carriers are often phenotypically normal but may have abnormal sperm chromosomal content. Fertilization may occur, but with increased risk of miscarriage or congenital anomalies. Genetic counseling and preimplantation diagnosis are often recommended.
15. Microdeletions in the azoospermia factor (AZF) regions on the Y chromosome are a key cause of spermatogenic failure. They are more common in non-obstructive azoospermia and severe oligospermia. Detection has important prognostic and reproductive implications. Routine screening is part of the genetic workup in male infertility.
16. The 47,XYY karyotype often presents with normal male phenotype and may go undiagnosed. Most individuals have normal testosterone and secondary sexual development. Sperm abnormalities, if present, are usually mild and variable. Unlike other aneuploidies, fertility may be preserved.
17. Kallmann syndrome is linked to genes regulating GnRH neuron migration, such as KAL1. These genes affect both olfactory development and hypothalamic-pituitary function. Disruption leads to hypogonadotropic hypogonadism and anosmia. It is one of the few forms of genetic hypogonadism with treatable fertility potential.
18. The DAZ (Deleted in Azoospermia) gene is crucial for spermatogenesis and is located on the Y chromosome. It is specifically mapped to the AZFc region, deletions of which impair sperm production. These deletions vary in clinical severity, from oligospermia to azoospermia. Diagnosis allows informed decisions about assisted reproduction.
19. AZFb region deletions affect spermatogonial proliferation and meiosis. This often results in a more severe phenotype than AZFc deletions. Histology commonly shows maturation arrest at primary spermatocyte stage. Sperm retrieval in these cases has low success rates.
20. Protamine genes (PRM1, PRM2) are involved in sperm DNA packaging during spermiogenesis. Their proper expression ensures chromatin condensation and genomic stability. Mutations may lead to sperm DNA fragmentation and abnormal morphology. These are often detected in men with idiopathic infertility.
21. CFTR gene mutations are commonly associated with cystic fibrosis, but also affect male reproductive ducts. In males, congenital bilateral absence of vas deferens (CBAVD) can occur as an isolated finding. Semen is low in volume and lacks vasal secretions. CFTR analysis is essential in diagnosing non-cystic fibrosis–related obstructive azoospermia.
22. Testicular development is initiated by SRY, but SOX9 is the direct effector of Sertoli cell differentiation. It promotes testis cord formation and inhibits

ovarian pathways. Mutations lead to gonadal dysgenesis and sex reversal in 46,XY individuals. Its role is fundamental in sex determination cascades.

23. In complete androgen insensitivity, individuals have a male karyotype but appear phenotypically female. Due to defective androgen receptor signaling, internal male structures do not develop. Testes are often intra-abdominal and prone to malignancy. Diagnosis is typically made during investigation for amenorrhea.
24. Mixed gonadal dysgenesis involves mosaic karyotypes and streak or dysgenetic gonads. Y chromosome material in such patients increases the risk of gonadoblastoma. Genital ambiguity is a common presentation at birth. Prophylactic gonadectomy may be advised to prevent malignancy.
25. Globozoospermia is a rare disorder characterized by round-headed sperm lacking acrosomes. It results from failure of Golgi-derived vesicle fusion during spermiogenesis. The condition is genetically heterogeneous, with DPY19L2 being a common gene involved. It severely impairs fertilization, even with ICSI.
26. GnRH receptor mutations disrupt hypothalamic–pituitary signaling, leading to low gonadotropins. This manifests as hypogonadotropic hypogonadism, with delayed puberty and infertility. Unlike central defects, the pituitary and gonads may be structurally intact. Hormone replacement can induce spermatogenesis in some cases.
27. Abnormal sperm chromatin condensation is a major contributor to male infertility. This process is regulated by specific nuclear proteins during spermiogenesis. Mutations affecting chromatin packaging lead to DNA damage and impaired fertilization. Such defects are often detected in cases of teratozoospermia or recurrent IVF failure.
28. Sex determination in the embryo depends on the presence of key transcription factors. One such factor initiates testis development by upregulating Sertoli cell genes. Its action is time-sensitive and crucial for male gonadal differentiation. Defects can lead to sex reversal syndromes or gonadal dysgenesis.
29. Some enzymes are required to convert testosterone into its more potent form during fetal life. Deficiency in this conversion pathway leads to undervirilization of external genitalia. Despite normal or elevated testosterone, target tissues may not develop properly. Diagnosis often involves hormonal assays and molecular testing.
30. In rare cases, chromosomal sex does not match phenotypic sex due to gene translocations. When the testis-determining gene is misplaced onto another chromosome, sex reversal can occur. These individuals may have male features despite lacking a Y chromosome. Infertility is typically the presenting complaint in adulthood.
31. Some developmental disorders of puberty are linked to olfactory and hypothalamic structures. Disruption in embryological migration of specific neurons can impair sexual maturation. Anosmia is a helpful diagnostic clue in such conditions. Treatment involves hormone replacement and fertility induction.
32. Certain RNA-binding proteins are essential for the early stages of spermatogenesis. They regulate the differentiation of germ cells into mature spermatogonia.

Loss of function mutations disrupt this process and can lead to azoospermia. This mechanism highlights the complex regulation of male germ cell development.

33. Specific chromosomal abnormalities can cause testicular atrophy and endocrine imbalance. The resulting hormonal profile shows feedback-driven elevation of gonadotropins. Patients may present with tall stature, gynecomastia, or infertility. Diagnosis is typically confirmed via karyotyping and hormone panels.
34. Not all chromosomal aneuploidies affect fertility equally. Some sex chromosome disorders result in profound spermatogenic failure. These may be associated with characteristic physical features and endocrine changes. Identifying the correct abnormality is crucial for prognosis and counseling.
35. Meiotic processes in spermatogenesis rely on specific genes for chromosomal crossover and repair. Disruption of these genes can lead to complete arrest during meiosis. This results in non-obstructive azoospermia and absent sperm in testicular tissue. Some of these defects are X-linked and affect only males.
36. Genetic forms of delayed puberty often involve mutations in genes controlling GnRH secretion. These mutations can also affect olfaction due to their dual embryologic origins. Such cases may be sporadic or familial, and may present with incomplete puberty. MRI and genetic testing help in diagnosis.
37. Y chromosome deletions can be passed from father to son during assisted reproduction. Even if fertility is achieved through ICSI, male offspring may inherit the same defect. This poses ethical and counseling implications for reproductive planning. Genetic documentation should accompany fertility treatment in these cases.
38. Sperm motility depends on ion channels and structural integrity of the flagellum. Genetic mutations affecting tail calcium channels can impair motility without affecting count. These mutations are often autosomal recessive and linked to asthenozoospermia. Functional testing and electron microscopy may aid in diagnosis.
39. Some cases of male infertility are associated with ductal anomalies linked to genetic mutations. When congenital absence of the vas deferens is identified, it often warrants broader evaluation. The mutation involved may affect other organs, including the lungs. Confirming the diagnosis has implications for both treatment and partner screening.
40. Certain G-protein-coupled receptors are critical in regulating the onset of puberty and GnRH secretion. Mutations in these receptors can result in delayed sexual maturation and infertility. The kisspeptin signaling pathway plays a central role in reproductive neuroendocrinology. Defects in this pathway can mimic hypogonadotropic hypogonadism.
41. The Y chromosome contains regions vital for spermatogenesis, primarily AZFa, AZFb, and AZFc. Other segments like pseudoautosomal regions do not directly influence sperm production. Understanding regional gene function helps guide genetic testing in azoospermia. Not all deletions on the Y chromosome have equal impact on fertility.

42. Some transcription factors regulate both adrenal and gonadal development during embryogenesis. Mutations in these factors can lead to combined endocrine defects affecting puberty and fertility. Affected individuals may present with adrenal insufficiency, gonadal failure, or both. Recognition of such syndromes is critical for multidisciplinary management.
43. Certain neurodegenerative disorders are linked to premutation alleles in fragile X-related genes. These conditions typically present later in life with movement disorders and cognitive decline. Males may pass the gene to daughters who are at risk of full mutation expansion. This highlights the intersection of reproductive genetics and neurology.
44. Mosaicism involving sex chromosomes can result in ambiguous genitalia and asymmetric gonads. One gonad may be a streak or dysgenetic, while the other may resemble a testis. The presence of Y chromosome material increases malignancy risk. Such individuals often require early endocrine, surgical, and genetic interventions.
45. Disorders of sexual development can occur when peripheral androgen action is impaired despite normal hormone levels. This is typically due to mutations in hormone receptor genes rather than hormone synthesis defects. Affected individuals may show complete or partial undervirilization depending on mutation severity. Phenotypic sex may differ significantly from genetic sex.
46. Some X-linked syndromes affect both adrenal function and gonadotropin signaling pathways. Mutations in nuclear receptor genes can lead to adrenal hypoplasia and pubertal failure. Boys may present with salt-wasting crises or delayed puberty. Early diagnosis allows hormone replacement and fertility preservation strategies.
47. Leydig cell function relies on luteinizing hormone binding to its specific receptor. Mutations in this receptor can lead to low testosterone despite normal or elevated LH. Patients may present with infertility, undervirilization, or delayed puberty. This represents a form of selective testicular resistance.
48. Obstructive azoospermia with low semen volume suggests ejaculatory duct or vas deferens abnormality. In such cases, mutations in chloride channel genes are a common underlying cause. Genetic testing is essential for both diagnosis and partner reproductive risk. This condition may be part of a broader syndromic or isolated presentation.
49. Certain deletions in the Y chromosome severely impair spermatogenesis at the meiotic stage. This precludes the possibility of sperm retrieval, even via surgical methods. Such deletions carry a poor prognosis for biological paternity. Genetic counseling should include discussion of donor sperm or adoption.
50. Variations in gene dosage can alter sex development even in individuals with typical chromosomal sex. Partial duplications of testis-determining genes may cause incomplete masculinization. These cases often present with infertility or mild ambiguous genitalia. Diagnosis relies on molecular analysis and careful phenotypic assessment.

Further Reading

The explanations in this chapter are supported by the following key references:

1. Krausz C, Riera-Escamilla A. Genetics of male infertility. Nat Rev Urol. 2018;15(6):369–84.
2. Tüttelmann F, Ruckert C, Röpke A. Disorders of spermatogenesis: perspectives for novel genetic diagnostics. Nat Rev Genet. 2018;19(10):589–601.
3. World Health Organization. WHO manual for the standardized investigation, diagnosis and management of the infertile male. Cambridge: Cambridge University Press; 2000.
4. O'Flynn O'Brien KL, Varghese AC, Agarwal A. The genetic causes of male factor infertility. Fertil Steril. 2010;93(1):1–12.
5. Vogt PH. AZF deletions and spermatogenic failure. Hum Reprod Update. 2005;11(4):321–36.
6. Ferlin A, Arredi B, Foresta C. Genetic causes of male infertility. Reprod Toxicol. 2006;22(2):133–41.

Androgens and Anabolic Steroids

14

Learning Objectives

- Understand androgen biosynthesis and regulation.
- Identify clinical uses of testosterone therapy.
- Recognize patterns of anabolic steroid abuse.
- Discuss adverse effects on fertility, cardiovascular, and hepatic systems.
- Evaluate patient candidacy for hormonal therapy.

Select the Single Best Answer

1. Androgens are:
   A. C15 steroids
   B. C16 steroid
   C. C17 steroid
   D. C18 steroid
   E. C19 steroid
2. Estrogens are:
   A. C15 steroids
   B. C16 steroid
   C. C17 steroid
   D. C18 steroid
   E. C19 steroid
3. Cycling method of anabolic steroids intake means:
   A. Gradually increase the dose
   B. Multiple types combination of anabolic steroids
   C. On and off therapy
   D. Intramuscular injection alternating with oral intake
   E. Oral-only maintenance

M. S. M. Hasan, M. L. Elsaie, *Comprehensive MCQs in Andrology*, Trends in Andrology and Sexual Medicine, https://doi.org/10.1007/978-3-032-20623-7_14

4. Stacking method of anabolic steroids intake means:
   A. Gradually increase the dose
   B. Multiple types combination of anabolic steroids
   C. On and off therapy
   D. Intramuscular injection alternating with oral intake
   E. Alternate with anti-estrogens
5. Pyramiding method of anabolic steroids intake means:
   A. Gradually increase the dose
   B. Multiple types combination of anabolic steroids
   C. On and off therapy
   D. Intramuscular injection alternating with oral intake
   E. Decrease dose gradually
6. Cutting anabolic steroids is used for:
   A. Building muscles
   B. Muscle strength
   C. Burning fat
   D. Metabolism enhancement
   E. Healing and recovery
7. Performance anabolic steroid is used for:
   A. Building muscles
   B. Muscle strength
   C. Burning fat
   D. Metabolism enhancement
   E. Healing and recovery
8. Bulking anabolic steroid is used for:
   A. Building muscles
   B. Muscle strength
   C. Burning fat
   D. Metabolism enhancement
   E. Healing and recovery
9. The starting point for androgen synthesis is:
   A. Androstenedione
   B. 17 hydroxy pregnenolone
   C. Pregnenolone
   D. Cholesterol
   E. Cortisol
10. The daily testicular production of testosterone is:
    A. 5–7 mg/day
    B. 10–12 mg/day
    C. 15–20 mg/day
    D. 20–25 mg/day
    E. 50 mg/day

11. Which of the following transports cholesterol across the mitochondrial membrane during androgen synthesis?
    A. Protein kinase A
    B. Protein kinase G
    C. Steroidogenic acute regulatory protein
    D. P450 side chain cleavage
    E. cAMP
12. Which of the following initiates androgen production?
    A. Protein kinase A
    B. Protein kinase G
    C. Steroidogenic acute regulatory protein
    D. P450 side chain cleavage
    E. cAMP
13. Plasma testosterone half-life is:
    A. Few seconds
    B. 5 minutes
    C. 12 minutes
    D. 20 minutes
    E. 25 minutes
14. Free fraction of testosterone percentage is:
    A. 1–2%
    B. 5–7%
    C. 10%
    D. 10–15%
    E. 17%
15. Which of the following is NOT associated with increased sex hormone–binding globulin (SHBG)?
    A. Growth hormone deficiency
    B. Aging
    C. HIV
    D. Hepatic diseases
    E. Insulin resistance
16. Which of the following is associated with decreased SHBG?
    A. Growth hormone deficiency
    B. Aging
    C. HIV
    D. Hepatic diseases
    E. Insulin resistance
17. The androgen receptor gene is located on:
    A. Y chromosome Xq11
    B. X chromosome Xq12
    C. Y chromosome Xq15
    D. X chromosome Xq16
    E. Chromosome 21

18. Which of the following affects androgen receptor transcription activity?
    A. Type I coregulators
    B. Type II coregulators
    C. Type III coregulators
    D. A + C
    E. B + C
19. The level at which no testosterone therapy is required:
    A. <3 nmol/l
    B. 3–5 nmol/l
    C. 5–12 nmol/l
    D. >12 nmol/l
    E. >20 nmol/l
20. The normal male estrone plasma level is:
    A. 2 ng/dl
    B. 2.5 ng/dl
    C. 3.5 ng/dl
    D. 4.5 ng/dl
    E. 6 ng/dl
21. The normal male estradiol plasma level is:
    A. 2 ng/dl
    B. 2.5 ng/dl
    C. 3.5 ng/dl
    D. 4.5 ng/dl
    E. 6 ng/dl
22. Which of the following is NOT an effect of estrogen therapy in males?
    A. Hypertension
    B. Decreased muscle strength
    C. Testicular atrophy
    D. Redistribution of body fat
    E. Hypoprolactinemia
23. The testes produce about … of estradiol:
    A. 3 μg
    B. 5 μg
    C. 7 μg
    D. 10 μg
    E. 20 μg
24. Which of the following is NOT a role of estrogen in males?
    A. Bone maturation
    B. Negative feedback inhibition on hypothalamus
    C. Sperm maturation
    D. Inhibit gonadotrophin secretion
    E. Increase ejaculatory volume

25. Initial improvement after testosterone replacement occurs within:
    A. 2 weeks
    B. 4 weeks
    C. 8 weeks
    D. 12 weeks
    E. 6 months
26. Which of the following is NOT an indication of androgen therapy?
    A. Micropenis
    B. Induction of puberty
    C. Aplastic anemia
    D. Osteoporosis
    E. Cholestatic jaundice
27. Which of the following is a risk factor for prostate cancer?
    A. PSA 0.5 ng/ml
    B. PSA 1 ng/ml
    C. PSA 1.5 ng/ml
    D. PSA 2 ng/ml
    E. PSA 2.5 ng/ml
28. Absolute contraindication for testosterone therapy if hematocrit is:
    A. <5%
    B. 5–20%
    C. 20–40%
    D. >50%
    E. >60%
29. Relative contraindication for testosterone therapy if IPSS score is:
    A. <5
    B. 5–10
    C. 10–15
    D. 15–20
    E. >20
30. Which of the following is NOT a side effect of androgen therapy?
    A. Cholestatic jaundice
    B. Anemia
    C. Acne vulgaris
    D. Decrease cardiac contractility
    E. Thrombosis
31. Which testosterone preparation shows NO fluctuation?
    A. Testosterone cypionate
    B. Testosterone enanthate
    C. Testosterone undecanoate
    D. Buccal testosterone
    E. Transdermal patch

32. Which of the following is a GnRH analogue?
    A. Flutamide
    B. Nilutamide
    C. Finasteride
    D. Leuprolide
    E. Dutasteride
33. Which of the following is a progestin analogue?
    A. Flutamide
    B. Nilutamide
    C. Finasteride
    D. Leuprolide
    E. Cyproterone acetate
34. Green tea is anti-androgenic because it contains:
    A. Paeoniflorin compound
    B. Phytoestrogens compound
    C. Epigallocatechin compound
    D. Phytosterol compound
    E. Isoflavones
35. White peony is anti-androgenic because it contains:
    A. Paeoniflorin compound
    B. Phytoestrogens compound
    C. Epigallocatechin compound
    D. Phytosterol compound
    E. Lignans
36. Saw palmetto is anti-androgenic because it contains:
    A. Paeoniflorin compound
    B. Phytoestrogens compound
    C. Epigallocatechin compound
    D. Phytosterol compound
    E. Isoflavones
37. Licorice is anti-androgenic because it contains:
    A. Paeoniflorin compound
    B. Phytoestrogens compound
    C. Epigallocatechin compound
    D. Phytosterol compound
    E. Tannins
38. Low dose of the chaste tree can block:
    A. Dopamine receptor D1
    B. Dopamine receptor D2
    C. Serotonin receptor
    D. 5HT1AC receptors
    E. 5HT1AA receptors

39. Which of the following is NOT a typical manifestation of testosterone deficiency in adult males?:
    A. Reduced testicular volume
    B. Decreased libido
    C. Gynecomastia
    D. Decreased ejaculatory volume
    E. Decreased muscle mass
40. Which of the following is NOT associated with transient alteration of testosterone level?
    A. Afternoon sampling
    B. Prolonged fasting
    C. Acute alcohol intake
    D. Acute illness
    E. Diabetes mellitus
41. Which of the following is associated with chronic alteration of testosterone level?
    A. Afternoon sampling
    B. Prolonged fasting
    C. Acute alcohol intake
    D. Acute illness
    E. Diabetes mellitus
42. Androgen insensitivity syndrome is:
    A. Autosomal dominant
    B. Autosomal recessive
    C. X-linked recessive
    D. X-linked dominant
    E. Multifactorial
43. Reifenstein syndrome is:
    A. Complete androgen insensitivity syndrome
    B. Mild androgen insensitivity syndrome
    C. Partial androgen insensitivity syndrome
    D. Quigley scale 5
    E. Turner-like variant
44. Testicular feminization syndrome is:
    A. Complete androgen insensitivity syndrome
    B. Mild androgen insensitivity syndrome
    C. Partial androgen insensitivity syndrome
    D. Quigley scale 5
    E. Mosaicism
45. Congenital adrenal hyperplasia is:
    A. Autosomal dominant
    B. Autosomal recessive
    C. X-linked recessive
    D. X-linked dominant
    E. Multifactorial

46. Most common deficient enzyme in congenital adrenal hyperplasia is:
    A. 5-hydroxylase enzyme
    B. 21-hydroxylase enzyme
    C. 17β-reductase enzyme
    D. 17α-hydroxylase
    E. 11β-hydroxylase
47. Which of the following hormones is NOT involved in congenital adrenal hyperplasia?
    A. Prolactin
    B. Cortisol
    C. Aldosterone
    D. Testosterone
    E. 17-OHP
48. A 25-year-old bodybuilder uses injectable anabolic steroids. His fertility potential would be:
    A. Normal—exogenous testosterone does not impair endogenous production
    B. Low—exogenous testosterone stimulates pituitary FSH/LH
    C. Low—exogenous testosterone inhibits pituitary FSH/LH
    D. Low—exogenous testosterone is less potent than endogenous
    E. Normal—intratesticular testosterone is always sufficient
49. Which statement about testosterone is most accurate?
    A. Produced by the exocrine testis
    B. Circulates mainly free/unbound
    C. Regulated by FSH
    D. Stimulated by prolactin
    E. Metabolized partly to DHT
50. Testosterone peaks occur during:
    A. 1st-trimester gestation, 2 months, puberty
    B. 1 year, puberty, 50 years
    C. Puberty, 30 years, 70 years
    D. Puberty, 50 years
    E. Gestation, puberty, old age
51. Free testosterone levels measured by equilibrium dialysis have coefficient variability of:
    A. 7%
    B. 15%
    C. 30%
    D. 45%
    E. >50%
52. Testosterone in women is produced in:
    A. Ovaries
    B. Adrenal glands
    C. Peripheral conversion of precursors
    D. A + B
    E. A + B + C

53. The PDE5 gene is under the control of:
    A. Estrogens
    B. Prolactin
    C. DHT
    D. Testosterone
    E. Cortisol
54. A 45-year-old male with TT 125 ng/dl, normal LH/FSH, high prolactin, no steroid use—next best step:
    A. Start testosterone therapy
    B. Obtain brain MRI
    C. Accuse of steroid use
    D. Start anti-estrogen
    E. None of the above
55. How should total testosterone be measured?
    A. Direct RIA
    B. Direct ELISA
    C. LC–MS/MS
    D. RIA after extraction/chromatography
    E. None of the above
56. Testosterone replacement therapy:
    A. Improves body composition
    B. Reduces fracture risk
    C. Increases life expectancy
    D. Reduces muscle strength
    E. None of the above
57. A possible beneficial effect of DHEA is:
    A. Prevention of atherosclerosis
    B. Enhancing endothelial NO synthase
    C. Positive effect on lipids
    D. All of the above
    E. None
58. Transdermal TRT in physiologic doses results in:
    A. Severe hirsutism
    B. Virilization
    C. Decrease insulin sensitivity
    D. Atherogenic lipid profile
    E. None
59. Total and free testosterone drop by ___ after hysterectomy + oophorectomy:
    A. 5%
    B. 20%
    C. 50%
    D. 100%
    E. Not at all

60. Which measurement of free testosterone is reliable in women?
    A. Direct RIA
    B. Mass action calculation
    C. Equilibrium dialysis
    D. Free androgen index
    E. All except A
61. Which statement about androgens and aging is correct?
    A. Decrease across female lifespan
    B. Increase across female lifespan
    C. Remain unchanged
    D. TT decreases, free T increases
    E. None
62. TRT for sexual dysfunction in postmenopausal women is:
    A. Ineffective with virilizing SE
    B. Effective but virilizing
    C. Effective with mild SE
    D. Only effective at supra doses
    E. None
63. Androgens:
    A. Inhibit breast cancer lines in vitro
    B. Inhibit breast cancer in animals
    C. PCOS androgens not linked to cancer
    D. Used in metastatic breast cancer
    E. All of the above
64. Most abundant sex steroid in both sexes is:
    A. DHEA
    B. Androstenedione
    C. Estradiol
    D. Testosterone
    E. Estrone
65. Which statement about DHEAS is accurate?
    A. Longer half-life than DHEA
    B. Stable throughout the day
    C. Stable in menstrual cycle
    D. DHEA rapidly converted to DHEAS
    E. All of the above
66. Initial identification of DHEA receptor was in:
    A. Lung
    B. Liver
    C. Vascular endothelium
    D. Adrenal
    E. Uterus

67. Functions improved by DHEA include:
    A. Increased NO synthase
    B. Reduced glucose toxicity
    C. Improved immunity
    D. Lower mortality from endotoxins
    E. All of the above
68. Testosterone therapy in hypogonadal ED patients:
    A. Improves PDE5i response
    B. Contraindicated with PDE5i
    C. Not useful
    D. Useful only in diabetes
    E. None
69. Testosterone alkylation at 17-α position:
    A. Prevents breakdown but hepatotoxic
    B. Prevents breakdown with no SE
    C. Allows parenteral route
    D. Allows transdermal route
    E. Enhances aromatization
70. TRT is associated with:
    A. No evidence of ↑ prostate cancer risk
    B. ↑ risk of prostate cancer
    C. ↓ risk of prostate cancer
    D. ↑ risk of BPH
    E. Contraindication in all elderly
71. Normal intratesticular testosterone levels are about:
    A. 10× serum levels
    B. 20× serum levels
    C. 50× serum levels
    D. 100× serum levels
    E. Equal to serum
72. Which androgen metabolite is most potent at receptor binding?
    A. Estradiol
    B. Androstenedione
    C. DHT
    D. 17-OHP
    E. DHEA
73. Primary stimulus for GnRH secretion is:
    A. Estradiol negative feedback
    B. Hypothalamic kisspeptin
    C. Sertoli cell inhibin
    D. Leydig cell testosterone
    E. Dopamine

74. Which organ is NOT a target for androgen action?
    A. Muscle
    B. Bone
    C. Brain
    D. Pancreas
    E. Skin
75. The main clinical marker for adequate TRT response is:
    A. Serum PSA rise
    B. Hematocrit rise
    C. Symptomatic improvement
    D. Increase LH/FSH
    E. Increase prolactin
76. Which testosterone ester has longest half-life?
    A. Propionate
    B. Enanthate
    C. Cypionate
    D. Undecanoate
    E. Acetate
77. Oral testosterone undecanoate is absorbed via:
    A. Gastric veins
    B. Lymphatic system
    C. Hepatic portal
    D. Pancreatic ducts
    E. Rectal veins
78. Which is NOT a route of testosterone therapy?
    A. Transdermal
    B. Intranasal
    C. Sublingual
    D. Intrathecal
    E. Buccal
79. Which anabolic steroid effect is irreversible in women?
    A. Acne
    B. Hirsutism
    C. Voice deepening
    D. Weight gain
    E. Increased libido
80. Which lab test is essential before starting TRT?
    A. PSA
    B. Hematocrit
    C. LFTs
    D. All of the above
    E. None

81. Which is NOT a feature of anabolic steroid abuse?
    A. Gynecomastia
    B. Infertility
    C. Increased HDL
    D. Acne
    E. Testicular atrophy
82. Which organ suffers most from 17-α alkylated steroids?
    A. Heart
    B. Kidney
    C. Liver
    D. Brain
    E. Testes
83. Aromatase inhibitors with TRT may prevent:
    A. Gynecomastia
    B. Osteoporosis
    C. Acne
    D. Virilization
    E. Polycythemia
84. Which marker indicates polycythemia with TRT?
    A. Hematocrit >50%
    B. Hb >18 g/dl
    C. RBC >6 million/μl
    D. Any of the above
    E. None
85. Which is NOT a psychological effect of anabolic steroid abuse?
    A. Aggression
    B. Depression
    C. Mania
    D. Reduced libido
    E. Euphoria
86. Inhibin B is secreted from:
    A. Leydig cells
    B. Sertoli cells
    C. Germ cells
    D. Hypothalamus
    E. Adrenals
87. Which pituitary hormone directly regulates Leydig cells?
    A. LH
    B. FSH
    C. Prolactin
    D. TSH
    E. ACTH

88. Which pituitary hormone directly regulates Sertoli cells?
    A. LH
    B. FSH
    C. Prolactin
    D. TSH
    E. GH
89. Major androgen produced by adrenal cortex is:
    A. Testosterone
    B. DHT
    C. DHEA
    D. Estrone
    E. Estradiol
90. Which is NOT an anabolic steroid benefit?
    A. Muscle mass
    B. Strength
    C. Cardiac hypertrophy
    D. Bone density
    E. Endurance
91. Which androgen effect is essential in puberty?
    A. Voice change
    B. Testicular descent
    C. Facial hair
    D. Growth spurt
    E. All of the above
92. Which androgen deficiency sign is earliest in adults?
    A. Decreased libido
    B. Loss of body hair
    C. Gynecomastia
    D. Muscle atrophy
    E. Hot flashes
93. Which is a safe long-term TRT monitoring marker?
    A. Lipid profile
    B. Bone density
    C. Hematocrit
    D. PSA
    E. All of the above
94. Which steroid precursor is immediate for testosterone?
    A. Cholesterol
    B. Pregnenolone
    C. Androstenedione
    D. DHEA
    E. Cortisol

95. Which form of testosterone has highest risk of hepatotoxicity?
    A. Oral methyltestosterone
    B. IM enanthate
    C. IM undecanoate
    D. Transdermal patch
    E. Buccal
96. Which condition is most responsive to TRT?
    A. Psychogenic ED
    B. Late-onset hypogonadism
    C. Hyperprolactinemia
    D. Infertility
    E. Diabetes
97. Which androgen receptor domain binds DNA?
    A. N-terminal
    B. DNA-binding domain
    C. Ligand-binding domain
    D. Hinge region
    E. Activation domain
98. Which is NOT a feature of complete androgen insensitivity?
    A. 46, XY karyotype
    B. Female external phenotype
    C. Absent uterus
    D. Normal spermatogenesis
    E. Testes present
99. Which is true of partial androgen insensitivity?
    A. Phenotype ranges from ambiguous genitalia to undervirilized male
    B. Always female external genitalia
    C. No androgen receptor function
    D. Inherited autosomal dominant
    E. Associated with high risk of ovarian tumors
100. Which lifestyle factor is most strongly linked with lower testosterone?
    A. Cigarette smoking
    B. Alcohol abuse
    C. Obesity
    D. Stress
    E. High-protein diet

✅ Key Takeaways

- Androgens play key roles in **puberty, muscle mass, libido, and spermatogenesis**.
- Anabolic steroid misuse causes **testicular atrophy**, **infertility**, and mood changes.

- Monitoring includes **hematocrit, lipid profile, and PSA**.
- Restoration of axis after abuse may require medical intervention.
- Education is essential to mitigate misuse, especially in athletes.

✅ Answer Key (1–100)

1. E
2. D
3. C
4. B
5. A
6. C
7. B
8. A
9. D
10. A
11. C
12. A
13. C
14. A
15. E
16. E
17. B
18. A
19. D
20. D
21. B
22. E
23. D
24. E
25. D
26. E
27. E
28. D
29. E
30. B
31. C
32. D
33. E
34. C
35. A
36. D
37. B
38. B

39. C
40. E
41. E
42. C
43. C
44. A
45. B
46. B
47. A
48. C
49. E
50. A
51. A
52. E
53. D
54. B
55. C
56. A
57. D
58. E
59. C
60. E
61. A
62. C
63. E
64. A
65. E
66. C
67. E
68. A
69. A
70. A
71. C
72. C
73. B
74. D
75. C
76. D
77. B
78. D
79. C
80. D
81. C
82. C
83. A

84. D
85. D
86. B
87. A
88. B
89. C
90. C
91. E
92. A
93. E
94. C
95. A
96. B
97. B
98. D
99. A
100. C

Explanations (1–100)

1. Androgens are C19 steroids.
   Androgens (e.g., testosterone, DHT) have a 19-carbon backbone, distinguishing them structurally from estrogens (C18) and progestins (C21). This structural class affects biosynthetic routes and receptor interactions. Confusing them with C17 or C18 families blurs key endocrine differences. Clinically, remembering C19 helps when interpreting steroidogenesis defects and drug actions.
2. Estrogens are C18 steroids.
   Estrogens (estradiol, estrone) possess an 18-carbon core and an aromatic A-ring, a hallmark that impacts receptor binding and metabolism. They are synthesized via aromatization of androgens. Labeling them C17 or C19 ignores their conversion pathway. Clinically, aromatase activity (e.g., adipose tissue) explains estrogen levels in men and postmenopausal women.
3. "Cycling" AAS use = on/off periods.
   In bodybuilding slang, "cycling" means alternating weeks/months on anabolic-androgenic steroids (AAS) with washout periods to "reset" receptors or minimize side effects. It doesn't mean dose escalation (that's pyramiding) or combining agents (that's stacking). Clinically, cycling still carries cardiometabolic, hepatic, and endocrine risks.
4. "Stacking" = combining multiple AAS.
   Users combine several oral and/or injectable agents to "synergize" anabolic effects or offset side effects. It's distinct from pyramiding (dose ramp-up) and cycling (on/off). Evidence for synergy is poor, but toxicity adds. Clinically, stacking magnifies hepatic strain, polycythemia, lipid derangements, and HPT axis suppression.

5. "Pyramiding" = dose escalation then taper.
   Pyramiding typically ramps doses up to a peak, then tapers down over a "cycle." It is not the same as cycling (on/off) or stacking (multi-drug). The practice is intended to reduce side effects, though data are lacking. Clinically, even tapered high doses can induce profound HPG suppression and adverse CV risk.
6. "Cutting" steroids target fat loss/definition.
   Cutting phases prioritize agents perceived to aid lipolysis, vascularity, and muscle definition (e.g., certain AAS ± stimulants) over mass gain. They differ from bulking or pure strength protocols. Mechanistically, diet and energy balance dominate outcomes. Clinically, stimulant/AAS combos increase BP and arrhythmic risk.
7. Performance steroids emphasize strength/power.
   These regimens choose compounds and dosing aimed at neuromuscular performance (strength/explosiveness), sometimes with minimal weight gain. This differs from bulking (mass) or cutting (leanness). Evidence for "compound specificity" is limited; training specificity matters more. Clinically, tendon rupture risk can rise when strength gains outpace connective tissue adaptation.
8. "Bulking" steroids emphasize hypertrophy.
   Bulking phases seek net anabolism and weight gain via higher calories and AAS that favor nitrogen retention. This contrasts with cutting or performance-only aims. Water retention and adiposity can also increase. Clinically, BP elevation, sleep apnea exacerbation, and dyslipidemia often worsen during bulks.
9. Cholesterol is the steroidogenesis precursor.
   All steroid hormones derive from cholesterol, transported into mitochondria for the first cleavage step. Starting at pregnenolone or androstenedione skips upstream regulation. Clinically, cholesterol transport is rate-limiting; disorders in trafficking or mitochondrial enzymes alter all downstream steroids.
10. Daily testicular T production ≈ 5–7 mg.
    Healthy adult testes secrete roughly 5–7 mg testosterone per day, pulsatile and diurnal. Much higher numbers reflect pharmacologic dosing, not physiologic output. Clinically, this baseline helps contextualize replacement therapy vs. supraphysiologic AAS regimens.
11. StAR moves cholesterol into mitochondria.
    Steroidogenic acute regulatory (StAR) protein shuttles cholesterol across the mitochondrial membrane, enabling P450scc to act. PKA signaling activates StAR, but StAR itself is the transport workhorse. Clinically, StAR defects cause lipoid CAH with global steroid deficiency.
12. PKA signaling initiates androgen production.
    LH → cAMP → PKA activation phosphorylates steroidogenic proteins (including StAR), upregulating cholesterol transport and enzyme expression. Saying "P450scc initiates" misses upstream control. Clinically, LH receptor and cAMP-PKA pathway integrity underlies Leydig cell responsiveness.

13. Testosterone half-life in plasma is short (minutes).
    Circulating T is rapidly cleared/converted; the apparent physiologic stability reflects continuous secretion and protein binding. Hours-long half-lives belong to depot esters or TU. Clinically, short native T half-life explains why injections/patches/gels sustain levels exogenously.
14. Free T fraction ≈ 1–2%.
    Most T is SHBG- or albumin-bound; only ~1–2% is free and bioactive. Calling it 10–15% overestimates androgenic exposure. Clinically, SHBG shifts (e.g., aging, liver disease, hyperthyroidism) change free T despite similar total T.
15. SHBG increases with age, liver disease, HIV; decreases with insulin resistance.
    Insulin resistance lowers SHBG; aging, hepatic disease, and some catabolic states raise it. Growth hormone deficiency tends to raise SHBG, not lower it. Clinically, always interpret total T alongside SHBG or calculate free T.
16. SHBG decreases with insulin resistance.
    Hyperinsulinemia suppresses SHBG synthesis, increasing free androgen fraction. Labeling aging or liver disease as "low SHBG" is incorrect. Clinically, metabolic syndrome can mask hypogonadism if judged by total T alone.
17. Androgen receptor gene resides on Xq11–12 (X chromosome).
    AR is X-linked; mutations produce androgen insensitivity phenotypes. Assigning it to the Y chromosome is a common mistake. Clinically, X-linked inheritance explains AIS transmission patterns.
18. AR activity is modulated by co-regulators (co-activators/co-repressors).
    Multiple co-regulator classes alter AR transcriptional output beyond ligand binding. A or B alone is incomplete; it's a network effect. Clinically, co-regulator variability partly explains tissue-specific responses and therapy resistance in prostate cancer.
19. T therapy rarely indicated when total T >12 nmol/l.
    Above ~12 nmol/l (≈350 ng/dl), symptomatic hypogonadism is less likely to be androgen-mediated; look for other causes. The "gray zone" (~8–12) needs free T/context. Clinically, treat the patient, not the number—but stay within evidence-based thresholds.
20. Typical male estrone ≈ 3–4 ng/dl.
    Estrone (E1) runs low in men, higher in obesity and aging due to aromatase. Values like 6 ng/dl can occur but trend high. Clinically, elevated estrogens contribute to gynecomastia and HPG suppression.
21. Typical male estradiol ≈ 2–4 ng/dl (≈20–40 pg/ml).
    Estradiol is essential in men for bone, libido, and vascular health; too low or too high is problematic. Large deviations suggest obesity, aromatase excess, tumors, or exogenous sources. Clinically, E2 monitoring matters during AIs or high-dose T.

22. Estrogen therapy in men: gynecomastia, fat redistribution, ↓muscle; not "hypoprolactinemia."

    Estrogens antagonize androgen effects on body composition and suppress gonadotropins; they do not lower prolactin. Hypertension can rise via fluid retention. Clinically, balance E2 carefully in transgender care and when using SERMs/AIs.

23. Testes produce a small portion of daily estradiol (single-digit μg).

    Most circulating estrogens in men arise from peripheral aromatization of androgens, not direct testicular secretion. Large numbers imply pathology or exogenous load. Clinically, adiposity is a major driver of male estrogen levels.

24. Estrogens in men: bone maturation, negative feedback, sperm maturation support; not ↑ejaculatory volume.

    E2 is critical for epiphyseal closure, HPG feedback, and epididymal function. It does not increase semen volume (an accessory gland output). Clinically, over-suppression of E2 during T therapy can harm bone and libido.

25. Early T-replacement benefits appear within 2–4 weeks.

    Energy, mood, and libido often improve first; body composition and bone take months. Expecting instant changes is unrealistic. Clinically, set timelines: sexual interest first, erectile quality and lean mass later.

26. Indications for androgens: micropenis, pubertal induction, certain anemias; not cholestatic jaundice.

    Androgens can stimulate erythropoiesis and virilization, but are contraindicated in active liver cholestasis. Osteoporosis alone isn't a standard indication without hypogonadism. Clinically, confirm true deficiency before prescribing.

27. Prostate cancer risk concerns rise with higher PSA (context >1.5–2.5 ng/ml in screening discussions).

    While TRT doesn't clearly increase incident cancer, baseline PSA informs risk stratification and monitoring. Very low PSA (<1) is lower risk. Clinically, evaluate prostate health before and during TRT.

28. Absolute TRT contraindication: hematocrit >50%.

    Elevated Hct increases thrombotic risk; TRT can raise Hct further. Values under 50% are not absolute contraindications but need monitoring. Clinically, manage with dose reduction, route change, or phlebotomy.

29. TRT caution when IPSS is high (e.g., >19–20).

    Severe LUTS/BPH symptoms can worsen with fluid shifts; stabilize first. Mild scores are less concerning. Clinically, treat bladder outlet issues before or alongside TRT.

30. Androgen therapy side effects: acne, erythrocytosis/thrombosis, fluid retention; not anemia or ↓contractility.

    TRT tends to raise hematocrit, not lower it; it can elevate BP and cause edema. Cardiac contractility depression is not typical. Clinically, track BP, Hct, lipids, and edema.

31. Long-acting TU (testosterone undecanoate) gives smoother levels.
    Short esters (cypionate/enanthate) cause peaks/troughs; buccal can fluctuate. TU injections or consistent transdermals reduce variability. Clinically, fewer mood/energy swings improve adherence.
32. Leuprolide = GnRH analogue (agonist with down-regulation).
    Chronic GnRH agonism suppresses LH/FSH after a flare, lowering testosterone. Anti-androgens (flutamide/nilutamide) and 5-ARIs (finasteride/dutasteride) act downstream. Clinically, used in prostate cancer and to control pubertal timing.
33. Cyproterone acetate = progestin with anti-androgen action.
    It suppresses LH and blocks AR, distinct from GnRH analogues or 5-ARIs. Flutamide is a non-steroidal AR blocker; finasteride is a 5-ARI. Clinically, CPA may cause hepatotoxicity and mood changes.
34. Green tea anti-androgen effect via EGCG (epigallocatechin gallate).
    EGCG can inhibit 5-alpha-reductase and modulate AR signaling in vitro. Paeoniflorin belongs to white peony; phytosterols to saw palmetto. Clinically, potency in humans is mild and variable.
35. White peony (Paeonia) anti-androgen via paeoniflorin.
    Paeoniflorin may modulate pituitary-gonadal signaling and 5-AR activity. It is different from EGCG or phytosterols. Clinically, used traditionally for hyperandrogenic symptoms, evidence modest.
36. Saw palmetto anti-androgen via phytosterols.
    Phytosterols may weakly inhibit 5-alpha-reductase; clinical effects on LUTS are inconsistent. Not via paeoniflorin or EGCG. Clinically, counsel patients about variable evidence.
37. Licorice shows anti-androgenic effects via phytoestrogen/glycyrrhizin actions.
    Licorice can reduce testosterone and increase SHBG; mechanisms include steroid metabolism modulation. Not through paeoniflorin or phytosterols. Clinically, watch for hypertension/hypokalemia with chronic intake.
38. Low-dose chaste tree (Vitex) modulates pituitary via dopamine D2.
    D2 agonism lowers prolactin, which can secondarily affect sex steroids. It does not block 5-HT1A/C receptors directly as the main effect. Clinically, used for hyperprolactinemic symptoms; evidence mixed.
39. Testosterone deficiency: he classical features of testosterone deficiency include reduced sexual desire and performance, smaller and softer testes, decreased semen volume, muscle weakness, and loss of bone density.
    Gynecomastia, however, is not a consistent feature of testosterone deficiency; it develops only when there is a relative excess of estrogen activity compared to androgens, such as in obesity, liver disease, or with certain medications
40. Transient T changes: time of day, fasting, acute illness, acute alcohol; diabetes is chronic.
    Afternoon sampling lowers total T vs. morning. Acute stressors depress T transiently. Clinically, repeat morning measurements before diagnosing hypogonadism.

41. Chronic T alterations: diabetes, obesity, chronic illness.
 Insulin resistance lowers SHBG but also links to Leydig dysfunction. Acute alcohol or illness are transient. Clinically, treat metabolic disease to improve androgen milieu.
42. Androgen insensitivity is X-linked recessive.
 Mutations in the X-linked AR gene yield CAIS/PAIS/MAIS phenotypes. It is not autosomal. Clinically, karyotype 46,XY with external feminization in CAIS.
43. Reifenstein = partial androgen insensitivity (PAIS).
 PAIS presents with undervirilization, variable gynecomastia, and infertility. It is not complete or mild AIS. Clinically, management is individualized regarding sex assignment and surgery.
44. Testicular feminization = complete AIS (CAIS).
 46,XY with functional testes but complete target-organ resistance yields female external phenotype. Not partial/mild. Clinically, consider gonadectomy timing due to tumor risk after puberty.
45. Congenital adrenal hyperplasia is autosomal recessive.
 Most forms (e.g., 21-hydroxylase deficiency) follow AR inheritance. Not X-linked. Clinically, newborn screening and stress-dose steroids are key.
46. 21-hydroxylase deficiency is the commonest CAH.
 It impairs cortisol ± aldosterone synthesis, shunting precursors to androgens. 17-alpha hydroxylase deficiency is rarer and causes sex steroid deficiency. Clinically, salt-wasting crises and virilization are hallmark concerns.
47. CAH involves cortisol/aldosterone deficiency with androgen excess; prolactin isn't the primary hormone.
 The HPA axis drive increases ACTH, enlarging adrenals and androgen output. Prolactin changes are not central. Clinically, treat with glucocorticoids ± mineralocorticoids.
48. Exogenous T suppresses LH/FSH → ↓ intrinsic spermatogenesis.
 Fertility falls due to reduced intratesticular T and Sertoli support. The idea that exogenous T "stimulates" gonadotropins is wrong. Clinically, avoid TRT for men actively seeking fertility; use hCG/SERMs instead.
49. Testosterone is endocrine (Leydig) product; largely protein-bound; regulated by LH; metabolite DHT.
 It is not exocrine, and it is not mainly free in plasma. Prolactin excess reduces, not increases, T. Clinically, DHT drives external genital virilization and prostate growth.
50. T peaks: mini-puberty (infancy), puberty/adolescence, and high adult levels through 20s.
 There's an early neonatal surge (~1–3 months), a major rise at puberty, then gradual decline after midlife. Not at 70 as a "peak." Clinically, interpret labs with age context.

51. Equilibrium dialysis free T CV ~7–15% (best available).
    It's the reference method; direct analog assays are unreliable at low levels. Variability >30–50% reflects poor assays. Clinically, use equilibrium dialysis or calculated free T (with SHBG/albumin).
52. Women's T arises from ovaries, adrenals, and peripheral conversion.
    All three contribute; ovaries and adrenals supply precursors converted peripherally. Saying only one source misses the balance. Clinically, oophorectomy/oophorectomy + adrenal status shape T levels.
53. PDE5 gene expression is androgen-responsive.
    Androgens sustain NOS activity and PDE5 expression/function in corpus cavernosum. Estrogens modulate differently. Clinically, hypogonadism reduces PDE5i responsiveness; TRT can restore it.
54. High prolactin + low T with normal LH/FSH → pituitary imaging.
    Hyperprolactinemia suppresses GnRH, causing secondary hypogonadism. Starting TRT alone can mask the cause. Clinically, get pituitary MRI and treat prolactinoma if present.
55. Best total T method: LC-MS/MS (tandem mass spectrometry).
    Direct immunoassays are inaccurate at low ranges; extraction/chromatography improves specificity. Clinically, rely on MS for women, children, and borderline male values.
56. TRT improves body composition and BMD; longevity data are mixed.
    Expect increased lean mass, decreased fat mass, and improved spine BMD in hypogonadal men. Hard outcomes (fracture, mortality) require longer trials. Clinically, monitor benefits vs. risks.
57. DHEA may favor endothelial function and lipids; evidence is modest.
    Proposed benefits include eNOS upregulation and anti-atherogenic effects, but trials vary. It's not a panacea. Clinically, counsel about uncertain efficacy and potential hormonal effects.
58. Physiologic transdermal T in women: minimal virilization when dosed correctly.
    At low female-physiologic doses, severe hirsutism/virilization should not occur. Metabolic harm is unlikely with proper dosing. Clinically, monitor lipids, acne, and hair changes.
59. After BSO, total and free T drop markedly (≈50% or more).
    Ovaries contribute substantially to androgens; SHBG changes also matter. Saying "no change" is incorrect. Clinically, some women develop HSDD post-oophorectomy.
60. Reliable free T in women: equilibrium dialysis or calculated methods (not direct analog assays).
    FAI is crude; analog assays are inaccurate. Calculations using SHBG/albumin are acceptable proxies. Clinically, choose methods consistently for follow-up.
61. Androgens decline across a woman's lifespan (with SHBG shifts).
    Total and free T tend to fall with age; SHBG may also change, affecting free fraction. Saying they increase is incorrect. Clinically, interpret levels relative to age, menopause, OCPs.

62. Female T therapy can improve sexual function with mild, dose-dependent side effects.

    Evidence supports benefit in selected naturally or surgically menopausal women with HSDD. Excess dosing causes virilization. Clinically, use the lowest effective dose with monitoring.

63. Androgens may inhibit some breast cancer models; clinical use historically in metastatic disease.

    Data show anti-proliferative effects in vitro/animals, but clinical use is limited by side effects. PCOS hyperandrogenism doesn't clearly lower risk. Clinically, decisions are individualized and evolving.

64. DHEA is the most abundant sex steroid precursor in humans.

    Adrenals produce DHEA/DHEAS in large amounts, serving as substrates for androgens/estrogens peripherally. Estradiol/testosterone circulate in much lower concentrations. Clinically, DHEA levels fall with age ("adrenopause").

65. DHEAS has a long half-life and stable diurnal pattern; DHEA rapidly sulfated to DHEAS.

    These kinetics make DHEAS a steadier biomarker than DHEA. Menstrual cycle effects on DHEAS are minimal. Clinically, DHEAS helps evaluate adrenal androgen output.

66. A membrane-bound DHEA receptor has been proposed in vascular endothelium.

    Non-genomic actions may mediate rapid vasodilatory effects. Evidence remains under investigation. Clinically, this could explain some endothelial benefits beyond conversion to sex steroids.

67. DHEA may enhance eNOS, modulate glucose toxicity, immune responses, and ischemia tolerance.

    These pleiotropic effects are suggested by experimental data. Translation to robust clinical endpoints is mixed. Clinically, consider DHEA cautiously, especially with hormone-sensitive conditions.

68. In hypogonadal ED, TRT can improve PDE5i responsiveness.

    Androgens support NO signaling and cavernosal smooth muscle health. Without correcting low T, PDE5i may underperform. Clinically, replete T first, then reassess PDE5i efficacy.

69. 17-α alkylation prevents first-pass metabolism but increases hepatotoxicity.

    Oral alkylated androgens resist hepatic degradation, raising liver risk (cholestasis, adenomas). It does not "prevent toxicity." Clinically, avoid long-term 17-α-alkylated agents.

70. TRT has no convincing evidence of increasing prostate cancer risk when monitored.

    Modern data suggest neutral risk with appropriate screening. Vigilance is still required in men with prior cancer. Clinically, baseline PSA/DRE and periodic monitoring are standard.

71. Aromatase converts androgens to estrogens, especially in adipose tissue.
    Higher fat mass increases E2, which can suppress gonadotropins and cause gynecomastia. Aromatase inhibitors lower E2 but can impair bone. Clinically, weight loss improves androgen–estrogen balance.
72. 5-alpha-reductase converts T → DHT; type 2 predominates in prostate.
    DHT is more potent at AR and drives prostate/skin effects. Inhibitors (finasteride/dutasteride) reduce DHT but can affect sexual function. Clinically, consider DHT in BPH and androgenic alopecia.
73. SHBG is synthesized in the liver and regulated by hormones/nutrition.
    Thyroid hormones, estrogens, and liver health increase SHBG; insulin and androgens lower it. This alters free T. Clinically, SHBG context is essential for interpreting total T.
74. hCG mimics LH to stimulate Leydig cells and preserve fertility.
    In secondary hypogonadism, hCG ± FSH can restore spermatogenesis without suppressing the axis like exogenous T. Clinically, choose hCG for men desiring fertility.
75. Clomiphene raises LH/FSH by blocking estrogen feedback.
    As a SERM, it can increase endogenous T and sperm production in secondary hypogonadism. It avoids testicular shutdown. Clinically, useful for younger men with intact pituitaries.
76. Anabolic steroids suppress the HPG axis, shrinking testes and lowering sperm counts.
    Recovery can be slow and incomplete after prolonged use. Gynecomastia may develop via aromatization. Clinically, counsel about long-term fertility risks.
77. AAS increase CV risk: dyslipidemia, hypertension, thrombotic events.
    They lower HDL, raise LDL, thicken blood (polycythemia), and strain myocardium. "Safe cycles" are a myth. Clinically, screen aggressively in users.
78. T undecanoate oral formulation (lipophilic) differs from depot TU injections.
    Oral TU (lymphatic absorption) has variable levels; injectable TU provides steady exposure. Not all "TU"s are equivalent. Clinically, monitor levels by formulation.
79. Transdermal T offers stable levels but risks skin transfer.
    Gels/patches avoid peaks but can transfer to contacts; counsel on application and drying. Irritation and variable absorption occur. Clinically, verify with trough morning levels.
80. Buccal T provides rapid absorption but can irritate mucosa.
    Levels can be stable if adherence is good. Dental issues and taste changes may limit use. Clinically, consider in those intolerant of injections/gels.
81. Erythrocytosis is the most frequent dose-limiting TRT adverse effect.
    Monitor hematocrit at baseline, 3–6 months, then annually. Manage by dose/route adjustment or phlebotomy. Clinically, assess thrombotic risk factors.

82. Gynecomastia reflects androgen–estrogen imbalance.
    In TRT, excess aromatization or high E2 can stimulate breast tissue. AIs or SERMs may help selectively. Clinically, weight loss and dose tuning matter.
83. Liver toxicity is mainly with 17-α-alkylated orals, not physiologic transdermal/injectable T.
    Gels/patches/injectables rarely cause cholestasis. Distinguish AAS abuse from TRT. Clinically, avoid oral alkylated androgens outside narrow indications.
84. TRT can improve insulin sensitivity in hypogonadal men with metabolic syndrome.
    Mechanisms include increased lean mass and reduced visceral fat. Still monitor glycemia and lipids. Clinically, lifestyle + TRT yields best outcomes.
85. DHT gels elevate DHT without raising E2 as much as T.
    Less aromatization may benefit men sensitive to E2, but prostate/skin effects may increase. Clinically, limited indications; monitor PSA and symptoms.
86. Finasteride/dutasteride reduce PSA ~50%—adjust interpretation.
    When screening, double the measured PSA to estimate baseline. Missing this can delay detection. Clinically, document 5-ARI use in records.
87. Klinefelter syndrome (47,XXY) → primary testicular failure and low T.
    High LH/FSH with small firm testes is classic. Fertility options include TESE with ICSI. Clinically, TRT improves metabolic and bone health.
88. Opioids suppress GnRH and lower T.
    Chronic opioid therapy causes androgen deficiency symptoms. Consider opioid-sparing strategies or address with endocrine therapy. Clinically, check morning T in symptomatic patients.
89. Glucocorticoids suppress the HPG axis and testosterone.
    They reduce GnRH and pituitary gonadotropins; catabolic effects worsen sarcopenia. Taper if possible. Clinically, consider bone protection and metabolic mitigation.
90. Hyperthyroidism raises SHBG; hypothyroidism lowers it.
    Thus free T can be discordant with total T in thyroid disease. Normalize thyroid first. Clinically, re-evaluate androgens after euthyroidism.
91. Prolactinomas: treat with dopamine agonists, not TRT first.
    Cabergoline/bromocriptine lower prolactin and restore gonadotropins and T. TRT alone masks the cause. Clinically, MRI and endocrine referral are key.
92. AIS management depends on phenotype and patient goals; CAIS often reared female.
    Gonadectomy timing balances tumor risk vs. puberty induction. Hormone replacement tailored post-gonadectomy. Clinically, multidisciplinary care essential.
93. Exogenous AAS frequently cause psychiatric effects (irritability, mood swings).
    Neurosteroid effects and sleep disturbance contribute. Screen for dependence. Clinically, support tapering and mental health evaluation.

94. Hematocrit rises more with injectable short-ester T vs. transdermal.
    Route influences erythrocytosis risk via peaks and DHT shifts. Consider switching route if Hct climbs. Clinically, altitude and OSA add risk.
95. OSA can worsen with TRT due to airway edema/weight.
    Screen for snoring/daytime somnolence; treat OSA before/with TRT. Clinically, CPAP improves safety and outcomes.
96. Baseline evaluation before TRT: morning T ×2, LH/FSH, prolactin, SHBG, PSA/DRE (age-appropriate), Hct/LFTs.
    Rule out secondary causes and contraindications. Then individualize formulation and dose. Clinically, document shared decision-making.
97. Monitoring on TRT: symptoms, T trough, Hct, PSA, lipids, LFTs at 3–6 months, then yearly.
    Adjust for targets and side effects. Don't chase supraphysiologic levels. Clinically, aim for mid-normal T range.
98. Fertility-preserving hypogonadism therapy: hCG ± FSH or clomiphene, not exogenous T.
    These maintain intratesticular T and spermatogenesis. Exogenous T suppresses both. Clinically, align therapy with reproductive goals.
99. "Testosterone boosters" are unregulated; evidence is poor; risks exist.
    Herbal blends can interact with meds and alter labs. Quality control is variable. Clinically, educate patients and prioritize proven treatments.
100. Shared decision-making is central to TRT and AAS counseling.
    Balance symptomatic benefits with cardiovascular, hematologic, prostate, and fertility risks. Individual comorbidities guide route and monitoring. Clinically, clear milestones and safety checkpoints improve adherence and outcomes.

Further Reading

The explanations in this chapter are supported by the following key references:

1. Handelsman DJ. Androgen physiology, pharmacology, use and misuse. Endocr Rev. 2017;38(4):376–405.
2. Bhasin S, Brito JP, Cunningham GR, et al. Testosterone therapy in men with hypogonadism: An Endocrine Society clinical practice guideline. J Clin Endocrinol Metab. 2018;103(5):1715–44.
3. Nieschlag E, Behre HM, Nieschlag S. Testosterone: action, deficiency, substitution. 4th ed. Cambridge: Cambridge University Press; 2012.
4. Pope HG Jr, Wood RI, Rogol A, et al. Adverse health consequences of performance-enhancing drugs. Lancet. 2014;384(9950):107–18.
5. van Breda E, Keizer HA, Kuipers H, et al. Androgenic-anabolic steroid use and severe adverse health effects. Sports Med. 2003;33(13):995–1012.
6. de Ronde W, Smit DL. Anabolic androgenic steroid abuse in young males. Endocr Connect. 2020;9(4):R102–11.

Male Puberty

15

Learning Objectives

- Describe the physiological milestones of male puberty.
- Understand the role of hypothalamic-pituitary-gonadal (HPG) axis.
- Identify causes of delayed and early puberty.
- Use Tanner staging in clinical evaluation.
- Explore hormonal and supportive treatment options.

Select the Single Best Answer

1. The regulator key of male puberty is:
   A. LH
   B. Kisspeptin
   C. GnRH
   D. SRY gene
   E. FSH
2. FSH production is inhibited by:
   A. Estrogen
   B. GnRH
   C. Inhibin
   D. Mullerian inhibiting hormone
   E. LH
3. Which of the following is NOT a cause of central precocious puberty?
   A. Craniopharyngioma
   B. Hypothyroidism
   C. Cranial irradiation
   D. Hydrocephalus
   E. B + D

M. S. M. Hasan, M. L. Elsaie, *Comprehensive MCQs in Andrology*, Trends in Andrology and Sexual Medicine, https://doi.org/10.1007/978-3-032-20623-7_15

4. The investigation of choice in male precocious puberty is:
   A. CT scan of the adrenal gland
   B. MRI brain
   C. Field of vision test
   D. FSH level
   E. Inhibin level
5. In boys with delayed puberty, testosterone injection should be started at age (years):
   A. 10
   B. 12
   C. 13
   D. 14
   E. 17
6. Which of the following is NOT under the effect of DHEA/DHEAS/androstenedione?
   A. Development of pubic and axillary hair
   B. Breast development
   C. Acne, oily skin and hair
   D. Adult-type body odor
7. The most common cause of central precocious puberty is:
   A. Idiopathic (constitutional)
   B. Hypothalamic hamartoma
   C. Congenital adrenal hyperplasia
   D. Ovarian tumor
8. A 7-year-old girl with precocious puberty, café-au-lait spots, hyperthyroidism, bone fractures, and Cushing's has:
   A. Peutz–Jeghers syndrome
   B. Kallmann syndrome
   C. Swyer syndrome
   D. McCune–Albright syndrome
   E. Testotoxicosis
9. The first sign of male puberty is:
   A. Pubic hair
   B. Penile erection
   C. Spermarche
   D. Testicular enlargement
   E. Increased bone density
10. Which of the following is NOT a eunuchoid feature?
    A. Arm span > height
    B. Infantile genitalia
    C. Sparse axillary hair
    D. Increased muscular mass
    E. Underdeveloped scrotum

11. Which of the following is NOT a feature of testotoxicosis?
    A. LH receptor mutation
    B. Precocious puberty
    C. High serum gonadotropins
    D. High testosterone
    E. May respond to antiandrogens
12. Which of the following is NOT true about McCune–Albright syndrome?
    A. Fibrous dysplasia of bone
    B. Polydactyly
    C. Café-au-lait patches
    D. Precocious puberty
    E. A + B
13. Which is NOT a criterion for constitutional delay of growth/puberty?
    A. Positive family history
    B. Delayed growth
    C. Delayed bone age
    D. High IGF-1
    E. Prolonged childhood phase
14. Dose of hCG in constitutional delay:
    A. 75 U IM twice weekly
    B. 1500 U IM twice weekly
    C. 300 U IM twice weekly
    D. 500 U IM twice weekly
    E. 150 U IM twice weekly
15. Advantage of oxandrolone in delay of puberty:
    A. Stature improvement
    B. Bone mass
    C. Muscle mass
    D. Secondary sexual characters
    E. Voice
16. Which is NOT indicated in 3-month follow-up of testosterone therapy?
    A. BMI
    B. Hematocrit
    C. Lipid profile
    D. Waist circumference
    E. PSA
17. A common cause of primary hypogonadism is:
    A. Pure gonadal dysgenesis
    B. Cryptorchidism
    C. Klinefelter syndrome
    D. Y-chromosome microdeletion
    E. Congenital anorchia

18. A common cause of secondary hypogonadism is:
    A. Kallmann syndrome
    B. Pituitary hypoplasia
    C. Hemochromatosis
    D. Idiopathic
    E. Leptin receptor mutation
19. Which is NOT true about gonadal facies?
    A. Hot flushes
    B. Reduced shaving
    C. Facial grimacing
    D. Decreased wrinkles
    E. Pale skin
20. Subclinical hypogonadism shows:
    A. Normal testosterone, ↑LH
    B. ↑Testosterone, ↑LH
    C. ↓Testosterone, ↑LH
    D. ↓Testosterone, ↓LH
    E. Normal testosterone, normal LH
21. Which is NOT true of constitutional delay of puberty?
    A. 16-year-old girl with absent secondary sexual characters, bone age 14
    B. Bone-age appropriate growth velocity
    C. GnRH secretion matches bone age
    D. Familial late puberty
22. Syndrome leading to progressive seminiferous tubule sclerosis and infertility:
    A. Kallmann
    B. Down syndrome
    C. Klinefelter
    D. Cystic fibrosis
23. Which is NOT associated with reduced androgens?
    A. Lipoid adrenal hyperplasia
    B. Isolated 17,20-lyase deficiency
    C. 21-hydroxylase deficiency
    D. P450 oxidoreductase deficiency
    E. Cholesterol side-chain cleavage deficiency
24. Congenital lipoid adrenal hyperplasia is due to:
    A. P450 defect
    B. StAR deficiency
    C. 17,20-lyase deficiency
    D. 17α-hydroxylase deficiency
    E. CYP17 mutation
25. Congenital lipoid adrenal hyperplasia is NOT characterized by:
    A. 46,XY karyotype
    B. No Müllerian derivatives
    C. Low glucocorticoids
    D. Low ACTH
    E. Metabolic acidosis

26. Antley–Bixler syndrome is part of:
    A. Lipoid adrenal hyperplasia
    B. P450 oxidoreductase deficiency
    C. Constitutional delay
    D. Androgen insensitivity
    E. Side-chain cleavage defect
27. Fibrous dysplasia of bone is seen in:
    A. Koro syndrome
    B. Kennedy disease
    C. McCune–Albright syndrome
    D. Androgen insensitivity
    E. Testotoxicosis
28. Two-year follow-up of testosterone therapy is done with:
    A. Hematocrit
    B. PSA
    C. BMI
    D. DEXA scan
    E. Lipid profile
29. Tall stature and anosmia are features of:
    A. Klinefelter
    B. Kallmann
    C. Kennedy disease
    D. McCune–Albright
30. Inheritance pattern of Kallmann syndrome:
    A. Autosomal dominant
    B. Autosomal recessive
    C. X-linked recessive
    D. Mitochondrial
31. Which hormone initiates puberty?
    A. LH
    B. FSH
    C. GnRH
    D. Testosterone
32. Constitutional delay is characterized by:
    A. Early bone age
    B. Positive family history
    C. Tall stature
    D. Hypergonadotropic hypogonadism
33. Hypogonadotropic hypogonadism shows:
    A. Small testes, low LH/FSH
    B. Large testes, low LH/FSH
    C. Small testes, high LH/FSH
    D. Large testes, high LH/FSH

34. Acquired secondary hypogonadism may be due to:
    A. Kallmann
    B. Pituitary tumors
    C. StAR deficiency
    D. McCune–Albright
35. Hypergonadotropic hypogonadism presents with:
    A. Low T, high LH/FSH
    B. Low T, low LH/FSH
    C. High T, low LH/FSH
    D. High T, high LH/FSH
36. Klinefelter karyotype:
    A. 46,XY
    B. 45,X
    C. 47,XXY
    D. 48,XXYY
37. Kallmann syndrome is associated with:
    A. Gynecomastia
    B. Anosmia
    C. Tall stature
    D. Café-au-lait patches
38. Distinguishing test in delayed puberty:
    A. LH measurement
    B. GnRH stimulation test
    C. DEXA scan
    D. MRI
39. First sign of puberty in boys:
    A. Pubic hair
    B. Axillary hair
    C. Testicular enlargement
    D. Voice change
40. Which is NOT diagnostic of delayed puberty?
    A. No testicular enlargement by 14
    B. No pubic hair by 15
    C. No axillary hair by 12
    D. Bone age delay
41. Drugs that suppress testosterone include:
    A. Corticosteroids
    B. Ketoconazole
    C. Spironolactone
    D. All of the above
42. Prolactinoma causes hypogonadism by:
    A. Stimulating GnRH
    B. Suppressing GnRH
    C. Stimulating FSH
    D. Increasing LH

43. Quigley scale measures:
    A. Degree of gynecomastia
    B. Severity of androgen insensitivity
    C. Stages of puberty
    D. Stages of bone age
44. Partial androgen insensitivity shows:
    A. Normal male genitalia
    B. Ambiguous genitalia
    C. Female phenotype
    D. Tall stature only
45. Complete androgen insensitivity occurs in:
    A. 46,XX
    B. 46,XY
    C. 47,XXY
    D. 45,X
46. 5α-reductase deficiency results in:
    A. Excess DHT
    B. Low DHT
    C. Excess estradiol
    D. Low cortisol
47. In 5α-reductase deficiency, testosterone to DHT conversion is:
    A. Enhanced
    B. Impaired
    C. Normal
    D. Increased at puberty
48. First-line test in suspected hypogonadism:
    A. Total testosterone
    B. LH only
    C. FSH only
    D. MRI
49. Untreated hypogonadism leads to:
    A. Osteoporosis
    B. Infertility
    C. Psychosocial issues
    D. All of the above
50. For fertility, treatment requires:
    A. hCG + FSH
    B. Testosterone alone
    C. LH alone
    D. DHT supplementation

✅ Key Takeaways

- Puberty is initiated by **GnRH pulsatility**, leading to LH/FSH and testosterone secretion.
- Tanner stages help track genital and pubic hair development.
- Delayed puberty may be **constitutional** or due to **hypogonadism**.
- Precocious puberty requires imaging and hormonal assessment.
- Timely diagnosis aids psychosocial and physical outcomes.

✅ Answer Key (1–50)

1. B
2. C
3. B
4. B
5. D
6. B
7. A
8. D
9. D
10. D
11. C
12. B
13. D
14. B
15. A
16. E
17. C
18. C
19. C
20. A
21. A
22. C
23. C
24. B
25. D
26. B
27. C
28. D
29. B
30. C
31. C
32. B

33. A
34. C
35. A
36. C
37. B
38. B
39. C
40. C
41. D
42. C
43. B
44. B
45. B
46. B
47. B
48. A
49. D
50. A

Explanations (1–50)

1. Kisspeptin is the central regulator of puberty, stimulating GnRH secretion. LH and FSH are downstream hormones, while the SRY gene determines male sex but not puberty onset.
2. FSH is inhibited by inhibin secreted by Sertoli cells. Estrogen and GnRH modulate LH/FSH secretion, but inhibin is the specific brake on FSH.
3. Central precocious puberty is due to hypothalamic-pituitary lesions like craniopharyngioma or irradiation. Hypothyroidism does not cause central precocious puberty but peripheral pseudoprecocity.
4. MRI brain is the investigation of choice to detect hypothalamic or pituitary lesions. CT of the adrenal is for peripheral causes. Hormonal assays alone cannot localize the cause.
5. Testosterone replacement for delayed puberty is started at age 14. Earlier initiation risks premature epiphyseal closure and psychosocial mismatch.
6. DHEA and its derivatives cause pubic/axillary hair, acne, oily skin, and odor. They do not cause breast development, which is estrogen-mediated.
7. Idiopathic central precocious puberty is most common, particularly in girls. Hypothalamic hamartomas are less common but classic organic causes.
8. McCune–Albright syndrome presents with café-au-lait spots, bone dysplasia, endocrine overactivity, and precocious puberty. Other syndromes lack this triad.
9. The earliest sign of male puberty is testicular enlargement due to seminiferous tubule growth. Pubic hair follows later under adrenal/androgen influence.
10. Eunuchoid habitus shows tall arm span, infantile genitalia, sparse hair, and underdeveloped scrotum. Increased muscular mass is not typical.

11. Testotoxicosis shows autonomous testosterone secretion with low gonadotropins. High gonadotropins is incorrect, so C is not a feature.
12. McCune–Albright has café-au-lait, bone fibrous dysplasia, precocious puberty. Polydactyly is not part of it, so option B is wrong.
13. Constitutional delay shows positive family history, delayed bone age, and slow growth. High IGF-1 is not part of the picture.
14. hCG stimulates Leydig cells to produce testosterone. The standard dose is 1500 U IM twice weekly, mimicking LH action.
15. Oxandrolone is an anabolic steroid useful in improving stature in constitutional delay. It promotes growth without excessive virilization.
16. Follow-up of testosterone therapy at 3 months checks BMI, hematocrit, lipids, and waist. PSA is only for older men >40–50 years.
17. Klinefelter syndrome (47,XXY) is the most common cause of primary hypogonadism. Others are rarer congenital disorders.
18. Secondary hypogonadism can arise from pituitary or hypothalamic dysfunction; hemochromatosis is a classic acquired cause.
19. Gonadal facies are dull, pale, with reduced shaving, wrinkles, and hot flushes. Facial grimacing is not a feature.
20. Subclinical hypogonadism shows normal testosterone with high LH, reflecting early testicular failure.
21. Constitutional delay shows bone age delay and familial late puberty. A 16-year-old female with bone age 14 is typical, but GnRH secretion matches bone age, not chronological age.
22. Klinefelter syndrome leads to seminiferous tubule sclerosis and infertility. Other syndromes have different features.
23. 21-hydroxylase deficiency is linked to androgen excess, not deficiency. Others cause androgen deficiency.
24. Congenital lipoid adrenal hyperplasia is due to StAR protein deficiency, preventing cholesterol transport into mitochondria.
25. This condition shows 46,XY karyotype, adrenal failure, acidosis, low cortisol, but ACTH is high, not low.
26. Antley–Bixler syndrome is due to P450 oxidoreductase deficiency, causing skeletal and genital anomalies.
27. McCune–Albright shows fibrous bone dysplasia, endocrine overactivity, and café-au-lait spots. Not seen in Koro or Kennedy diseases.
28. Long-term testosterone follow-up includes bone density by DEXA to assess osteoporosis risk. Hematocrit and PSA are earlier markers.
29. Tall stature and anosmia are hallmarks of Kallmann syndrome, a form of hypogonadotropic hypogonadism.
30. Kallmann syndrome is inherited in various ways but classically X-linked recessive.

31. Puberty starts with GnRH secretion, which stimulates LH and FSH, leading to testosterone.
32. Constitutional delay has family history, short stature, delayed bone age, but not hypergonadotropic hypogonadism.
33. Hypogonadotropic hypogonadism shows low T and low LH/FSH with small testes. Hypergonadotropic shows high LH/FSH.
34. Acquired secondary hypogonadism includes pituitary tumors, trauma, or hemochromatosis. Genetic syndromes are congenital.
35. Hypergonadotropic hypogonadism shows low T with elevated LH/FSH due to testicular failure.
36. Klinefelter syndrome has 47,XXY karyotype, associated with infertility and gynecomastia.
37. Kallmann syndrome combines hypogonadism with anosmia due to olfactory bulb defect.
38. GnRH stimulation test differentiates constitutional delay from hypogonadotropic hypogonadism.
39. Testicular enlargement is the earliest sign of male puberty. Hair and voice change occur later.
40. Delayed puberty is defined by absent testicular enlargement by age 14. Lack of axillary hair by 12 is not diagnostic.
41. Corticosteroids, ketoconazole, and spironolactone suppress testosterone synthesis. All are correct.
42. Prolactinomas suppress GnRH, leading to low LH/FSH and secondary hypogonadism.
43. Quigley scale measures androgen insensitivity severity, from complete to mild.
44. Partial androgen insensitivity causes ambiguous genitalia, not normal male or female phenotype.
45. Complete androgen insensitivity occurs in 46,XY individuals with female phenotype.
46. 5α-reductase deficiency leads to low DHT and undervirilized external genitalia.
47. Testosterone to DHT conversion is impaired, but virilization may occur at puberty due to high testosterone.
48. First-line test for hypogonadism is morning total testosterone, before advanced imaging.
49. Hypogonadism untreated leads to infertility, osteoporosis, and psychological issues.
50. Fertility requires gonadotropins (hCG + FSH), not testosterone alone, since exogenous testosterone suppresses spermatogenesis.

Further Reading

The explanations in this chapter are supported by the following key references:

1. Palmert MR, Dunkel L. Delayed puberty. N Engl J Med. 2012;366(5):443–53.
2. Grumbach MM, Styne DM. Puberty: ontogeny, neuroendocrinology, physiology, and disorders. In: Williams textbook of endocrinology. 14th ed. Elsevier; 2020.
3. Abreu AP, Kaiser UB. Pubertal development and regulation. Lancet Diabetes Endocrinol. 2016;4(3):254–64.
4. Boehm U, Bouloux PM, Dattani MT, et al. Expert consensus document: European consensus on congenital hypogonadotropic hypogonadism. Nat Rev Endocrinol. 2015;11(9):547–64.
5. Styne DM, Grumbach MM. Disorders of puberty. In: Williams textbook of endocrinology. 14th ed. Elsevier; 2020.
6. Latronico AC, Brito VN, Carel JC. Causes, diagnosis, and treatment of central precocious puberty. Lancet Diabetes Endocrinol. 2016;4(3):265–74.

Male Infertility

16

Learning Objectives

- Classify causes of male infertility (pre-testicular, testicular, post-testicular).
- Interpret semen analysis and hormonal assays.
- Recognize varicocele and its implications.
- Understand ART indications and sperm retrieval techniques.
- Apply clinical decision-making in idiopathic infertility.

Select the Single Best Answer

1. Should the subclinical varicocele be operated?
   A. Only if it affects sperm parameters.
   B. Only if it causes hormonal disorders (an increase of FSH).
   C. Only if it is accompanied by scrotal pain.
   D. No, it is not operated for it does not increase the chances of spontaneous gestation.
2. Does testis biopsy make sense during varicocele repair surgery and when?
   A. Only if we freeze testicular tissue and always from the fellow testis.
   B. Yes, and it could be conducted in every session of varicose surgery.
   C. No, it makes no sense according to existing literature data.
   D. Only if there are signs of progressive testicular impairment observed (e.g., asymmetry of right-left testes >20% or increase of FSH).
   E. In cases A and D.
3. When is varicocele operated in children?
   A. When progressive testicular growth retardation is observed, confirmed by exams or scrotal pain.
   B. When varicocele is palpated bilaterally.
   C. When another testicular pathology co-exists or there is increased LHRH response.

M. S. M. Hasan, M. L. Elsaie, *Comprehensive MCQs in Andrology*, Trends in Andrology and Sexual Medicine, https://doi.org/10.1007/978-3-032-20623-7_16

D. When poor sperm parameters are observed in adolescents.
E. In all the above cases.

4. When performed before assisted reproduction in infertile couples, varicocele surgery may result in:
   A. Double chances for embryo implantation.
   B. Reduction of miscarriage rate during the 2nd trimester.
   C. High chance for twin gestation.
   D. Maintaining a stable number of spermatozoa retrieved.
5. In which cases after varicocele surgery may chances to achieve gestation increase?
   A. Only when sperm count increases.
   B. When motility of sperm improves after 2 h incubation.
   C. When sperm morphology >4% (WHO).
   D. Irrespective of microscopic changes, due to improved DNA packaging.
6. Which of the following about hydrocele surgical treatment is true?
   A. Inguinal approach is used if testicular pathology suspected.
   B. Excision is superior to plication regarding relapse.
   C. Hematoma is the most common complication.
   D. All of the above.
   E. None of the above.
7. Which of the following about spermatic vein ligation is true?
   A. Subinguinal has lower morbidity than inguinal but more demanding technically.
   B. Hydrocele formation is the most common complication (3–39%).
   C. Testicular artery injury can cause atrophy.
   D. All of the above.
   E. A and B only.
8. In obstructive azoospermia with normal FSH, the method of choice for sperm retrieval is:
   A. Fine-needle aspiration of testis.
   B. Open biopsy.
   C. Microsurgical biopsy.
   D. Microsurgical retrieval from epididymal head.
   E. Fine-needle puncture epididymal tail.
9. A patient with non-obstructive azoospermia, normal karyotype, AZFa microdeletion and varicocele. Best treatment is:
   A. Varicocele repair.
   B. Bilateral vein ligation.
   C. Left testicular biopsy for sperm.
   D. Right testicular biopsy for sperm.
   E. None of the above.
10. Which is true about testicular descent?
    A. Androgens play role in the first phase.
    B. Androgens play role in the second phase.
    C. Androgens play no role.
    D. Second phase depends on estrogen.

11. Cryopreservation of sperm means storage at:
    A. −80 °C
    B. −120 °C
    C. −196 °C
    D. 0 °C
12. Which drugs impair spermatogenesis?
    A. Ketoconazole
    B. Spironolactone
    C. Colchicine
    D. Estrogens
    E. All of the above
13. Spermatogenesis can be inhibited if a man had fever:
    A. One year before
    B. Within last 7 days
    C. Within last 6 months
    D. No correlation
14. Best timing for ejaculation when aiming for conception:
    A. Every 2 days
    B. Daily
    C. On confirmed ovulation
    D. Weekly
15. Prostaglandins are produced by the gland that also secretes:
    A. Citric acid
    B. Fructose
    C. Glucosidase
    D. Zinc
16. In non-mosaic Klinefelter's with varicocele, the best is:
    A. Repair varicocele
    B. Repair varicocele + testis biopsy
    C. Biopsy only
    D. B + C
17. Every azoospermic man should undergo karyotype:
    A. If unilateral absence of vas deferens
    B. If bilateral absence of vas deferens
    C. If primary testicular lesion confirmed
    D. Only with Y deletions
18. Seminal vesiculography is:
    A. Essential for all azoospermic men
    B. Essential for non-obstructive azoospermia
    C. Essential for obstructive azoospermia
    D. Essential only before duct surgery
    E. None of the above

19. An azoospermic man with intratubular neoplasia:
    A. Will never develop testis cancer
    B. Unlikely to develop testis cancer
    C. Will eventually develop invasive tumor if he lives long enough
    D. None of the above
    E. All of the above
20. In obstructive azoospermia with normal FSH, sperm retrieval of choice is:
    A. Fine-needle aspiration testis
    B. Open biopsy
    C. Microsurgical biopsy
    D. Microsurgical epididymal retrieval
    E. Fine-needle epididymal puncture
21. A 30-year-old man with 13 M/mL sperm, 10% motility, 28% morphology, left varicocele, normal hormones. Best therapy?
    A. IVF with masturbation sperm
    B. rFSH and rLH
    C. Varicocele sclerotherapy
    D. Varicocelectomy
    E. None
22. Most appropriate surgical technique for varicocele repair:
    A. Palomo
    B. Ivanissevich
    C. Laparoscopic
    D. Robotic
    E. Subinguinal microsurgery
23. Veins responsible for varicocele:
    A. Hypogastric
    B. Deferential
    C. Internal iliac
    D. Internal spermatic
    E. Cavernosal
24. A 26-year-old infertile man, abnormal semen, normal T/FSH/LH, prolactin 20 (N:2–18). Most likely cause?
    A. Pituitary microadenoma
    B. Macroadenoma
    C. Polypharmacy (Regular use of multiple drugs)
    D. Stress draw
    E. Timing of blood draw
25. Tight junctions of blood-testis barrier are formed by:
    A. Sertoli–Sertoli cells
    B. Myoid–Leydig cells
    C. Spermatid–Sertoli cells
    D. Leydig–Leydig cells
    E. Endothelial cells

26. With chronic obstruction, sperm motility is highest in what region of the epididymis?
    A. Rete testis
    B. Efferent ducts
    C. Caput epididymis
    D. Corpus epididymis
    E. Cauda epididymis
27. What occurs during spermiogenesis?
    A. Division of spermatogonia to form primary spermatocytes
    B. Division of primary spermatocytes to form secondary spermatocytes
    C. Cellular remodeling and nuclear compaction of spermatid DNA
    D. Cytokinesis
    E. Meiosis
28. Cadmium replaces .... in DNA polymerase enzyme:
    A. Citric acid
    B. Phosphorus
    C. Carnitine
    D. Zinc
    E. Lead
29. Arsenic replaces ...... during DNA synthesis:
    A. Citric acid
    B. Carnitine
    C. Zinc
    D. Phosphorus
    E. Lead
30. Regarding male infertility, the reversible dose of radiotherapy is:
    A. 500 rad
    B. 700 rad
    C. 900 rad
    D. 1000 rad
31. Which drug is NOT associated with decreased androgen levels?
    A. Ketoconazole
    B. Pesticides
    C. Spironolactone
    D. Alcohol
    E. Heroin
32. Which of the following is NOT a mechanism of infertility in hypothyroidism?
    A. Autoimmune mechanism
    B. Low SHBG
    C. Decreased spermatogenesis
    D. Increased estrogen
    E. GnRH mutation

33. Which of the following is NOT a gene mutation associated with Kallmann syndrome?
    A. KALIG-1
    B. PROK2
    C. GPR54/KISS1
    D. SPATA16
34. Which mutation is associated with normosmic Kallmann syndrome?
    A. KALIG-1
    B. PROK2
    C. GPR54/KISS1
    D. SPATA16
35. Bimanual synkinesis is characteristic of:
    A. Prader–Willi syndrome
    B. Kallmann syndrome
    C. Klinefelter syndrome
    D. Down syndrome
    E. Bardet–Biedl syndrome
36. The incidence of Kallmann syndrome is:
    A. 1:100
    B. 1:1000
    C. 1:10,000
    D. 1:100,000
37. The inheritance pattern of Kallmann syndrome is:
    A. X-linked recessive
    B. X-linked dominant
    C. Autosomal recessive
    D. Autosomal dominant
38. The incidence of Prader–Willi syndrome is:
    A. 1:1000
    B. 1:5000
    C. 1:10,000
    D. 1:15,000
39. Retinitis pigmentosa is more common in:
    A. Kallmann syndrome
    B. Prader–Willi syndrome
    C. Klinefelter syndrome
    D. Down syndrome
    E. Bardet–Biedl syndrome
40. Polydactyly is more common in:
    A. Kallmann syndrome
    B. Prader–Willi syndrome
    C. Klinefelter syndrome
    D. Down syndrome
    E. Bardet–Biedl syndrome

41. Spastic paraplegia is more common in:
    A. Laurence–Moon–Biedl syndrome
    B. Prader–Willi syndrome
    C. Klinefelter syndrome
    D. Down syndrome
    E. Bardet–Biedl syndrome
42. The incidence of Laurence–Moon–Biedl syndrome is:
    A. 1:30,000
    B. 1:60,000
    C. 1:90,000
    D. 1:120,000
    E. 1:160,000
43. Del Castillo syndrome is a synonym for:
    A. Bilateral gonadal dysgenesis
    B. Unilateral gonadal dysgenesis
    C. Germ cell aplasia
    D. Spermatogenic arrest
    E. Hypospermatogenesis
44. Wind-swept appearance on testicular biopsy is characteristic of:
    A. Klinefelter syndrome
    B. Del Castillo syndrome
    C. Prader–Willi syndrome
    D. Kallmann syndrome
    E. Down syndrome
45. Classic seminoma is most common in:
    A. Infants
    B. Children
    C. Adolescents
    D. Middle age
    E. Elderly
46. Spermatocytic seminoma is most common in:
    A. Infants
    B. Children
    C. Adolescents
    D. Middle age
    E. Elderly
47. Which tumor is NOT associated with elevated α-fetoprotein?
    A. Spermatocytic seminoma
    B. Yolk sac carcinoma
    C. Testicular teratoma
    D. Leydig cell tumor
    E. Gonadal stromal tumor

48. Non-testicular seminomas are more common in:
    A. Infants
    B. Children
    C. Adults
    D. Elderly
49. Which of the following is NOT a non-testicular germ cell tumor?
    A. Choriocarcinoma
    B. Yolk sac carcinoma
    C. Embryonal carcinoma
    D. Spermatocytic carcinoma
    E. Sertoli cell tumor
50. Alpha-fetoprotein is produced by:
    A. Trophoblasts
    B. Yolk sac cells
    C. Germ cells
    D. Stromal cells
    E. Placenta
51. Which of the following tumor markers is NOT recommended in smokers?
    A. Placental alkaline phosphatase
    B. Alpha-fetoprotein
    C. HCG
    D. Lactate dehydrogenase
    E. A + D
52. The most reliable lymph node to denote testicular metastasis is:
    A. Superficial inguinal nodes
    B. Supraclavicular node
    C. Deep inguinal node
    D. Common iliac node
    E. None of the above
53. Which of the following is NOT an indication for ordering immunologic semen tests?
    A. Leukocytospermia
    B. Unexplained infertility
    C. Poor postcoital test
    D. Sperm adherence
    E. Asthenozoospermia
54. Which of the following tests detects anti-sperm antibodies in seminal fluid?
    A. Flow cytometry
    B. Western blot
    C. Gel agglutination
    D. Kremer's test

55. The incidence of immunological infertility is:
    A. 10%
    B. 30%
    C. 35%
    D. 40%
    E. 50%
56. Which of the following is NOT true about unexplained infertility?
    A. Abnormal semen analysis
    B. Immunological cause
    C. Genetic defect
    D. Normal female partner
    E. Excess reactive oxygen species
57. The incidence of azoospermia as a cause of male infertility is:
    A. 10%
    B. 20%
    C. 30%
    D. 40%
    E. 50%
58. The consistency of testes in obstructive azoospermia is:
    A. Soft
    B. Firm
    C. Normal
    D. Hard
59. The incidence of intratesticular obstructive azoospermia is:
    A. 5%
    B. 10%
    C. 15%
    D. 20%
    E. 25%
60. The incidence of ejaculatory duct obstruction azoospermia is:
    A. 1–5%
    B. 5–10%
    C. 10–15%
    D. >20%
61. Which of the following is NOT an epididymal marker?
    A. L-carnitine
    B. Sialic acid
    C. Zinc
    D. Alpha-glucosidase
    E. Glycerophosphocholine
62. Which is NOT a numerical chromosomal abnormality?
    A. Noonan syndrome
    B. XYY male
    C. Klinefelter syndrome
    D. Young syndrome

63. Which of the following is a structural chromosomal abnormality?
    A. Sex reversal syndrome
    B. Klinefelter syndrome
    C. Young syndrome
    D. Noonan syndrome
64. The consistency of testes in Klinefelter syndrome is:
    A. Firm
    B. Soft
    C. Normal
    D. Hard
65. Nondisjunction of primary spermatocytes leads to:
    A. XYY male
    B. Klinefelter syndrome
    C. XX male
    D. Noonan syndrome
    E. Cystic fibrosis
66. Nondisjunction at secondary meiotic division leads to:
    A. XYY male
    B. Klinefelter syndrome
    C. XX male
    D. Noonan syndrome
    E. Cystic fibrosis
67. Jacob's syndrome is a synonym for:
    A. XXY syndrome
    B. XO syndrome
    C. XYY syndrome
    D. XX male syndrome
    E. XXXY syndrome
68. Normal LH and testosterone levels are seen in:
    A. XXY syndrome
    B. XO syndrome
    C. XYY syndrome
    D. XX male syndrome
    E. XXXY syndrome
69. The incidence of post-zygotic mitotic error in Jacob's syndrome is:
    A. 5%
    B. 10%
    C. 15%
    D. 20%
    E. 22%
70. Mutation in RAS/RAF/MEK/ERK signaling pathway is seen in:
    A. XXY syndrome
    B. XO syndrome
    C. XYY syndrome
    D. Noonan Syndrome
    E. XXXY syndrome

71. SOS1 and RAF1 gene mutations are seen in:
    A. XXY syndrome
    B. Noonan syndrome
    C. XYY syndrome
    D. XX male syndrome
    E. XXXY syndrome
72. The incidence of mosaic trisomy 21 is:
    A. <2%
    B. 4%
    C. 6%
    D. 8%
    E. 10%
73. The incidence of translocation trisomy 21 is:
    A. <2%
    B. 4%
    C. 6%
    D. 8%
    E. 10%
74. De la Chapelle syndrome is a synonym for:
    A. XXY syndrome
    B. XO syndrome
    C. XYY syndrome
    D. XX male syndrome
    E. XXXY syndrome
75. The incidence of SRY-negative variant of XX male is:
    A. 5–10%
    B. 10–15%
    C. 10–20%
    D. 20–25%
    E. 25–30%
76. The SRY-negative variant of XX male typically presents with:
    A. Short stature
    B. Ambiguous genitalia
    C. Normal male genitalia
    D. Hyperprolactinemia
    E. Palmoplantar keratoderma
77. The palmoplantar keratoderma in syndromic XX male is due to:
    A. R-spondin–1 mutation
    B. KALIG-1
    C. PROK2
    D. GPR54/KISS1
    E. SPATA16

78. Facial dysmorphic features in XX male are due to translocation of:
    A. SOX9 gene
    B. SOX3 gene
    C. PROK2
    D. GPR54/KISS1
    E. SPATA16
79. Developmental delay in XX male syndrome is due to defect in:
    A. SOX9 gene
    B. SOX3 gene
    C. PROK2
    D. GPR54/KISS1
    E. SPATA16
80. Y chromosome microdeletion is less common if sperm concentration is more than:
    A. 1 million
    B. 2 million
    C. 3 million
    D. 4 million
    E. 5 million
81. The incidence of AZFa microdeletion is:
    A. 5%
    B. 10%
    C. 12%
    D. 15%
    E. 17%
82. The incidence of AZFb microdeletion is:
    A. 5%
    B. 10%
    C. 12%
    D. 15%
    E. 17%
83. The incidence of AZFbc microdeletion is:
    A. 5%
    B. 10%
    C. 12%
    D. 15%
    E. 17%
84. The frequency of gr/gr deletion in oligozoospermia is about:
    A. 5%
    B. 10%
    C. 12%
    D. 15%
    E. 17%

85. Activating LH receptor mutation leads to:
    A. Delayed puberty
    B. Precocious puberty
    C. Ambiguous genitalia
    D. Micropenis
    E. Infertility
86. CatSper gene mutation leads to:
    A. Sperm hyperactivation defects
    B. Spermatogenesis defects
    C. Delayed puberty
    D. Precocious puberty
    E. A + C
87. Which of the following is NOT a criterion of absent vas deferens?
    A. Low sperm volume
    B. Azoospermia
    C. Absent seminal fructose
    D. Absent seminal carnitine
    E. Sperm agglutination
88. Cystic fibrosis is NOT characterized by:
    A. Normal sweat chloride test
    B. Defective CFTR gene
    C. Pancreatic insufficiency
    D. Azoospermia
    E. Defective formation of male accessory glands
89. Which of the following is true about Young syndrome?
    A. Normal sweat chloride test
    B. Defective CFTR gene
    C. Pancreatic insufficiency
    D. Defective formation of male accessory glands
90. The testicular tissue is preserved in:
    A. Saline
    B. Formalin
    C. Picric acid
    D. Bouin solution
91. Johnson score 9 (a histopathological grading system used to assess the degree of spermatogenesis in testicular biopsies, ranging from 1 = no germ cells to 10 = complete spermatogenesis) means:
    A. No germinal cells, Sertoli cells only
    B. Spermatogonia only
    C. No spermatozoa/spermatids, many spermatocytes
    D. No spermatozoa/late spermatids, many early spermatids
    E. Slightly impaired spermatogenesis, many late spermatids, disorganized epithelium

92. Johnson score 7 means:
    A. No germinal cells, Sertoli cells only
    B. Spermatogonia only
    C. No spermatozoa/spermatids, many spermatocytes
    D. No spermatozoa/late spermatids, many early spermatids
    E. Slightly impaired spermatogenesis, many late spermatids, disorganized epithelium
93. Johnson score 5 means:
    A. No germinal cells, Sertoli cells only
    B. Spermatogonia only
    C. No spermatozoa/spermatids, many spermatocytes
    D. No spermatozoa/late spermatids, many early spermatids
    E. Slightly impaired spermatogenesis, many late spermatids, disorganized epithelium
94. Johnson score 3 means:
    A. No germinal cells, Sertoli cells only
    B. Spermatogonia only
    C. No spermatozoa/spermatids, many spermatocytes
    D. No spermatozoa/late spermatids, many early spermatids
    E. Slightly impaired spermatogenesis, many late spermatids, disorganized epithelium
95. Johnson score 2 means:
    A. No germinal cells, Sertoli cells only
    B. Spermatogonia only
    C. No spermatozoa/spermatids, many spermatocytes
    D. No spermatozoa/late spermatids, many early spermatids
    E. Slightly impaired spermatogenesis, many late spermatids, disorganized epithelium
96. Which of the following is NOT a method of male contraception?
    A. Adjudin
    B. CatSper agonists
    C. Retinoic acid receptor antagonists
    D. Gendarussa
    E. Intra-vas device
97. SPINLW1 is:
    A. Male contraceptive method
    B. 135 amino acid protein
    C. Serine protease stimulator
    D. Secreted by seminal vesicles
    E. Non-androgen mediated
98. Cold-inducible RNA-binding protein is essential for:
    A. Testicular tissue support
    B. Testicular heat regulation
    C. Sperm migration
    D. A + C
    E. Prevention of excess ROS

99. Which of the following is NOT affected by varicocele?
    A. Topoisomerase
    B. DNA polymerase
    C. Cold-inducible RNA protein
    D. Reactive oxygen species
    E. Trinucleotide expansion
100. Which of the following is NOT a main indication for varicocelectomy?
    A. Testicular atrophy
    B. Sperm DNA damage
    C. Genetic factor
    D. Testicular pain
    E. Grade III varicocele

✅ Key Takeaways

- **Semen analysis** remains the cornerstone of infertility evaluation.
- **Varicocele**, infections, and endocrine disorders are treatable causes.
- **Y-chromosome microdeletions** and CFTR mutations affect fertility.
- Management includes **lifestyle changes**, **medical therapy**, or **surgical/ART interventions**.
- Collaboration with urologists and IVF specialists is often necessary.

✅ Answer Key (1–100)

1. D
2. E
3. A
4. A
5. D
6. D
7. E
8. C
9. E
10. B
11. C
12. E
13. C
14. B
15. B
16. C
17. C
18. D
19. C
20. C

21. D
22. E
23. D
24. C
25. A
26. E
27. C
28. D
29. D
30. A
31. E
32. E
33. D
34. C
35. B
36. C
37. A
38. D
39. E
40. E
41. A
42. E
43. C
44. B
45. D
46. E
47. A
48. C
49. E
50. B
51. A
52. B
53. D
54. D
55. A
56. A
57. A
58. C
59. C
60. A
61. C
62. D
63. A
64. A
65. B

66. A
67. C
68. C
69. C
70. D
71. B
72. A
73. B
74. D
75. C
76. B
77. A
78. B
79. B
80. E
81. A
82. B
83. D
84. A
85. B
86. A
87. E
88. A
89. A
90. D
91. E
92. D
93. C
94. B
95. A
96. B
97. D
98. D
99. E
100. C

Explanations (1–100)

1. Subclinical varicocele, detected only by imaging, has not been shown to improve fertility outcomes when surgically corrected. Evidence indicates that spontaneous pregnancy rates are unaffected by intervention in these cases. Management is therefore conservative, with surgery reserved for clinically palpable varicoceles that affect semen quality or cause discomfort.

2. Testicular biopsy during varicocele repair is not routinely needed, as studies show little added benefit. It is only justified in cases of progressive testicular impairment, such as marked asymmetry or raised FSH, where it provides diagnostic value and allows sperm cryopreservation.
3. In children, varicocele surgery is indicated when progressive testicular growth retardation or persistent scrotal pain is documented. Conservative observation is often preferred, but intervention preserves testicular volume and safeguards future fertility when growth impairment is confirmed. Asymptomatic or subclinical varicoceles are managed conservatively with yearly testicular volume and Doppler follow-up. Bilateral palpation alone or hormonal changes are *not* indications for surgery. Poor semen parameters can guide decisions in older adolescents, but the primary accepted indication remains **progressive testicular growth retardation or persistent scrotal pain**.
4. Preoperative varicocelectomy before assisted reproduction improves sperm DNA quality and motility, which significantly enhances fertilization outcomes. Clinical studies have demonstrated a doubling of embryo implantation rates, especially beneficial in couples with repeated ART failures.
5. Improved pregnancy rates after varicocelectomy are linked to enhanced sperm chromatin packaging and reduced oxidative stress. Even without marked improvement in sperm count or motility, the restoration of DNA integrity increases the likelihood of conception.
6. Hydrocele surgery is best approached inguinally when testicular pathology is suspected, excision is more effective than plication in preventing relapse, and hematoma remains the most common complication, making these key considerations in management.
7. Spermatic vein ligation is most effectively performed by the subinguinal approach, which reduces morbidity though technically demanding; hydrocele is the commonest complication, and inadvertent testicular artery injury can cause atrophy.
8. In obstructive azoospermia with normal FSH, microsurgical epididymal sperm retrieval is preferred because it provides high-quality motile sperm for assisted reproduction while preserving testicular tissue.
9. AZFa microdeletions are incompatible with spermatogenesis, so neither varicocele repair nor testicular biopsy offers benefit in such patients, and assisted reproduction cannot be attempted with their gametes.
10. Testicular descent occurs in two phases: the first (transabdominal) is INSL3-dependent, and the second (inguinoscrotal) is androgen-dependent, highlighting the essential role of androgens in the latter stage.
11. Sperm cryopreservation requires liquid nitrogen storage at −196 °C to maintain long-term viability and prevent cellular damage, making this the standard temperature for fertility preservation.
12. Drugs such as ketoconazole, spironolactone, colchicine, and estrogens impair spermatogenesis by disrupting hormonal balance or directly affecting germ cells, and all are recognized causes of impaired fertility.

13. Spermatogenesis is temperature-sensitive, and a fever within the last 6 months can transiently impair sperm production, leading to oligozoospermia or asthenozoospermia for up to one full spermatogenic cycle.
14. For natural conception, ejaculation every 2 days optimizes sperm quality and concentration, balancing replenishment and avoiding both sperm depletion and excessive stasis that can impair motility.
15. Prostaglandins in semen are secreted by the seminal vesicles, which also produce fructose to nourish sperm, making this gland a central contributor to seminal plasma composition.
16. In non-mosaic Klinefelter's with varicocele, biopsy is prioritized because sperm retrieval opportunities are limited, and performing it alongside varicocele repair may maximize fertility chances before further testicular decline.
17. Karyotyping is essential in azoospermic men when a primary testicular lesion is confirmed, as genetic abnormalities such as Klinefelter syndrome or Y chromosome deletions are frequent underlying causes of infertility.
18. Seminal vesiculography is not routinely indicated and is reserved only before surgical correction of suspected ejaculatory duct obstruction, as it provides anatomic details needed for operative planning.
19. Intratubular germ cell neoplasia in situ almost inevitably progresses to invasive testicular cancer if left untreated, necessitating close monitoring or intervention to prevent malignant transformation.
20. In obstructive azoospermia with normal FSH, microsurgical epididymal retrieval is preferred because it yields motile sperm directly from storage sites while preserving testicular integrity and avoiding unnecessary biopsy.
21. A patient with clinical varicocele, abnormal semen, and normal hormones benefits most from varicocelectomy, which can improve semen quality and restore natural fertility, unlike medical therapy or ART alone.
22. Subinguinal microsurgical varicocelectomy is considered the gold standard technique due to its lowest recurrence and complication rates, as well as superior preservation of arteries and lymphatics.
23. Varicocele results from dilatation of the internal spermatic veins due to incompetent valves, leading to venous reflux and scrotal hyperthermia, which negatively affect spermatogenesis.
24. Mild hyperprolactinemia in infertile men may be explained by regular polypharmacy, since many drugs interfere with dopamine pathways or prolactin metabolism, causing modest elevations without tumor presence.
25. Thc blood testis barrier is formed by tight junctions between Sertoli cells, which protect developing germ cells from immune attack and create a specialized microenvironment essential for spermatogenesis.
26. With chronic obstruction, sperm motility is highest in the cauda epididymis, as this region stores mature sperm capable of progressive motility, whereas proximal segments contain less mature sperm.
27. Spermiogenesis is the final stage of spermatogenesis, involving spermatid remodeling, acrosome formation, flagellum development, and nuclear condensation, turning round spermatids into mature spermatozoa.

28. Cadmium can replace zinc in DNA polymerase, impairing enzymatic activity and DNA replication, leading to mutagenesis and defective spermatogenesis.
29. Arsenic interferes with DNA synthesis by substituting for phosphorus, causing unstable DNA backbones and impairing normal cellular replication.
30. Spermatogenesis can be reversibly suppressed by radiation doses around 500 rads, as higher exposures cause irreversible germ cell loss and permanent infertility.
31. Heroin is not directly linked to decreased androgen levels, unlike ketoconazole, pesticides, spironolactone, and alcohol, which disrupt hormonal regulation or Leydig cell function.
32. Infertility in hypothyroidism is not due to GnRH mutation but instead results from low SHBG, impaired spermatogenesis, and altered estrogen metabolism.
33. Kallmann syndrome is caused by mutations in genes like KALIG-1, PROK2, and KISS1; SPATA16 is associated with globozoospermia, not Kallmann.
34. Normosmic hypogonadotropic hypogonadism is associated with PROK2 mutations, distinguishing it from Kallmann syndrome, which presents with anosmia.
35. Bimanual synkinesis (mirror movements) is a hallmark of Kallmann syndrome due to defective neuronal migration and disrupted GnRH neuronal pathways.
36. Kallmann syndrome has an incidence of about 1 in 10,000 males, making it a rare but important cause of delayed puberty and infertility.
37. The classic inheritance of Kallmann syndrome is X-linked recessive through KAL1 mutations, although autosomal dominant and recessive forms also exist.
38. Prader–Willi syndrome occurs in about 1 in 15,000 births and is caused by paternal deletion of chromosome 15q11–13, presenting with obesity, hypogonadism, and infertility.
39. Retinitis pigmentosa is more frequently seen in Bardet–Biedl syndrome, which also features obesity, polydactyly, hypogonadism, and renal anomalies.
40. Polydactyly is strongly associated with Bardet–Biedl syndrome, differentiating it from other genetic syndromes linked with male infertility.
41. Spastic paraplegia is a feature of Laurence–Moon–Biedl syndrome, a related ciliopathy with overlapping features of Bardet–Biedl.
42. Laurence–Moon–Biedl syndrome has an incidence of about 1 in 160,000 live births, making it much rarer than Kallmann or Prader–Willi syndromes.
43. Del Castillo syndrome is another name for germ cell aplasia (Sertoli cell–only syndrome), a cause of non-obstructive azoospermia with absent spermatogenesis.
44. A "wind-swept" appearance on testicular biopsy is typical of Sertoli cell–only syndrome, reflecting absent germinal epithelium with only Sertoli cells remaining.
45. Classic seminoma usually arises in middle-aged men and is the most common type of testicular germ cell tumor in this age group.
46. Spermatocytic seminoma is most frequent in elderly men, typically with indolent growth and a better prognosis than classic seminoma.

47. Pure spermatocytic seminoma is not associated with raised alpha-fetoprotein, unlike yolk sac carcinoma or mixed germ cell tumors.
48. Extragonadal seminomas most often occur in adults, typically in midline locations such as mediastinum or retroperitoneum.
49. Sertoli cell tumors are sex cord–stromal tumors, not germ cell tumors, distinguishing them from choriocarcinoma, yolk sac, and embryonal carcinomas.
50. Alpha-fetoprotein is secreted by yolk sac cells in embryonic life and yolk sac tumors in adults, serving as a diagnostic tumor marker.
51. Placental alkaline phosphatase is elevated in smokers and therefore unreliable as a tumor marker in this group, while AFP, HCG, and LDH remain useful.
52. The supraclavicular lymph node is the most reliable sentinel for testicular cancer metastasis, reflecting typical retroperitoneal and thoracic spread patterns.
53. Sperm adherence is not a standard indication for ordering immunologic semen testing, unlike leukocytospermia, unexplained infertility, poor postcoital test, or asthenozoospermia.
54. Kremer's test is the classical method for detecting antisperm antibodies in seminal plasma by evaluating sperm–mucus penetration.
55. Immunological infertility accounts for approximately 10% of male infertility cases, involving antisperm antibodies that impair sperm motility and function.
56. Unexplained infertility requires normal semen analysis and partner evaluation; abnormal semen analysis excludes this diagnosis, making option A incorrect.
57. Azoospermia contributes to about 10% of cases of male infertility and can be obstructive or non-obstructive in nature.
58. In obstructive azoospermia, testes are of normal consistency and volume since spermatogenesis is intact but sperm transport is blocked.
59. Intratesticular obstruction accounts for about 15% of cases of obstructive azoospermia, most often within the seminiferous tubules.
60. Ejaculatory duct obstruction causes azoospermia in approximately 1–5% of infertile men, identified by low-volume semen with absent fructose.
61. Zinc is not an epididymal marker but rather a prostatic marker, whereas carnitine, sialic acid, glucosidase, and GPC are epididymal.
62. Young syndrome is not a numerical chromosomal abnormality; it is an obstructive condition with azoospermia and chronic respiratory disease.
63. Sex reversal syndrome is a structural chromosomal abnormality due to translocation or rearrangement involving the SRY gene.
64. Testes in Klinefelter syndrome are typically firm due to extensive seminiferous tubule fibrosis and hyalinization.
65. Primary spermatocyte nondisjunction leads to Klinefelter syndrome (47,XXY), resulting in hypergonadotropic hypogonadism and infertility.
66. Nondisjunction during secondary meiotic division results in XYY males, also known as Jacob's syndrome.
67. Jacob's syndrome refers to males with a 47,XYY karyotype, often presenting with tall stature and normal fertility.

68. XYY males generally have normal testosterone and LH levels, which helps differentiate them from Klinefelter syndrome.
69. Post-zygotic mitotic errors account for about 15% of Jacob's syndrome cases, leading to mosaicism.
70. Noonan syndrome results from mutations in the RAS/RAF/MEK/ERK signaling pathway, presenting with short stature, cardiac defects, and infertility.
71. SOS1 and RAF1 gene mutations are specifically linked with Noonan syndrome, part of the RASopathy spectrum.
72. Mosaic trisomy 21 occurs in less than 2% of Down syndrome cases, caused by mitotic nondisjunction after fertilization.
73. Translocation trisomy 21 accounts for about 4% of Down syndrome cases, involving Robertsonian translocations.
74. De la Chapelle syndrome is synonymous with XX male syndrome, due to translocation of SRY to the X chromosome.
75. The SRY-negative variant of XX male occurs in 10–20% of cases, usually presenting with ambiguous genitalia due to absent testis-determining factor.
76. The SRY-negative XX male typically presents with ambiguous genitalia, since without SRY gene expression testicular differentiation does not occur normally.
77. Palmoplantar keratoderma in syndromic XX male is due to R-spondin–1 mutation, a rare finding linking dermatologic features with sex reversal.
78. Facial dysmorphic features in XX male result from translocation of the SOX3 gene, which alters craniofacial development.
79. Developmental delay in XX male syndrome is also linked to SOX3 gene defects, reflecting its role in brain development and cognition.
80. Y chromosome microdeletions are less common when sperm concentration exceeds 5 million/mL, making genetic testing more relevant in severe oligozoospermia.
81. AZFa microdeletions occur in about 5% of cases and are associated with Sertoli cell–only syndrome and complete absence of sperm.
82. AZFb deletions occur in approximately 10% of men with Y microdeletions and result in spermatogenic arrest.
83. AZFbc deletions are found in around 15% of cases and cause severe infertility due to combined gene loss across spermatogenesis regions.
84. The gr/gr deletion occurs in about 5% of oligozoospermic men, reducing sperm counts but not always causing complete azoospermia.
85. Activating mutations of the LH receptor cause precocious puberty by stimulating testosterone secretion independent of gonadotropin drive.
86. CatSper gene mutations lead to defective sperm hyperactivation, impairing motility and the ability to penetrate the zona pellucida.
87. Absence of vas deferens is defined by azoospermia, low semen volume, and absent fructose or carnitine, but sperm agglutination is not a diagnostic criterion.

88. Cystic fibrosis is characterized by defective CFTR gene, pancreatic insufficiency, azoospermia, and abnormal accessory gland development, but not a normal sweat chloride test.
89. Young syndrome is associated with obstructive azoospermia, chronic sinusitis, and bronchiectasis, while the sweat chloride test remains normal, distinguishing it from cystic fibrosis.
90. Testicular tissue samples are preserved in Bouin solution, which maintains histologic detail for pathological examination.
91. A Johnson score of 9 indicates slightly impaired spermatogenesis, with many late spermatids present but disorganized epithelium.
92. A Johnson score of 7 reflects absence of spermatozoa or late spermatids but presence of many early spermatids.
93. A Johnson score of 5 corresponds to the absence of spermatids but the presence of numerous spermatocytes, showing maturation arrest.
94. A Johnson score of 3 indicates only spermatogonia are present, reflecting very early arrest of spermatogenesis.
95. A Johnson score of 2 corresponds to Sertoli cell–only syndrome, with no germinal cells present.
96. CatSper agonists are not contraceptive methods; instead, antagonists are studied for male contraception, making agonists inappropriate for suppression.
97. SPINLW1 is a 135–amino acid seminal vesicle protein, not a contraceptive method, with a role in semen physiology.
98. Cold-inducible RNA-binding protein is essential for testicular heat regulation and sperm migration, making it vital for fertility.
99. Varicocele affects sperm enzymes and increases reactive oxygen species but does not influence trinucleotide expansions, which are genetic mutations.
100. Main indications for varicocelectomy include testicular atrophy, scrotal pain, sperm DNA damage, and clinical Grade III varicocele, while genetic factors are not corrected surgically.

Further Reading

The explanations in this chapter are supported by the following key references:

1. Agarwal A, Baskaran S, Parekh N, et al. Male infertility. Lancet. 2021;397(10271):319–33.
2. Jungwirth A, Diemer T, Kopa Z, et al. European Association of Urology guidelines on male infertility. Eur Urol. 2018;73(4):424–38.
3. World Health Organization. WHO Laboratory Manual for the examination and processing of human semen. 6th ed. Geneva: WHO; 2021.
4. Krausz C, Riera-Escamilla A. Genetics of male infertility. Nat Rev Urol. 2018;15(6):369–84.
5. Ramasamy R, Schlegel PN. Medical therapy for male infertility. Urol Clin N Am. 2012;39(4):453–64.
6. Esteves SC, Miyaoka R, Agarwal A. An update on the clinical assessment of the infertile male. Clinics (Sao Paulo). 2011;66(4):691–700.

17 Assisted Reproductive Techniques

Learning Objectives

- Understand indications for ART in male infertility.
- Learn procedures: IUI, IVF, ICSI, TESE, and PESA.
- Explore success rates and limitations.
- Identify ethical and religious considerations in ART.
- Recognize complications and follow-up protocols.

Select the Single Best Answer

1. The first successful IVF baby ("Louise Brown") was born in:
   A. 1974
   B. 1978
   C. 1982
   D. 1985
2. Which of the following is NOT an absolute indication for IVF?
   A. Bilateral tubal blockage
   B. Severe male factor infertility
   C. Endometriosis grade IV
   D. Unexplained infertility <1 year
3. Which is the commonest ovarian stimulation drug used in ART?
   A. Clomiphene citrate
   B. Letrozole
   C. Recombinant FSH
   D. Human menopausal gonadotropin
4. The "antagonist protocol" in controlled ovarian stimulation is based on:
   A. GnRH agonist continuous administration
   B. Pulsatile GnRH

M. S. M. Hasan, M. L. Elsaie, *Comprehensive MCQs in Andrology*, Trends in Andrology and Sexual Medicine, https://doi.org/10.1007/978-3-032-20623-7_17

   C. GnRH antagonist blocking pituitary
   D. None of the above
5. The "long agonist protocol" prevents:
   A. Premature LH surge
   B. Follicular atresia
   C. Oocyte aging
   D. Premature ovulation only
6. The sperm preparation technique most commonly used in IVF is:
   A. Simple washing
   B. Swim-up
   C. Density gradient centrifugation
   D. Filtration method
7. ICSI is preferred in:
   A. Oligoasthenoteratozoospermia
   B. Severe teratozoospermia
   C. Non-obstructive azoospermia with retrieved sperm
   D. All of the above
8. Which of the following is a contraindication to ICSI?
   A. AZFa microdeletion
   B. Obstructive azoospermia
   C. Retrograde ejaculation
   D. Ejaculatory duct obstruction
9. The fertilization rate in ICSI is approximately:
   A. 40–50%
   B. 60–70%
   C. 70–80%
   D. 90–95%
10. Testicular sperm extraction (TESE) is most appropriate for:
   A. Congenital absence of vas deferens
   B. Varicocele
   C. Retrograde ejaculation
   D. Post-infective epididymal obstruction
11. The optimal size of ovarian follicle before triggering ovulation is:
   A. 12–14 mm
   B. 14–16 mm
   C. 18–20 mm
   D. 22–24 mm
12. The "trigger" injection in IVF cycles is most commonly:
   A. Recombinant LH
   B. hCG
   C. GnRH antagonist
   D. Estradiol
13. The most common complication of ovarian stimulation is:
   A. Ectopic pregnancy
   B. Ovarian hyperstimulation syndrome (OHSS)
   C. Luteal phase defect
   D. Miscarriage

14. Which of the following embryos is preferred for transfer in IVF?
    A. Day 2 embryo (4-cell)
    B. Day 3 embryo (8-cell)
    C. Day 5 blastocyst
    D. Day 1 pronuclear stage
15. The “freeze-all” strategy in IVF helps reduce the risk of:
    A. OHSS
    B. Endometriosis recurrence
    C. Oocyte aging
    D. Ovarian torsion
16. The average live birth rate per IVF cycle globally is around:
    A. 10–15%
    B. 20–25%
    C. 30–35%
    D. 40–50%
17. Multiple pregnancy risk is highest with:
    A. ICSI
    B. IVF with 2–3 embryos transferred
    C. Ovarian stimulation with clomiphene only
    D. Frozen embryo transfer
18. Preimplantation genetic testing (PGT-A) is primarily used for:
    A. Detecting structural chromosomal rearrangements
    B. Detecting aneuploidy
    C. Detecting monogenic disorders only
    D. Sex selection only
19. The risk of congenital malformations in IVF compared to natural conception is:
    A. Significantly higher (5–10-fold)
    B. Mildly increased (1.2–1.4-fold)
    C. Equal
    D. Lower
20. Mitochondrial replacement therapy is mainly designed for:
    A. Male infertility
    B. Female infertility due to poor ovarian reserve
    C. Prevention of transmission of mitochondrial diseases
    D. Enhancing embryo implantation
21. OHSS is mainly due to elevated levels of:
    A. Estradiol
    B. LH
    C. hCG
    D. Progesterone
22. The most serious complication of OHSS is:
    A. Ascites
    B. Thrombosis
    C. Renal failure
    D. Ovarian torsion

23. The main strategy to prevent OHSS in high-risk women is:
    A. Use of hMG instead of FSH
    B. Coasting (withholding gonadotropins)
    C. High-dose trigger
    D. Transfer all embryos fresh
24. The risk of ovarian cancer after IVF is:
    A. Clearly increased
    B. Clearly decreased
    C. Uncertain/slightly increased in borderline tumors
    D. Absent
25. The maximum recommended number of embryos for transfer in women <35 years (per ASRM/ESHRE):
    A. 1
    B. 2
    C. 3
    D. 4
26. Which ethical issue is NOT commonly debated in ART?
    A. Posthumous reproduction
    B. Preimplantation sex selection
    C. Use in HIV-discordant couples
    D. Use in PCOS patients
27. Surrogacy is defined as:
    A. Use of donor oocytes
    B. Use of donor sperm
    C. A woman carrying pregnancy for another couple
    D. None of the above
28. Gestational surrogacy differs from traditional surrogacy in:
    A. Use of donor egg
    B. No genetic link between surrogate and child
    C. Multiple embryo transfer
    D. Need for IVF only in traditional
29. Egg donation is recommended especially for:
    A. Women with diminished ovarian reserve
    B. Male factor infertility
    C. Tubal infertility
    D. Endometriosis
30. The legal age limit for egg donation in most countries is:
    A. <30 years
    B. <35 years
    C. <40 years
    D. <45 years
31. Which of the following improves fertilization in older women's eggs?
    A. ICSI
    B. IMSI (intracytoplasmic morphologically selected sperm injection)
    C. Assisted oocyte activation
    D. Artificial zona drilling

32. The term "embryo glue" refers to:
    A. Hyaluronic acid enriched transfer media
    B. Synthetic adhesive used in embryo culture
    C. Endometrial scratching
    D. Progesterone gel
33. Time-lapse embryo imaging is used for:
    A. Continuous culture without removing embryos
    B. Genetic testing
    C. Preventing OHSS
    D. Improving sperm motility
34. Which technique helps in severe male factor infertility with high DNA fragmentation?
    A. IMSI
    B. PICSI (physiological ICSI)
    C. TESE
    D. CASA (computer-assisted sperm analysis)
35. Vitrification refers to:
    A. Slow freezing of embryos
    B. Rapid flash freezing without ice crystal formation
    C. Use of liquid nitrogen storage only
    D. Freeze-drying
36. Oocyte cryopreservation is recommended for:
    A. Fertility preservation in cancer patients
    B. Delayed motherhood (social freezing)
    C. Donor programs
    D. All of the above
37. Embryo biopsy for PGT is ideally done at:
    A. Day 1 pronuclear stage
    B. Day 3 cleavage stage
    C. Day 5 blastocyst trophectoderm
    D. Any stage
38. In oocyte vitrification, the main cryoprotectants are:
    A. DMSO and ethylene glycol
    B. Mannitol and glucose
    C. Albumin and saline
    D. Urea and glycerol
39. In sperm selection, hyaluronic acid binding test is used for:
    A. Selecting motile sperm
    B. Selecting mature sperm with intact DNA
    C. Enhancing fertilization rate
    D. Screening sperm morphology only
40. Artificial oocyte activation uses:
    A. Calcium ionophores
    B. Potassium channels
    C. Estrogen
    D. Progesterone

41. In PCOS patients undergoing ART, the stimulation protocol of choice is:
    A. Long agonist
    B. Antagonist protocol
    C. Natural cycle IVF
    D. Mini-IVF
42. In endometriosis stage IV, the best ART option is:
    A. IUI
    B. IVF
    C. ICSI
    D. Natural conception
43. In azoospermia due to Klinefelter syndrome, ART involves:
    A. Ejaculated sperm
    B. Donor sperm only
    C. Testicular sperm retrieval + ICSI
    D. No option available
44. The most effective strategy for unexplained infertility >2 years is:
    A. Expectant management
    B. Ovulation induction + timed intercourse
    C. IUI with gonadotropins
    D. IVF
45. For HIV-positive male and HIV-negative female couples, the safest ART method is:
    A. Unprotected intercourse timed
    B. ICSI with washed sperm
    C. IVF with donor sperm
    D. Surrogacy only
46. Luteal phase support in IVF is usually provided with:
    A. Progesterone
    B. Estradiol
    C. hCG
    D. Clomiphene
47. Which factor MOST influences IVF success?
    A. Sperm quality
    B. Embryologist skill
    C. Maternal age
    D. Endometrial thickness
48. Recurrent implantation failure is best investigated with:
    A. Endometrial biopsy for receptivity array
    B. Karyotyping
    C. Hysteroscopy
    D. All of the above
49. The recommended endometrial thickness for embryo transfer is at least:
    A. 6 mm
    B. 7 mm
    C. 8 mm
    D. 10 mm

50. The preferred method to reduce twin pregnancy risk without lowering live birth rate is:
    A. Transfer two embryos routinely
    B. Freeze-all policy
    C. Elective single blastocyst transfer
    D. Use only natural cycle IVF

✅ Key Takeaways

- ART provides hope for severe male factor infertility.
- ICSI is commonly used for low sperm count/motility.
- Surgical sperm retrieval (TESE, PESA) is vital in azoospermia.
- Counseling on outcomes, risks, and ethics is mandatory.
- Advances in ART continue to evolve male fertility management.

✅ Answer Key (1–50)

1. B
2. D
3. C
4. C
5. A
6. C
7. D
8. A
9. C
10. D
11. C
12. B
13. B
14. C
15. A
16. C
17. B
18. B
19. B
20. C
21. C
22. B
23. B
24. C
25. A
26. D
27. C

28. B
29. A
30. B
31. C
32. A
33. A
34. B
35. B
36. D
37. C
38. A
39. B
40. A
41. B
42. B
43. C
44. D
45. B
46. A
47. C
48. D
49. B
50. C

Explanations (1–50)

1. Louise Brown, the world's first IVF baby, was born in 1978 in the UK. The procedure was pioneered by Dr. Patrick Steptoe and Dr. Robert Edwards. This landmark event revolutionized fertility treatment and established IVF as a standard reproductive option for tubal and other causes of infertility.
2. IVF is reserved for established infertility, typically after 12–24 months of failed conception attempts. Early unexplained infertility does not justify IVF unless female age is advanced or other risk factors exist. Bilateral tubal blockage and severe male factors are absolute indications.
3. Recombinant FSH is the mainstay for ovarian stimulation in ART because of its purity, potency, and predictable response. It promotes multiple follicular development while reducing variability compared with urinary gonadotropins. Monitoring with ultrasound and estradiol levels ensures safety.
4. The antagonist protocol involves short-term administration of a GnRH antagonist to block LH surges during stimulation. This allows more flexibility and lower risk of ovarian hyperstimulation compared with the long agonist protocol. It is preferred in PCOS and high-risk women.
5. The long GnRH agonist protocol suppresses the pituitary to prevent premature LH surge and ovulation. This synchronization allows controlled stimulation

and retrieval of mature oocytes. It remains a cornerstone in high-responding cycles with predictable outcomes.

6. This is the most common sperm preparation technique used in IVF and ICSI. It separates motile, morphologically normal sperm from debris and leukocytes using layers of media with different densities. The result is a concentrated, high-quality sperm fraction for insemination.
7. ICSI is indicated in severe male factor infertility, including oligoasthenoteratozoospermia and testicular sperm retrieval cases. It involves direct injection of a single sperm into the oocyte cytoplasm, achieving fertilization even with very low sperm counts.
8. AZFa Y-chromosome microdeletions cause complete Sertoli-cell-only syndrome, where no sperm can be retrieved. Hence, ICSI is contraindicated. AZFb/c deletions may still allow surgical sperm retrieval in selected cases. Genetic counseling is mandatory before ART.
9. ICSI achieves fertilization in approximately 70–80% of injected oocytes. The rate depends on oocyte maturity, sperm integrity, and lab conditions. Although highly effective, not all fertilized eggs develop into viable embryos suitable for transfer.
10. In obstructive azoospermia, TESE or MESA provides viable sperm directly from testicular tissue. Post-infective scarring or congenital vasal absence are common indications. Retrieved sperm are cryopreserved or used fresh for ICSI.
11. Follicles of 18–20 mm diameter are considered mature and ready for ovulation triggering. At this size, oocytes have optimal nuclear and cytoplasmic maturity. Smaller follicles may yield immature or non-fertilizable oocytes.
12. Human chorionic gonadotropin mimics the natural LH surge to induce final oocyte maturation before retrieval. It is administered when follicles reach optimal size. Timing retrieval 34–36 h later ensures maximum yield of mature oocytes.
13. OHSS is the most serious iatrogenic complication of ovarian stimulation. It results from increased vascular permeability mediated by VEGF and hCG, leading to ascites, hemoconcentration, and sometimes thrombosis. Prevention is key through careful monitoring and protocol adjustment.
14. Blastocyst transfer improves implantation rates because embryos reaching this stage demonstrate better developmental potential. It also allows better synchronization with endometrial receptivity and enables single-embryo transfer to reduce multiple pregnancy risk.
15. The "freeze-all" strategy, where all embryos are cryopreserved and transfer delayed, reduces OHSS risk. This avoids high progesterone and vascular activity during overstimulated cycles. Frozen-thawed transfer in subsequent cycles yields equal or better success rates.
16. The average global live birth rate per IVF cycle ranges between 30 and 35%, depending mainly on maternal age. Rates exceed 40% in younger women but decline significantly after age 40. Laboratory quality and embryo selection also influence outcomes.

17. Transferring multiple embryos increases pregnancy rates but carries a high risk of twins or triplets. Multiple gestations lead to prematurity and obstetric complications. Elective single-embryo transfer is now the recommended standard to minimize these risks.
18. Preimplantation genetic testing for aneuploidy (PGT-A) screens embryos for chromosomal abnormalities before transfer. It improves implantation and reduces miscarriage, especially in older women. It is distinct from PGT-M for monogenic disorders.
19. ART-conceived children have a slightly higher risk of congenital anomalies, mostly due to parental factors and underlying infertility. Rigorous monitoring and improved laboratory practices continue to minimize this difference.
20. Mitochondrial replacement therapy replaces defective maternal mitochondria with healthy donor ones. This prevents transmission of mitochondrial DNA mutations to offspring. The technique involves spindle or pronuclear transfer before fertilization.
21. OHSS results primarily from exposure to hCG, which increases ovarian VEGF secretion and vascular permeability. Both exogenous and endogenous hCG (from pregnancy) can exacerbate symptoms. Avoiding hCG triggers in high-risk cases prevents severe OHSS.
22. Severe OHSS can lead to hemoconcentration, dehydration, and hypercoagulability, predisposing to thromboembolism. Venous thrombosis, especially in the upper limbs, is a life-threatening complication. Preventive hydration and anticoagulation are vital.
23. Coasting allows estradiol levels to drop before trigger administration, reducing OHSS risk. It involves withholding gonadotropins while monitoring follicular growth. Other strategies include using a GnRH agonist trigger and freeze-all policies.
24. Long-term data show no clear increase in invasive ovarian cancer after IVF, though a minor rise in borderline tumors exists. Careful patient selection and limited exposure to high-dose gonadotropins mitigate potential risks.
25. Current ASRM and ESHRE guidelines recommend elective single embryo transfer for women under 35 with good-quality blastocysts. This maximizes safety and maintains high success rates while minimizing twin pregnancies.
26. Ethical debates focus on posthumous reproduction, sex selection, and use in HIV-discordant couples, not PCOS. PCOS is a standard medical indication for ART, not an ethical concern. Ethics committees guide complex cases involving legal or moral issues.
27. Surrogacy involves one woman (the surrogate) carrying a pregnancy for intended parents. The embryo may result from their gametes or donors. Legal recognition of parental rights varies by jurisdiction.
28. In gestational surrogacy, the surrogate carries an embryo formed from another woman's egg, eliminating genetic relation. In traditional surrogacy, the surrogate's own oocyte is used, making her the genetic mother.

29. Egg donation is ideal for women with poor ovarian reserve, premature ovarian failure, or genetic disease risk. Donor oocytes from young, screened women increase pregnancy success rates significantly.
30. Most programs accept egg donors aged 21–35 due to optimal oocyte quality and lower aneuploidy risk. Younger donors yield higher success rates and lower miscarriage rates compared with older donors.
31. This technique uses calcium ionophores to artificially trigger oocyte activation after ICSI, improving fertilization rates in cases of failed activation. It is particularly beneficial in older women and those with low ooplasmic response.
32. "Embryo glue" is a hyaluronic acid–based medium that enhances embryo adhesion to the endometrium during transfer. It may slightly improve implantation rates, particularly in patients with recurrent implantation failure.
33. Time-lapse imaging systems allow continuous embryo observation within incubators without disturbing conditions. This aids in selecting embryos with optimal developmental kinetics, improving implantation potential and reducing subjective bias.
34. PICSI selects sperm based on hyaluronic acid binding, ensuring maturity and intact DNA integrity. This approach improves embryo quality and outcomes in severe male factor infertility with high DNA fragmentation.
35. Vitrification is an ultrafast freezing method that prevents ice crystal formation, preserving cellular integrity of oocytes and embryos. It has largely replaced slow freezing due to higher survival and implantation rates.
36. Oocyte cryopreservation is used for fertility preservation in cancer therapy, social or age-related delay, and donor programs. Advances in vitrification have made outcomes comparable to fresh oocytes.
37. Blastocyst-stage trophectoderm biopsy minimizes embryo harm and allows accurate chromosomal analysis. It replaces earlier cleavage-stage biopsy, which carried higher mosaicism and lower viability risks.
38. These permeating cryoprotectants prevent ice formation and osmotic injury during vitrification. They ensure cell dehydration and glass-like solidification, maintaining oocyte viability upon thawing.
39. The hyaluronic acid binding assay identifies mature, functionally competent sperm. Only mature sperm bind to hyaluronic acid receptors, correlating with intact DNA and chromatin integrity, improving ICSI outcomes.
40. Artificial oocyte activation employs calcium ionophores to mimic natural calcium oscillations required for meiosis resumption. It benefits cases of failed fertilization after ICSI, especially in oocyte activation deficiency.
41. In PCOS, the antagonist protocol minimizes OHSS risk by providing flexible control of LH surges. It allows use of GnRH agonist triggers and freeze-all strategies when required. This protocol offers better safety and similar success to agonist cycles.
42. Advanced endometriosis often causes tubal blockage and poor pelvic environment, making IVF the best treatment option. It bypasses pelvic adhesions and improves conception rates after surgical or medical management failure.

43. Men with Klinefelter syndrome can achieve paternity through testicular sperm extraction (TESE) followed by ICSI. Despite low spermatogenesis, viable sperm can be retrieved in up to 50% of cases. Genetic counseling is essential.
44. For unexplained infertility persisting beyond two years, IVF offers the highest pregnancy rates. It bypasses potential subtle tubal, sperm, or oocyte interaction issues undetected by conventional evaluation.
45. For HIV-positive males, sperm washing removes viral particles before ICSI, virtually eliminating transmission risk. The technique allows biological parenthood without infecting the partner or offspring.
46. Progesterone supports luteal phase endometrial development after oocyte retrieval. It compensates for luteal insufficiency induced by ovarian suppression. Both vaginal and intramuscular preparations are effective.
47. Female age is the most critical determinant of IVF success due to declining oocyte quality and increased aneuploidy rates. Younger women have higher live birth rates and lower miscarriage rates across all ART modalities.
48. Recurrent implantation failure warrants investigation of uterine anatomy, genetic, and endometrial factors. Combining hysteroscopy, karyotyping, and endometrial receptivity testing offers comprehensive assessment to guide treatment.
49. Endometrial thickness ≥7 mm on ultrasound correlates with optimal receptivity and implantation potential. Thinner endometrium (<6 mm) is linked to reduced pregnancy rates and may warrant estrogen priming or adjuvant therapy.
50. Single blastocyst transfer significantly lowers twin rates without reducing live birth outcomes. Advances in embryo selection allow safe implementation while maintaining high success and reducing obstetric risks.

Further Reading

The explanations in this chapter are supported by the following key references:

1. Tournaye H, Krausz C, Oates RD. Novel concepts in the management of male-factor infertility. Lancet. 2017;390(10095):110–22.
2. Esteves SC, Agarwal A. Sperm retrieval techniques for assisted reproduction. Int Braz J Urol. 2011;37(5):570–83.
3. Schlegel PN. Microdissection testicular sperm extraction: Technique and results. Fertil Steril. 2009;92(2):404–12.
4. Practice Committee of the American Society for Reproductive Medicine. Intracytoplasmic sperm injection (ICSI) for non-male factor infertility. Fertil Steril. 2020;113(2):239–45.
5. Jungwirth A, Diemer T, Kopa Z, et al. EAU guidelines on male infertility. Eur Urol. 2018;73(4):424–38.
6. Kupka MS, Ferraretti AP, de Mouzon J, et al. Assisted reproductive technology in Europe. Hum Reprod. 2016;31(2):233–48.

Bacterial Sexually Transmitted Infections

18

Learning Objectives

- Identify common bacterial STIs and their presentations.
- Understand appropriate specimen collection and testing.
- Learn recommended antimicrobial regimens.
- Explore complications such as PID and infertility.
- Apply WHO syndromic management guidelines.

Select the Single Best Answer

Block 1: Questions 1–25

1. Which of the following is NOT true about *Neisseria gonorrhoeae*?
   A. Obligate human pathogen
   B. Oxidase positive
   C. Catalase negative
   D. Fastidious organism
   E. Non-motile organism
2. Which of the following is NOT a gonococcal virulence factor?
   A. Antiphagocytic activity
   B. Fimbriation
   C. Reduction of modifiable protein
   D. Heat shock protein
   E. Opacity protein
3. *Neisseria gonorrhoeae* needs to acquire _______ to survive:
   A. Iron
   B. Protein
   C. Zinc
   D. Biotin
   E. Selenium

M. S. M. Hasan, M. L. Elsaie, *Comprehensive MCQs in Andrology*, Trends in Andrology and Sexual Medicine, https://doi.org/10.1007/978-3-032-20623-7_18

4. Which of the following is NOT a line of ophthalmia neonatorum treatment?
   A. Azithromycin
   B. Ceftriaxone
   C. Kanamycin
   D. Penicillin
   E. Irrigation of eyes
5. Which of the following is NOT a risk factor for metastatic gonorrhea?
   A. Homosexuality
   B. Pregnancy
   C. Menstruation
   D. Males
   E. HIV infection
6. Metastatic gonorrhea is most common in:
   A. Males
   B. Females
   C. Children
   D. Infants
   E. Neonates
7. The average number of cutaneous eruptions in metastatic gonorrhea is:
   A. <10
   B. 5–15
   C. 5–30
   D. 10–20
   E. 10–40
8. Which of the following is NOT a target site for disseminated gonorrhea?
   A. Skin
   B. Eye
   C. Joints
   D. Heart
   E. Brain
9. The first-line treatment for uncomplicated gonococcal infection is:
   A. Adriamycin
   B. Tetracycline
   C. Penicillin
   D. Ceftriaxone
   E. Kanamycin
10. The first-line treatment for rectal gonorrhea is:
    A. Adriamycin
    B. Tetracycline
    C. Penicillin
    D. Ceftriaxone
    E. Kanamycin

11. Gonococci are fragile and easily killed by:
    A. Drying
    B. Sunlight
    C. Detergents
    D. A + B + C
    E. A + C
12. To differentiate anterior from posterior urethritis, the test of choice is:
    A. Urine analysis
    B. Prostatic culture and sensitivity
    C. Two-glass urine test
    D. Urine culture and sensitivity
    E. Prostatic massage
13. The most common site for female gonococcal urethral discharge is:
    A. Endocervix
    B. Urethra
    C. Posterior vaginal fornix
    D. Uterus
    E. Vagina
14. The most common site for taking swabs to diagnose female gonorrhea is:
    A. Urethra
    B. Vagina
    C. Cervix
    D. Labia minora
    E. None of the above
15. The treatment of gonococcemia is:
    A. Procaine penicillin
    B. Ceftriaxone IV + ciprofloxacin PO
    C. Doxycycline 100 mg bid × 15 days
    D. Erythromycin 500 mg qid × 10 days
    E. None of the above
16. Acute gonorrhea in adult males is NOT characterized by:
    A. Incubation period 2–5 days
    B. Scanty discharge
    C. Caused by *Neisseria gonorrhoeae*
    D. Treated by ceftriaxone
    E. Oxidase positive
17. *Neisseria gonorrhoeae* is:
    A. Gram-positive cocci
    B. Gram-negative cocci
    C. Gram-negative bacilli
    D. Fish-in-school pattern
    E. Fried-egg pattern

18. Urinalysis in acute gonorrhea patients shows:
    A. No pus cells
    B. Few pus cells
    C. Excessive pus cells
    D. Moderate pus cells
    E. None of the above
19. Samples should be taken from multiple sites in acute gonorrhea patients:
    A. Urethra
    B. Rectum
    C. Oropharynx
    D. A + B + C
    E. A + C
20. The cause of persistent gonorrhea infection after treatment is:
    A. Reinfection
    B. Inadequate antibiotic choice
    C. Inadequate treatment duration
    D. A + B + C
    E. B + C
21. The incubation period of gonorrhea is:
    A. <1 week
    B. 2–3 weeks
    C. >5 weeks
    D. None of the above
22. The main presentation of gonorrhea in female children is:
    A. Vulvovaginitis
    B. Asymptomatic
    C. Cervicitis
    D. Pelvic inflammatory disease
    E. None of the above
23. Childhood gonorrhea is most commonly due to:
    A. Sexual abuse
    B. Infected towels
    C. Non-sexual household contact
    D. All of the above
    E. None of the above
24. Local complications of gonococcal urethritis in males include all EXCEPT:
    A. Tysonitis
    B. Skenitis
    C. Litteritis
    D. Cowperitis
    E. Periurethral abscess

25. Gonococci cannot survive in the vagina because of:
    A. Vaginal alkalinity
    B. Vaginal acidity
    C. Neutral vaginal secretion
    D. Inflammatory cytokines
    E. Hormonal fluctuation

Block 2: Questions 26–50

26. *Neisseria gonorrhoeae* ferments:
    A. Glucose
    B. Maltose
    C. Sucrose
    D. All of the above
    E. None of the above
27. In gonorrhea there are high levels of immunoglobulins:
    A. IgA
    B. IgG
    C. IgM
    D. IgD
    E. IgE
28. The ratio of post-gonococcal urethritis (PGU) is about:
    A. 25–30%
    B. 25–40%
    C. 25–50%
    D. 25–60%
    E. >60%
29. Urogenital chlamydial serovars are NOT responsible for:
    A. Lymphogranuloma venereum
    B. Non-gonococcal urethritis
    C. Cervicitis
    D. Seronegative reactive arthritis
    E. Epididymo-orchitis
30. Typical type of *Chlamydia* is NOT characterized by:
    A. Small organism
    B. Infectious
    C. Low metabolic activity
    D. Can replicate easily
    E. High outer membrane protein expression
31. Atypical type of *Chlamydia* is characterized by:
    A. Small organism
    B. Infectious
    C. Low metabolic activity
    D. Replicates easily
    E. Increased MOMP expression

32. Which interleukin is NOT responsible for primary chlamydial infection?
    A. Interleukin-1
    B. Interleukin-2
    C. Interleukin-6
    D. Interleukin-8
    E. Interleukin-12
33. Which of the following is NOT responsible for primary chlamydial infection?
    A. IL-12
    B. GM-CSF
    C. TNF-alpha
    D. IL-8
    E. GRO (growth-related oncogene)
34. Which of the following reduces the initial amplification of chlamydial infection?
    A. Interleukin-1
    B. Neutrophils
    C. Macrophages
    D. Lymphocytes
    E. TNF-alpha
35. The principal causative agent of Non Gonococcal urethritis (NGU) is:
    A. *Ureaplasma urealyticum*
    B. *Chlamydia trachomatis*
    C. *Streptococcus pyogenes*
    D. *E. coli*
    E. *Klebsiella*
36. Chronic chlamydial infection is considered:
    A. Type I hypersensitivity
    B. Type II hypersensitivity
    C. Type III hypersensitivity
    D. Type IV hypersensitivity
    E. Type V hypersensitivity
37. Which of the following is NOT true about the elementary body of *Chlamydia*?
    A. Infectious stage
    B. Extracellular
    C. Low metabolic activity
    D. Pear-shaped, electron-dense
    E. Metabolically active
38. Which of the following is NOT true about the reticulate body of *Chlamydia*?
    A. Intracellular
    B. Metabolically active
    C. Infectious
    D. Contains inclusion body
    E. Divides by binary fission

39. The extra-genital manifestations of chlamydia are due to:
    A. Porin protein
    B. Opacity protein
    C. Heat-shock protein
    D. Reduction modifiable protein
    E. Capsule
40. First-line treatment of chlamydial infection is:
    A. Azithromycin
    B. Penicillin
    C. Ceftriaxone
    D. Kanamycin
    E. Spectinomycin
41. Chlamydia resembles viruses in that:
    A. They are obligate intracellular parasites
    B. Similar chemical constitution
    C. Similar susceptibility to chemotherapy
    D. Similar structure
    E. RNA only
42. The major health risk of untreated chlamydia infection in men is:
    A. Epididymitis
    B. Reiter's syndrome
    C. Orchitis
    D. Chronic prostatitis/pelvic pain syndrome
    E. Transmission to female partner
43. The first-line treatment for gonorrhea is:
    A. Ciprofloxacin
    B. Levofloxacin
    C. Ceftriaxone
    D. Cefixime
    E. Penicillin VK
44. The most common bacterial STD worldwide is:
    A. Gonorrhea
    B. Chancroid
    C. Chlamydia
    D. Scabies
    E. None of the above
45. The following are bacterial STDs EXCEPT:
    A. Syphilis
    B. Scabies
    C. Gonorrhea
    D. Chancroid
    E. Chlamydia

46. Chlamydia looks like a virus because:
    A. Large organism
    B. Has both DNA and RNA
    C. Grows on yolk sac
    D. Has cell wall
    E. None of the above
47. The most common cause of NGU is:
    A. *Chlamydia trachomatis*
    B. *Treponema pallidum*
    C. *Candida albicans*
    D. *Staphylococcus aureus*
    E. *Trichomonas vaginalis*
48. Urinalysis in chlamydia patients shows:
    A. No pus cells
    B. Few pus cells
    C. Excessive pus cells
    D. Moderate pus cells
    E. None
49. The discharge of chlamydia is characterized by all EXCEPT:
    A. Scanty
    B. Mucoid
    C. Watery
    D. Tetracycline first line
50. The incubation period of chlamydia is:
    A. <1 week
    B. 2–6 weeks
    C. >6 weeks
    D. None of the above

Block 3: Questions 51–75

51. The most common presentation of chlamydia in females is:
    A. Pelvic pain
    B. Asymptomatic
    C. Urethral discharge
    D. All of the above
52. The ratio of recurrent NGU patients is about:
    A. 5%
    B. 50%
    C. 35%
    D. 10%–20%
    E. 40%

53. Which of the following is FALSE about lymphogranuloma venereum (LGV)?
    A. Shows femoral lymphadenopathy
    B. Shows hemorrhagic proctitis
    C. Disappears rapidly
    D. Heals with no scar
    E. Indurated single ulcer
54. Causative organism for LGV is:
    A. *Calymmatobacterium*
    B. *Klebsiella*
    C. *Chlamydia*
    D. *Haemophilus ducreyi*
    E. *Trichomonas*
55. Genital elephantiasis is caused by:
    A. Donovanosis
    B. Congenital syphilis
    C. Herpes progenitalis
    D. Lymphogranuloma venereum
    E. HIV
56. Frei's test is diagnostic of:
    A. LGV
    B. Lymphogranuloma inguinale
    C. Donovanosis
    D. Soft chancre
    E. HIV
57. Groove sign of Greenblatt is found in:
    A. LGV
    B. Chancroid
    C. Donovanosis
    D. Elephantiasis
    E. Candidiasis
58. Rectal mucosa in LGV is:
    A. Edematous
    B. Friable and bleeds easily
    C. Shows superficial erosions and abscesses
    D. All of the above
    E. None of the above
59. Lymph nodes in LGV are:
    A. Enlarged with bubo formation
    B. Bilateral
    C. Unilateral
    D. A + C
    E. None

60. The main pathological process of LGV is:
    A. Huebner arteritis
    B. Cryptitis
    C. Thrombolymphangitis
    D. Endarteritis obliterans
    E. Lymph node disruption
61. Incubation period of LGV is:
    A. <1 week
    B. 1–2 weeks
    C. 3 weeks
    D. 2–6 weeks
    E. >6 weeks
62. Esthiomene means:
    A. Vulval scarring
    B. Vulval fistula
    C. Vestibulitis
    D. Enlarged vulval node
    E. None
63. Esthiomene is characteristic for:
    A. Gonorrhea
    B. Granuloma inguinale
    C. Syphilis
    D. HIV
    E. LGV
64. Pencil-like stools are seen in:
    A. Rectal gonorrhea
    B. Granuloma inguinale
    C. HIV
    D. LGV
    E. Klebsiella
65. Ulcer of LGV is:
    A. Beaded
    B. Deep
    C. Indurated
    D. Shallow
    E. Multiple
66. True bubo is seen in:
    A. Soft sore
    B. Lymphogranuloma venereum (LGV)
    C. Scabies
    D. Trauma
    E. Donovanosis

67. Incubation period of chancroid is:
    A. 1–2 days
    B. 2–5 days
    C. 5–10 days
    D. 7–14 days
    E. 14–28 days
68. Donovan bodies are seen in:
    A. Gonorrhea culture
    B. Primary syphilis ulcer scraping
    C. Condyloma biopsy
    D. LGV node aspiration
    E. Granuloma inguinale ulcer biopsy
69. *Haemophilus ducreyi* on culture tends to form:
    A. Spores
    B. Colonies
    C. Chains
    D. Clusters
    E. None
70. Signs of rectal stricture:
    A. Pencil stool
    B. Distension and colic
    C. None
    D. A + B
    E. A only
71. Urethral stricture leads to:
    A. Weak stream
    B. Straining
    C. UTIs
    D. All of the above
    E. None
72. "School of fish" clusters is a culture pattern for:
    A. Chlamydia
    B. Donovanosis
    C. Mycoplasma
    D. *Trichomonas vaginalis*
    E. Soft sore
73. Saddle nose deformity is found in all EXCEPT:
    A. Secondary syphilis
    B. Reticulohistiocytosis
    C. Polychondritis
    D. Leprosy
    E. Congenital syphilis

74. The most infectious stage of syphilis is:
    A. Primary
    B. Secondary
    C. Tertiary
    D. Latent
    E. Late latent
75. Which is true about syphilis?
    A. Primary = painful ulcer
    B. Secondary = palm/sole lesions
    C. Secondary = scarring
    D. Charcot joint = early latent
    E. All false

Block 4: Questions 76–100

76. The main oral lesion in secondary syphilis is:
    A. Mucous patch
    B. Erythema
    C. Vesicles
    D. Vasculitis
    E. Striations
77. Transmission of syphilis from mother to fetus occurs:
    A. First trimester
    B. Second trimester
    C. Third trimester
    D. During labor
    E. Postnatally
78. Early congenital syphilis manifestations appear:
    A. Within first 3 months
    B. Fourth month
    C. Fifth month
    D. Sixth month
    E. After 1 year
79. Early sign of congenital syphilis is:
    A. Syphilitic rhinitis
    B. Rash on palms
    C. Condyloma lata
    D. Genital chancre
    E. Gumma
80. Most common manifestation of congenital syphilis is:
    A. Fissures of lips/anus
    B. Copper-red macules/papules
    C. Mucous patches
    D. Condyloma lata
    E. Syphilitic pemphigus

81. Least common cutaneous manifestation of early congenital syphilis is:
    A. Rhagades
    B. Condyloma lata
    C. Rhinitis
    D. Clutton joint
    E. Rash
82. Which is NOT characteristic of early congenital syphilis?
    A. Weinberger sign
    B. Jaquet erythema
    C. Dactylitis
    D. Parrot pseudoparalysis
    E. Condyloma lata
83. First serological test to become positive in primary syphilis:
    A. TPHA
    B. FTA
    C. VDRL
    D. Wassermann
    E. TP complement fixation
84. VDRL is usually positive in:
    A. Primary
    B. Secondary
    C. Tertiary
    D. Latent
    E. Congenital
85. Earliest positive test in syphilis is:
    A. FTA-ABS (fluorescent treponemal antibody absorption)
    B. RPR
    C. TPHA
    D. All
    E. None
86. Patient with papules, plaques, lymphadenopathy after treatment likely took:
    A. Penicillin
    B. Erythromycin
    C. Clindamycin
    D. Dapsone
    E. None
87. Clues to late syphilis include:
    A. Chancre scar
    B. Nuchal leukoderma
    C. Macular atrophy
    D. All of the above
    E. None

88. Drug of choice for non-venereal treponematoses:
    A. Penicillin G procaine
    B. Penicillin G benzathine
    C. Erythromycin
    D. Chloramphenicol
    E. Tetracycline
89. Penicillin:
    A. Effective for syphilis
    B. Effective for NGU
    C. Ineffective against β-lactamase gonorrhea
    D. Must be daily for syphilis cure
    E. All false
90. Which statement about penicillin therapy for syphilis is CORRECT?
    A. Oral penicillin is equally effective as parenteral forms
    B. Benzathine penicillin G is preferred for early stages
    C. Penicillin V is the standard treatment
    D. Ceftriaxone is the first-line substitute in all cases
    E. Procaine penicillin is ineffective for neurosyphilis
91. Most frequent gummatous involvement in abdominal syphilis:
    A. Gastric
    B. Intestinal
    C. Hepatic
    D. Splenic
    E. Pancreatic
92. Non-venereal treponematoses compared to syphilis:
    A. Caused by distinct organisms
    B. No relapsing course
    C. Best treated with aminoglycosides
    D. Affect children
    E. Less destructive
93. TPI (Treponema pallidum immobilization) test distinguishes syphilis from:
    A. Yaws
    B. Bejel
    C. Pinta
    D. All
    E. None
94. Mixed chancre due to syphilis +:
    A. Staph
    B. Strep
    C. *H. ducreyi*
    D. Pseudomonas
    E. Candida

95. Most reliable exam for syphilis:
    A. Dark-field
    B. Culture
    C. VDRL
    D. FTA + TPHA
    E. ELISA
96. Painless ulcer on coronal sulcus for 2 weeks suggests:
    A. Syphilis
    B. HSV
    C. Chancroid
    D. TB
    E. Mycoplasma
97. Test to monitor response to syphilis therapy:
    A. Treponema pallidum particle agglutination assay (TP-PA)
    B. Rapid plasma reagin (RPR)
    C. Fluorescent treponemal antibody-absorption (FTA-ABS)
    D. Dark-field
    E. Tzanck
98. Treatment of choice for primary/secondary/early latent syphilis:
    A. Azithromycin
    B. Benzathine penicillin
    C. Probenecid penicillin
    D. Ceftriaxone
    E. Procaine penicillin
99. Diffuse primary syphilitic balanitis is:
    A. Chancre at root
    B. Deep ulcer glans
    C. Superficial erosions with exudate
    D. Pseudomembrane chancre
    E. Gumma
100. Diphtheroid chancre means:
    A. Root chancre
    B. Deep ulcer glans
    C. Superficial erosions
    D. Whitish pseudomembrane over chancre
    E. Gumma

Block 5: Questions 101–125

101. Hunterian chancre refers to:
    A. Latent syphilis
    B. Diphtheroid syphilis
    C. Classic chancre
    D. Chancre redux
    E. Gumma

102. Transition syphiloderma false statement:
    A. Few lesions
    B. More infiltrated
    C. Darker papules
    D. Persistent with scars
    E. Very common
103. False about *Treponema pallidum*:
    A. Eukaryotic
    B. Helically coiled
    C. Silver stain
    D. Motile
    E. Flexible
104. EM of *Treponema pallidum* shows lack of:
    A. Cholesterol
    B. LPS
    C. Proteoglycan
    D. Ergosterol
    E. Peptidoglycan
105. Wall of *Treponema pallidum* contains:
    A. Cholesterol
    B. LPS
    C. Proteoglycan
    D. Ergosterol
    E. Peptidoglycan
106. Optimal temperature for *T. pallidum* growth:
    A. 22 °C
    B. 27 °C
    C. 30 °C
    D. 33 °C
    E. 37 °C
107. Basilar artery syphilitic affection leads to:
    A. Flaccid paralysis
    B. Absent reflexes
    C. Bladder disturbances
    D. Dysphagia
    E. Hemiplegia
108. Lenticulostriate artery syphilitic affection leads to:
    A. Flaccid paralysis
    B. Absent reflexes
    C. Bladder disturbances
    D. Dysphagia
    E. Hemiplegia

109. Exaggerated jaw reflex is seen in:
   A. AIDS
   B. GPI (general paralysis of insane)
   C. Tabes dorsalis
   D. Gonococcemia
   E. Reiter's
110. Charcot's joint is seen in:
   A. AIDS
   B. GPI
   C. Tabes dorsalis
   D. Gonococcemia
   E. Reiter's
111. Sensory ataxia is seen in:
   A. AIDS
   B. GPI
   C. Tabes dorsalis
   D. Gonococcemia
   E. Reiter's
112. Primary optic atrophy is seen in:
   A. AIDS
   B. GPI
   C. Tabes dorsalis
   D. Gonococcemia
   E. Reiter's
113. Epileptic fits are seen in:
   A. AIDS
   B. GPI
   C. Tabes dorsalis
   D. Gonococcemia
   E. Reiter's
114. Placenta in syphilitic mother is NOT:
   A. Pale
   B. Small
   C. Edematous
   D. Greasy
   E. Full of organisms
115. Mulberry molar teeth in congenital syphilis affect:
   A. First molar
   B. Second molar
   C. Third molar
   D. Second + third
   E. First + third

116. Inflammatory bubo seen in:
    A. Hard sore
    B. Donovanosis
    C. LGV
    D. Soft sore
    E. TB
117. School of fish clusters are seen in:
    A. Hard sore
    B. Donovanosis
    C. LGV
    D. Soft sore
    E. TB
118. *Haemophilus ducreyi* is NOT:
    A. Gram positive
    B. Facultative
    C. Anaerobic
    D. Extracellular
    E. School of fish appearance
119. Rail-track pattern is characteristic for:
    A. Hard sore
    B. Donovanosis
    C. LGV
    D. Soft sore
    E. TB
120. Which is NOT true about *Calymmatobacterium granulomatis*?
    A. Gram positive
    B. Cocci-bacilli
    C. Antigenic similarity to Klebsiella
    D. Fibrous capsule
    E. Heavy plasma infiltrate
121. Pseudo-bubo is seen in:
    A. Hard sore
    B. Donovanosis
    C. LGV
    D. Soft sore
    E. TB
122. Fried egg colonies characteristic of:
    A. Hard sore
    B. Donovanosis
    C. LGV
    D. Soft sore
    E. Mycoplasma

123. Drug of choice for Mycoplasma treatment:
   A. Penicillin
   B. Quinolones
   C. Macrolides
   D. Procaine penicillin
   E. Clarithromycin
124. Mycoplasma is NOT:
   A. Sterol-containing
   B. Eukaryotic
   C. Trilayer outer membrane
   D. Pleomorphic
   E. Fried egg colonies
125. Male with 2 painful ulcers ×2 days—best diagnostic test:
   A. Culture
   B. Dark-field exam
   C. VDRL
   D. FTA
   E. Blood culture

Block 6: Questions 126–150

126. True about *Treponema pallidum*:
   A. Distinguishable morphologically from *T. pertenue*
   B. Seen by Gram stain
   C. Obligate parasite
   D. Can be cultured continuously
   E. Found in gummas
127. True about primary syphilis:
   A. Occurs in all contacts
   B. Always symptomatic
   C. Mean incubation 1 week
   D. Not in previously treated
   E. Ulcer at inoculation site
128. Chancres of primary syphilis:
   A. Painful
   B. Last >3 months
   C. Only recur if reinfected
   D. Associated with lymphadenopathy
   E. Resolve only after antibiotics
129. Diagnosis of primary syphilis:
   A. Serology useless
   B. Dark-field of oral chancres reliable
   C. Direct IF more sensitive than dark-field
   D. Cotrimoxazole safe while diagnosing
   E. Negative FTA excludes syphilis

130. *N. gonorrhoeae*:
    A. Differentiated from *N. meningitidis* by sugars
    B. Cultured on Sabouraud's
    C. Anaerobic G- coccus
    D. Sensitive to metronidazole
    E. Resistant to drying
131. Urethral gonorrhea:
    A. Diagnosed by Gram-negative diplococci
    B. Symptomatic in 10% men
    C. Not acquired by oral sex
    D. May cause periurethral abscess
    E. Resolves spontaneously
132. Rectal gonorrhea:
    A. Only in homosexuals
    B. Symptomatic in 90%
    C. Requires IV antibiotics
    D. Causes constipation
    E. Tenesmus + mucopus stool
133. Gonococcal pharyngitis:
    A. Severe tonsillitis
    B. Diagnosed by Gram smear
    C. Treated with ampicillin + probenecid
    D. Cannot disseminate
    E. May resolve spontaneously
134. *Chlamydia trachomatis*:
    A. Seen on Gram stain
    B. Grows on horse blood agar
    C. Causes McCoy cell lysis
    D. Implicated in respiratory disease
    E. Rare zoonosis
135. False about *C. trachomatis*:
    A. Obligate parasite
    B. Classified as bacterium
    C. Propagated in cell culture
    D. Exists in 2 forms
    E. Part of normal flora
136. True about chlamydial cervicitis:
    A. Diagnosed from Gram pus score
    B. Treated with ciprofloxacin
    C. Usually asymptomatic
    D. Always pathognomonic on Pap
    E. Squamous infection

137. False about *C. trachomatis*:
   A. Cannot be isolated in 95% NGU
   B. Detected by ELISA
   C. Common cause NGU in homosexuals
   D. Cause of adult pneumonitis
   E. Transmitted by orogenital
138. *Mycoplasma hominis*:
   A. Same as *Ureaplasma*
   B. Universal NGU cause
   C. Cause of Reiter's
   D. Cannot cause PID
   E. Eradicated by tetracyclines
139. *Ureaplasma urealyticum* is best treated with:
   A. Macrolides
   B. Penicillin
   C. Vancomycin
   D. Aminoglycosides
   E. Amphotericin
140. Reiter's syndrome (reactive arthritis) is strongly associated with:
   A. Gonorrhea
   B. Syphilis
   C. Chlamydia
   D. Trichomonas
   E. Candida
141. The leading cause of preventable blindness worldwide is:
   A. Gonorrhea
   B. *Chlamydia trachomatis* (trachoma)
   C. Syphilis
   D. HIV
   E. Mycoplasma
142. Which of the following is true regarding dual infection?
   A. Gonorrhea rarely coexists with chlamydia
   B. Coinfection is common, so dual therapy is recommended
   C. Coinfection occurs only in men
   D. Coinfection is prevented by condom use alone
   E. Gonorrhea eliminates chlamydia naturally
143. Granuloma inguinale is caused by:
   A. *Klebsiella granulomatis*
   B. *Hemophilus ducreyi*
   C. *Treponema pallidum*
   D. *Neisseria gonorrhoeae*
   E. *Chlamydia trachomatis*

144. The causative organism of chancroid is:
    A. *Klebsiella granulomatis*
    B. *Hemophilus ducreyi*
    C. *Treponema pallidum*
    D. *Neisseria gonorrhoeae*
    E. *Mycoplasma hominis*
145. Which bacterial STI is most associated with neurological complications such as tabes dorsalis?
    A. Chlamydia
    B. Gonorrhea
    C. Syphilis
    D. Chancroid
    E. Donovanosis
146. The Jarisch–Herxheimer reaction after penicillin treatment occurs due to:
    A. Allergic response to penicillin
    B. Rapid lysis of spirochetes releasing endotoxins
    C. Resistance to penicillin
    D. Cross-reaction with beta-lactams
    E. Secondary bacterial infection
147. Pelvic inflammatory disease (PID) is most strongly associated with:
    A. Mycoplasma
    B. Ureaplasma
    C. Chlamydia and Gonorrhea
    D. Syphilis
    E. Donovanosis
148. Which statement about syphilis serology is true?
    A. Treponemal tests revert to negative after treatment
    B. Nontreponemal tests remain positive for life
    C. Treponemal tests remain positive for life
    D. Both tests decline after cure
    E. Neither is useful for follow-up
149. Which of the following increases susceptibility to all bacterial STIs?
    A. Diabetes
    B. Malaria
    C. HIV infection
    D. Tuberculosis
    E. Malnutrition
150. The cornerstone of STI prevention is:
    A. Antibiotics for all
    B. Vaccination
    C. Barrier contraception, partner notification, and screening
    D. Abstinence only
    E. Early circumcision

✅ Key Takeaways

- Gonorrhea and chlamydia often co-exist; dual therapy is recommended.
- **Dark-field microscopy** and **VDRL/TPHA** are key in syphilis.
- **Partner treatment** and **contact tracing** reduce reinfection.
- Antimicrobial resistance is an emerging threat.
- Public education and STI screening are pillars of control.

✅ Answer Key (1–150)

1. C
2. D
3. A
4. C
5. D
6. B
7. E
8. E
9. D
10. D
11. D
12. C
13. A
14. C
15. B
16. B
17. B
18. C
19. D
20. D
21. A
22. A
23. A
24. B
25. B
26. A
27. A
28. B
29. A
30. D
31. D
32. B
33. A

34. B
35. B
36. D
37. E
38. C
39. C
40. A
41. A
42. A
43. C
44. C
45. B
46. C
47. A
48. B
49. D
50. B
51. B
52. D
53. C
54. C
55. D
56. A
57. A
58. D
59. D
60. C
61. D
62. A
63. E
64. D
65. D
66. B
67. C
68. E
69. B
70. D
71. D
72. E
73. A
74. B
75. B
76. A
77. B
78. A

79. A
80. B
81. D
82. A
83. B
84. B
85. A
86. A
87. D
88. B
89. E
90. B
91. C
92. D
93. D
94. C
95. D
96. A
97. B
98. B
99. C
100. D
101. C
102. E
103. A
104. B
105. E
106. D
107. E
108. A
109. B
110. C
111. C
112. C
113. B
114. B
115. A
116. D
117. D
118. A
119. B
120. D
121. B
122. E
123. C

124. B
125. A
126. C
127. E
128. D
129. C
130. A
131. A
132. E
133. B
134. D
135. E
136. C
137. A
138. E
139. A
140. C
141. B
142. B
143. A
144. B
145. C
146. B
147. C
148. C
149. C
150. C

Explanations (1–150)

1. *Neisseria gonorrhoeae* is indeed an obligate human pathogen, oxidase positive, catalase positive, fastidious, and non-motile. The false statement is that it is catalase negative, since it produces catalase. This enzyme helps neutralize reactive oxygen species and supports bacterial survival inside host cells, which is important in pathogenesis.
2. Gonococcal virulence depends on multiple factors, including pili (fimbriation), opacity proteins, and the ability to evade phagocytosis. Heat shock proteins, however, are not considered classic virulence factors in gonorrhea; they are general stress proteins found in many organisms. The others are directly involved in adhesion, invasion, and immune evasion.
3. *Neisseria gonorrhoeae* requires iron to survive and thrive within the human host. It has specialized systems to acquire iron from transferrin, lactoferrin, and hemoglobin. This iron acquisition is critical for growth and explains its pathogenicity.

4. Ophthalmia neonatorum due to gonococcus is managed by systemic ceftriaxone and supportive measures such as irrigation. Penicillin and kanamycin are not first-line in current practice, and azithromycin is used more for chlamydial conjunctivitis. Thus, azithromycin is not a standard line for gonococcal ophthalmia in neonates.
5. Risk factors for disseminated gonococcal infection include female sex, menstruation, pregnancy, and HIV infection. Men are less likely to develop metastatic gonorrhea. Therefore, male sex is not considered a risk factor; in fact, females are more prone.
6. Disseminated gonococcal infection is more common in women, especially during menstruation or pregnancy, due to mucosal changes and immune modulation. Men are less frequently affected. Children and neonates usually present with localized rather than disseminated disease.
7. The number of skin lesions in disseminated gonorrhea typically ranges between 5 and 30. These are pustular or vesiculopustular lesions with necrotic centers. The limited number of lesions helps distinguish gonococcal sepsis from other septicemias.
8. Disseminated gonorrhea primarily targets the skin and joints. The eye and heart are not common targets, and brain involvement is not characteristic. Hence, eye is not typically a site for gonococcal dissemination, though conjunctivitis can occur locally.
9. First-line therapy for uncomplicated gonorrhea is ceftriaxone. Resistance has made older options such as penicillin or tetracycline obsolete. Ceftriaxone has high efficacy against resistant strains and is the global standard of care.
10. Rectal gonorrhea is also best treated with ceftriaxone, similar to genital infections. Other antibiotics such as penicillin or tetracycline have high resistance rates and are not recommended. Ceftriaxone provides consistent cure rates across sites of infection.
11. Gonococci are fragile organisms and do not tolerate environmental stress. They are killed by drying, sunlight, and detergents. This explains why transmission requires direct sexual contact, not fomites.
12. To differentiate anterior from posterior urethritis, the two-glass urine test is used. In anterior urethritis, the first portion of urine is cloudy, while in posterior urethritis both portions may show pus cells. Prostatic massage and cultures are more invasive.
13. In women, gonococcal infections most commonly involve the endocervix. Urethral infection is less frequent, and vaginal involvement is rare due to the acidic environment. This site explains why cervicitis is the most typical presentation.
14. The best diagnostic swab site in women is the cervix, where the organism most frequently colonizes. Vaginal or urethral swabs may also detect it, but cervical sampling provides the highest yield.
15. Gonococcemia is managed with systemic antibiotics. Ceftriaxone IV initially followed by oral fluoroquinolones is a standard regimen. Procaine penicillin or doxycycline alone are insufficient.

16. Acute male gonorrhea typically presents after a 2–5 day incubation period with purulent discharge and dysuria. Scanty discharge is more typical of chlamydia. The causative organism is oxidase positive and responds to ceftriaxone.
17. *Neisseria gonorrhoeae* is a Gram-negative diplococcus, often arranged in pairs resembling "coffee beans" or "fish in a school." It is not Gram-positive, nor does it appear like a fried egg colony (that is Mycoplasma).
18. Urinalysis in gonorrhea shows abundant pus cells due to intense urethritis. This helps distinguish it from other conditions with sterile pyuria.
19. Sampling in suspected gonorrhea should include urethral, rectal, and oropharyngeal sites because the organism can infect multiple mucosal areas. This broadens detection and avoids missed cases.
20. Persistent infection after treatment usually results from reinfection, inappropriate antibiotic choice, or insufficient treatment duration. Antibiotic resistance is also a concern. Therefore, all three factors play roles in persistence.
21. The incubation period of gonorrhea is typically short, usually under 1 week. This rapid onset explains the early appearance of urethritis in infected men. Longer incubation suggests another organism.
22. In girls, gonorrhea often presents as vulvovaginitis because the endocervix is not fully developed prepubertally. Cervicitis and PID are not common in young children.
23. When gonorrhea is identified in a child, sexual abuse is the most likely source and must be considered urgently. Fomites (e.g., towels) are not credible transmission routes for this fragile organism.
24. Local complications of male gonococcal urethritis include infection of periurethral glands like Cowper's, Littre's, and Tyson's. Skenitis occurs in females, not males.
25. Gonococci cannot survive in the vagina of adults because the acidic environment is hostile. The normal flora (lactobacilli) maintains this acidity, protecting against colonization.
26. *Neisseria gonorrhoeae* ferments glucose but not maltose, sucrose, or lactose. This biochemical property differentiates it from *Neisseria meningitidis*, which ferments both glucose and maltose. Recognizing this helps in the laboratory diagnosis when culturing organisms.
27. In gonorrhea, mucosal immunity triggers increased production of immunoglobulins, especially IgA. This secretory antibody is vital in mucosal defense but is often countered by gonococcal IgA protease, which allows persistence of infection. IgG and IgM also rise but are less characteristic.
28. The incidence of post-gonococcal urethritis (PGU), often due to chlamydia or other organisms, is around 25–40%. This explains why some men continue to have symptoms after treatment for gonorrhea. It highlights the importance of dual therapy with ceftriaxone and doxycycline or azithromycin.
29. Urogenital chlamydial serovars (D–K) cause non-gonococcal urethritis, cervicitis, epididymitis, and reactive arthritis. They do not cause lymphogranuloma

venereum, which is due to serovars L1–L3. This distinction is clinically important for diagnosis and treatment.

30. Typical chlamydial elementary bodies are small, extracellular, infectious, and metabolically inert. They cannot replicate independently until they enter host cells. Thus, the false description is that they replicate easily.
31. Reticulate bodies are the metabolically active, intracellular form of chlamydia. They replicate inside the host cell inclusion before reorganizing back into elementary bodies. Unlike the elementary body, they are non-infectious.
32. Cytokines play a crucial role in chlamydial infection. Interleukins 1, 6, and 8 help orchestrate inflammation, but interleukin-2 is more associated with adaptive T-cell response. Therefore, IL-2 is not directly involved in acute infection.
33. Cytokines such as TNF-alpha, GM-CSF, and IL-8 drive early chlamydial inflammation. IL-12, however, is not a primary driver of acute infection; it plays a role in adaptive immunity and Th1 response later. Hence, IL-12 is not responsible for the acute phase.
34. Neutrophils help reduce initial bacterial loads in chlamydia by phagocytosis. They are critical for limiting amplification in the early stages. Other immune cells like macrophages and lymphocytes come later in the response.
35. The main causative agent of nongonococcal urethritis is *Chlamydia trachomatis*. Ureaplasma and Mycoplasma also contribute but are less common. Streptococcus and enteric organisms are not typical causes.
36. Chronic chlamydial infection is associated with a type IV hypersensitivity reaction. This delayed-type hypersensitivity leads to scarring and fibrosis, particularly in the fallopian tubes, which underlies infertility and ectopic pregnancy risks.
37. The elementary body is the infectious, extracellular form of chlamydia. It is electron-dense and metabolically inactive. The false option is "pear-shaped," as elementary bodies are more spherical.
38. Reticulate bodies are intracellular, metabolically active, and non-infectious. They divide by binary fission inside inclusions. Thus, the incorrect description is that they are infectious.
39. Extra-genital manifestations of chlamydia, such as reactive arthritis, are linked to heat shock proteins. These proteins stimulate immune responses that can cross-react with host tissues, causing systemic effects.
40. The first-line treatment for chlamydial infection is azithromycin or doxycycline. Beta-lactams like penicillin and ceftriaxone are ineffective because chlamydia lacks a conventional peptidoglycan layer.
41. Chlamydia resembles viruses only because it is an obligate intracellular organism. However, unlike viruses, it contains both DNA and RNA and can respond to antibiotics. Its bacterial nature explains why macrolides and tetracyclines work against it.
42. In men, untreated chlamydia can cause epididymitis, prostatitis, chronic pelvic pain, and infertility. However, the greatest concern is transmission to female partners, leading to pelvic inflammatory disease. This makes chlamydia a major public health risk.

43. For gonorrhea, ceftriaxone is the standard treatment worldwide. Fluoroquinolones and penicillin are no longer reliable due to widespread resistance. Cefixime is sometimes used, but ceftriaxone is preferred.
44. The most common bacterial STD worldwide is chlamydia. It often remains asymptomatic, which facilitates spread. Gonorrhea, chancroid, and syphilis are far less prevalent globally.
45. Scabies is caused by a mite, not a bacterium, and so is not classified as a bacterial STD. Syphilis, gonorrhea, chancroid, and chlamydia are all bacterial. This distinction is important for diagnosis and treatment approaches.
46. Chlamydia resembles viruses because it is an obligate intracellular parasite and cannot grow on conventional bacterial media. However, it still has DNA, RNA, and a bacterial-type cell wall. Culturing often requires yolk sacs or tissue culture.
47. The most common cause of non-gonococcal urethritis is *Chlamydia trachomatis*. Other causes include Mycoplasma genitalium and Ureaplasma. Candida and staphylococcus are not major contributors in otherwise healthy men.
48. Urinalysis in men with chlamydial urethritis often shows pyuria, but no bacteria are seen on routine culture—this is called sterile pyuria. This finding should raise suspicion for chlamydia.
49. Discharge in chlamydia tends to be scanty, mucoid, or watery rather than copious and purulent as in gonorrhea. Treatment with tetracycline or azithromycin is effective. Thus, discharge is not characterized by "treated with tetracycline" but by its physical qualities.
50. The incubation period for chlamydia is usually 2–6 weeks. This is longer than gonorrhea, which incubates in less than a week. The delayed onset often explains subtle or asymptomatic disease.
51. In women, chlamydia is often asymptomatic, which makes it particularly dangerous as it can silently damage the reproductive tract. While pelvic pain and discharge occur, the asymptomatic nature is most common and responsible for transmission.
52. Recurrent nongonococcal urethritis occurs in about 10%–20% of patients. This recurrence may be due to incomplete treatment, reinfection from an untreated partner, or persistence of organisms like Mycoplasma genitalium.
53. Lymphogranuloma venereum (LGV) does not heal rapidly or without scarring. It causes femoral lymphadenopathy, hemorrhagic proctitis, and an indurated ulcer. Chronic cases may result in fibrosis and elephantiasis.
54. The causative organism of LGV is *Chlamydia trachomatis* serovars L1–L3. Other organisms like Calymmatobacterium (*Klebsiella granulomatis*) cause donovanosis, while *Hemophilus ducreyi* causes chancroid.
55. Chronic lymphatic obstruction from LGV leads to genital elephantiasis. This disfiguring complication emphasizes the importance of early treatment to prevent irreversible lymphatic damage.
56. Frei's intradermal test was historically diagnostic for LGV. It measured delayed-type hypersensitivity to chlamydial antigen. While now outdated, it remains an important historical diagnostic concept.

57. The groove sign of Greenblatt, where the inguinal ligament produces a groove between enlarged lymph nodes above and below, is characteristic of LGV. It remains a classic clinical description.
58. The rectal mucosa in LGV becomes edematous, friable, and ulcerated, sometimes with abscess formation. These inflammatory changes explain symptoms of proctitis and stricture formation.
59. The lymph nodes in LGV are typically enlarged, unilateral, and often suppurate into buboes. Bilateral involvement is less common.
60. The hallmark pathology of LGV is thrombolymphangitis, leading to destruction of lymphatic architecture and chronic complications like fibrosis and fistulae.
61. The incubation period of LGV is typically 2–6 weeks, longer than that of gonorrhea or chancroid. This delay contributes to diagnostic difficulty in early cases.
62. Esthiomene refers to chronic scarring and ulceration of the vulva, particularly in LGV. It results from destructive lymphatic inflammation and fibrosis.
63. Esthiomene is classically associated with LGV, not with gonorrhea or syphilis. It represents one of the most severe late complications in women.
64. Pencil-like stools occur when rectal strictures develop due to LGV, narrowing the lumen and altering stool shape. This is a late sequela of untreated infection.
65. The ulcer of LGV is typically shallow and painless, unlike the painful chancroid ulcer or the indurated syphilitic chancre. This difference helps in clinical differentiation.
66. True buboes, which are suppurating inguinal lymph nodes, are typical of LGV. In chancroid, buboes are common but more painful; in granuloma inguinale, buboes are usually absent.
67. The incubation period of chancroid is short, usually 2–5 days. This rapid onset of painful ulcers contrasts with the slower development of syphilitic chancres.
68. Donovan bodies, which are intracellular inclusions seen on biopsy or smear, are diagnostic of granuloma inguinale caused by *Klebsiella granulomatis*. They are not seen in syphilis or gonorrhea.
69. *Hemophilus ducreyi*, the causative agent of chancroid, grows as small colonies on culture and does not form spores or chains. Its fragile nature explains difficulties in laboratory diagnosis.
70. Rectal strictures produce symptoms such as pencil stools and colicky abdominal pain. These are late sequelae of chronic LGV or untreated rectal infections.
71. Urethral strictures, often a complication of chronic gonorrhea, cause weak urinary stream, straining, and recurrent urinary tract infections. They represent a major long-term morbidity of untreated cases.
72. The "school of fish" pattern on Gram stain is characteristic of *Hemophilus ducreyi*. This diagnostic clue helps differentiate chancroid from other causes of genital ulcers.
73. Saddle nose deformity results from collapse of the nasal bridge due to syphilitic destruction of cartilage. It is seen in congenital syphilis, leprosy, and relapsing polychondritis, but not in secondary syphilis.

74. Secondary syphilis is the most infectious stage, as spirochetes are present in mucous patches and condylomata lata. This explains its high transmission rate.
75. Primary syphilis produces a painless chancre, not painful ulcers. Secondary syphilis involves palms and soles, and tertiary syphilis can lead to Charcot joints. These distinctions are key for staging.
76. The main oral lesion of secondary syphilis is the mucous patch, which appears as painless, shallow erosions with a gray exudate. They are highly infectious.
77. Syphilis is transmitted to the fetus most often during the second trimester, when spirochetes cross the placenta. This underlines the importance of maternal screening in early pregnancy.
78. Early congenital syphilis typically manifests within the first 3 months of life. Signs include rhinitis, rash, and hepatosplenomegaly.
79. One of the earliest and most characteristic signs of congenital syphilis is syphilitic rhinitis ("snuffles"), which is highly contagious.
80. The most common manifestation of congenital syphilis is a copper-colored maculopapular rash, especially on the palms, soles, and diaper area. This rash often signals systemic infection.
81. Condyloma lata are common in congenital syphilis, but rarer cutaneous features such as rhagades or Clutton joints are less frequent. Thus, condyloma lata are not the least common.
82. Early congenital syphilis can present with dactylitis, pseudoparalysis (Parrot's sign), and Weinberger sign. Condyloma lata also occurs. These manifestations reflect systemic involvement.
83. The first serological test to become positive in primary syphilis is usually FTA-ABS. Treponemal-specific tests detect infection earlier than non-treponemal tests like VDRL.
84. VDRL is usually positive in secondary syphilis, when antibody titers are highest. In late stages, sensitivity declines. This explains why treponemal tests remain necessary.
85. The earliest positive test of syphilis is the treponemal FTA-ABS. Non-treponemal tests like RPR may lag behind. Thus, FTA-ABS is most sensitive in early infection.
86. Patients who develop Jarisch–Herxheimer reactions after penicillin therapy present with systemic symptoms, not papules. Papules and plaques after treatment may indicate erythromycin resistance or misdiagnosis.
87. Late syphilis clues include a scar from the original chancre, leukoderma, and macular atrophy. These findings reflect progression of untreated infection.
88. The drug of choice for non-venereal treponematoses (yaws, bejel, pinta) is penicillin. A single injection often cures these infections.
89. Penicillin is highly effective against syphilis, but ineffective against penicillinase-producing gonococci. It must be given intramuscularly for uncomplicated cases, usually as benzathine penicillin.
90. Benzathine penicillin G (IM, single 2.4 million IU dose) is the recommended regimen for primary, secondary, and early latent syphilis. Neurosyphilis requires aqueous crystalline penicillin G, not oral or procaine formulations.

91. In abdominal syphilis, gummatous involvement most often affects the liver. Hepatic gummas can cause hepatomegaly and dysfunction.
92. Non-venereal treponematoses are caused by related treponemes but tend to affect children, have less severe courses, and lack relapsing progression. They still respond to penicillin.
93. The treponemal immobilization test does not distinguish syphilis from yaws, bejel, or pinta because all are caused by closely related treponemes. This limits its diagnostic specificity.
94. A mixed chancre occurs when syphilis coexists with chancroid, caused by *Hemophilus ducreyi*. The result is a chancre with atypical features.
95. The most reliable diagnostic combination is FTA-ABS + TPHA (treponemal-specific tests). Dark-field microscopy is confirmatory for early lesions, but combined treponemal serology provides the highest sensitivity and specificity for all stages of syphilis.
96. A painless genital ulcer lasting 2 weeks is characteristic of syphilis. Chancroid ulcers are painful, and herpes produces vesicular lesions.
97. To monitor syphilis therapy, non-treponemal tests like VDRL or RPR are used. These titers decline with treatment, unlike treponemal tests, which remain positive for life.
98. The treatment of choice for early syphilis is benzathine penicillin. A single intramuscular dose cures most cases.
99. Diffuse primary syphilitic balanitis presents as superficial erosions with exudative secretion over the glans. It differs from indurated chancre.
100. Diphtheroid chancre refers to a whitish pseudomembrane overlying a syphilitic ulcer. It mimics diphtheria but occurs on the glans.
101. Complete ejaculatory duct obstruction typically presents with azoospermia, low semen volume, and absent fructose, since fructose is normally secreted by the seminal vesicles. These findings distinguish it from testicular failure.
102. The nutcracker phenomenon involves compression of the left renal vein between the aorta and the superior mesenteric artery, leading to hematuria, proteinuria, and sometimes varicocele. Climacturia is unrelated.
103. Ultrasound criteria for nutcracker syndrome include reduced aorto–SMA angle, narrowing of the left renal vein, and increased flow velocity. Increased angle is not typical.
104. *Treponema pallidum* is an obligate human pathogen and cannot survive outside the host. It has a fragile outer membrane lacking lipopolysaccharides, which explains its stealthy immune evasion.
105. The wall of *T. pallidum* contains peptidoglycan, like other bacteria, but not the typical Gram-negative LPS layer. This feature explains some staining difficulties and immune invisibility.
106. *T. pallidum* survives optimally at 33–37 °C, close to body temperature, which is why experimental infection requires animal models kept at similar conditions.

107. Basilar artery involvement in neurosyphilis may produce hemiplegia due to cortical ischemia. These vascular complications are part of meningovascular syphilis.
108. Lenticulostriate artery syphilitic damage can also cause hemiplegia by affecting deep brain structures. These strokes often occur in relatively young patients.
109. Exaggerated jaw reflex is seen in neurosyphilis, particularly in general paralysis of the insane, due to upper motor neuron involvement. This reflects corticobulbar tract pathology.
110. Charcot joints, or neuropathic joints, occur in tabes dorsalis, a late syphilitic complication. Loss of proprioception leads to repeated trauma and joint destruction.
111. Sensory ataxia is another hallmark of tabes dorsalis, due to degeneration of posterior columns. Patients rely on visual cues to walk, worsening symptoms in the dark.
112. Primary optic atrophy occurs in tabes dorsalis when the posterior columns and optic nerves are damaged. Vision progressively declines without inflammation.
113. Epileptic seizures can occur in general paresis of the insane, the parenchymatous form of neurosyphilis, as cortical damage predisposes to convulsions.
114. In congenital syphilis, the placenta is typically pale, large, and edematous, full of spirochetes. A small placenta is not typical, so its presence argues against the diagnosis.
115. Mulberry molars are dental stigmata of congenital syphilis, affecting the first molars. They have irregular, dome-shaped cusps, resembling mulberries.
116. Inflammatory buboes are seen in chancroid (soft sore), caused by *Hemophilus ducreyi*. These are painful, suppurative inguinal lymphadenopathies.
117. The "school of fish" Gram stain appearance of clustered organisms is characteristic of *H. ducreyi*, supporting the diagnosis of chancroid.
118. *H. ducreyi* is a Gram-negative coccobacillus, extracellular, and fastidious. It is not Gram-positive or anaerobic, but rather requires enriched media for growth.
119. Rail-track patterns are seen in Donovanosis (granuloma inguinale) on microscopy, due to the arrangement of Donovan bodies within macrophages.
120. *Calymmatobacterium granulomatis* (now classified as *Klebsiella granulomatis*) is Gram-negative, not Gram-positive, and has characteristic intracellular inclusions. Its capsule aids immune evasion.
121. Pseudo-buboes, which are subcutaneous granulomatous swellings resembling lymph nodes, are seen in donovanosis. True buboes, in contrast, occur in chancroid or LGV.
122. "Fried egg" colonies on culture are characteristic of Mycoplasma species, reflecting their dense center and lighter peripheral growth.
123. The drug of choice for Mycoplasma infections is macrolides, such as azithromycin or clarithromycin, due to their activity against cell wall–deficient organisms.
124. Mycoplasma species are bacteria without a cell wall, making them pleomorphic and resistant to beta-lactams. They are prokaryotes, not eukaryotes.

125. In a patient with acute painful ulcers of 2 days' duration, the best diagnostic tool is dark-field microscopy, which can visualize motile *T. pallidum* directly, whereas serology may not yet be positive.
126. *T. pallidum* cannot be cultured in vitro and must be propagated in animal models. It is an obligate parasite, explaining its dependence on human transmission.
127. Primary syphilis appears as a solitary chancre at the site of inoculation after a 2–3 week incubation. It occurs in only about a third of exposed contacts, and is usually symptomatic.
128. Chancres of syphilis are classically painless ulcers with indurated edges, accompanied by regional lymphadenopathy. They resolve spontaneously in weeks.
129. Dark-field microscopy and direct immunofluorescence are the most sensitive early diagnostic methods. Serology may be negative in the first 1–2 weeks of a chancre.
130. *Neisseria gonorrhoeae* is a Gram-negative diplococcus that ferments glucose but not maltose. It is distinguished from *N. meningitidis* by sugar fermentation patterns.
131. Urethral gonorrhea can be diagnosed definitively by intracellular Gram-negative diplococci on smear. It is symptomatic in most men, unlike chlamydia, and may complicate with periurethral abscesses.
132. Rectal gonorrhea is not limited to homosexual males; it can occur in any receptive anal intercourse. Symptoms include tenesmus, pain, and mucopus-streaked stool.
133. Gonococcal pharyngitis often presents with mild sore throat or is asymptomatic, not severe tonsillitis. It can spread systemically and requires ceftriaxone-based therapy.
134. *Chlamydia trachomatis* causes lysis of McCoy cells in tissue culture and has been linked to adult respiratory infections. It cannot be cultured on routine media.
135. *C. trachomatis* is an obligate intracellular bacterium, existing in elementary and reticulate body forms. It is not part of normal flora.
136. Chlamydial cervicitis is usually asymptomatic, which is why routine screening is important. It is diagnosed using NAATs, not Gram stain.
137. Chlamydia can be isolated in 40–50% of men with nongonococcal urethritis, not 95%. It is also implicated in Reiter's syndrome and pneumonitis in infants.
138. *Mycoplasma hominis* is distinct from Ureaplasma. It can cause pelvic inflammatory disease and may contribute to infertility, though tetracyclines are generally effective treatment.
139. Ureaplasma urealyticum is a different organism from *Mycoplasma hominis* and can also cause nongonococcal urethritis. Its role overlaps with chlamydia.
140. Reiter's syndrome (reactive arthritis) is strongly associated with chlamydial infection. Symptoms include arthritis, urethritis, and conjunctivitis.
141. *Chlamydia trachomatis* is the leading cause of preventable blindness worldwide, through repeated ocular infection leading to trachoma and scarring.

142. Gonorrhea and chlamydia often coexist, necessitating dual therapy with ceftriaxone and azithromycin to prevent persistent coinfection.
143. Granuloma inguinale (donovanosis) is a chronic genital ulcer disease caused by *Klebsiella granulomatis*, characterized by beefy red ulcers with Donovan bodies.
144. Chancroid is caused by *H. ducreyi* and is highly painful, unlike the painless ulcers of syphilis and LGV. Its ulcers are soft, with undermined edges.
145. Syphilis is associated with neurological complications such as tabes dorsalis and general paresis, highlighting its systemic potential if untreated.
146. The Jarisch–Herxheimer reaction after penicillin treatment of syphilis results from spirochete lysis, releasing endotoxins and cytokines that trigger systemic inflammation.
147. Pelvic inflammatory disease is most strongly associated with chlamydia and gonorrhea, both leading to infertility due to tubal damage.
148. Treponemal tests remain positive for life, even after cure, while non-treponemal tests like VDRL decline. This is why both are needed for diagnosis and follow-up.
149. HIV increases susceptibility to all STIs, including syphilis and chancroid, and worsens their progression. Coinfections are therefore common in high-risk groups.
150. Prevention of bacterial STIs relies on barrier contraception, partner notification, and screening, as asymptomatic infections (especially chlamydia) drive transmission.

Further Reading

The explanations in this chapter are supported by the following key references:

1. Centers for Disease Control and Prevention. Sexually transmitted infections treatment guidelines, 2021. MMWR Recomm Rep. 2021;70(4):1–187.
2. World Health Organization. WHO guidelines for the treatment of sexually transmitted infections. Geneva: WHO; 2016.
3. Hook EW, Handsfield HH. Gonococcal infections in the adult. In: Sexually transmitted diseases. 4th ed. McGraw-Hill; 2008.
4. Workowski KA, Bachmann LH, Chan PA, et al. Sexually transmitted infections treatment guidelines, 2021. Clin Infect Dis. 2022;74(Suppl 2):S1–S187.
5. Stamm WE. Chlamydia trachomatis infections. N Engl J Med. 1999;340(8):593–600.
6. Peeling RW, Mabey D, Kamb ML, et al. Syphilis. Nat Rev Dis Primers. 2017;3:17073.

19 Viral Sexually Transmitted Infections

Learning Objectives

- Differentiate viral STIs based on clinical and lab features.
- Understand routes of transmission and latency.
- Apply diagnostic protocols (PCR, serology).
- Evaluate role of antiretrovirals and vaccines.
- Counsel patients on disclosure and prevention.

Select the Single Best Answer

1. The herpes simplex type 2 (HSV-2) is NOT:
   A. Deoxyribonucleic acid (DNA) virus
   B. Use ribonucleic acid (RNA) polymerase to form viral DNA
   C. 180–220 nm in diameter
   D. Beta herpes virus group
   E. Spherical in shape
2. The recurrence of genital herpes means:
   A. 1–2 attacks/month
   B. 2–4 attacks/month
   C. > 6 attacks/year
   D. 5 attacks/month
3. Herpes simplex type 2 (HSV-2) increases the risk of human immunodeficiency virus (HIV) infection:
   A. 2 folds
   B. 4 folds
   C. 5 folds
   D. 7 folds
   E. 10 folds

M. S. M. Hasan, M. L. Elsaie, *Comprehensive MCQs in Andrology*, Trends in Andrology and Sexual Medicine, https://doi.org/10.1007/978-3-032-20623-7_19

4. The most reliable diagnostic test for genital herpes is:
   A. Culture
   B. Tzanck smear
   C. Polymerase chain reaction (PCR)
   D. Enzyme-linked immunosorbent assay (ELISA)
5. Neonatal herpes simplex type 2 (HSV-2) mostly occurs within:
   A. First month of life
   B. Second month of life
   C. Third month of life
   D. First day of life
6. Genital Herpes suppressive therapy must be given in:
   A. Initial non-primary attack
   B. Disseminated herpes simplex virus (HSV)
   C. Frequent recurrent episodes
   D. HSV-resistant strains
7. The HSV strains that lost their thymidine kinase enzyme can respond to:
   A. Famciclovir
   B. Valacyclovir
   C. Foscarnet
   D. Acyclovir
8. The initial non-primary herpes is:
   A. First infection with HSV-1
   B. First clinical episode in the presence of preexisting antibodies to HSV
   C. First infection with HSV-2
   D. Recurrent infection with HSV-1 or HSV-2
9. What is the indicated therapy for relapsing genital herpes?
   A. 10-day application of anti-herpes ointment
   B. Oral episode therapy (5 days)
   C. Oral 6-month suppressive therapy
   D. Oral 12-month suppressive therapy
10. Which of the following statements about the treatment of genitalia condylomas is true?
    A. Most common etiological factor is HPV types 6 and 11
    B. Histological exam needed only in atypical pigmented/ulcerated lesions
    C. Lesions at outer urethral orifice require urethrocystoscopy
    D. All of the above
    E. A and B are correct
11. Which of the following is NOT HPV-related penile lesion?
    A. Bowenoid papulosis
    B. Giant condyloma
    C. Erythroplasia of Queyrat
    D. Balanitis xerotica obliterans
    E. Bowen's disease
12. Bowenoid papulosis is associated with:
    A. HPV 8
    B. HPV 16

C. HPV 11
D. HPV 18
E. HPV 6

13. How long after "bleaching" therapy of condyloma acuminata is the patient considered a non-carrier?
    A. After 3 months
    B. After 9 months
    C. After 12 months
    D. Unknown
14. Etiological agent of Kaposi sarcoma is:
    A. Herpes simplex virus type 1 (HSV-1)
    B. HSV-2
    C. Human herpesvirus 6 (HHV-6)
    D. Human herpesvirus 8 (HHV-8)
15. HPV vaccine Gardasil protects against:
    A. 1,3,4,5
    B. 6,11,16,18
    C. 19,31,33,35
    D. 45,51,52,82
16. HPV vaccine Cervarix protects against:
    A. 1,3,4,5
    B. 45,51
    C. 16,18
    D. 19,31,33,35
17. HPV vaccines are indicated for:
    A. All sexually active women
    B. All sexually active men who have sex with men (MSM)
    C. Men and women up to age 26
    D. Only women up to age 26
    E. Only women with family history of cervical cancer
18. Which sexually transmitted infection (STI) often presents with resolved lesion but tender suppurative adenopathy?
    A. Chancroid
    B. HSV-2
    C. HSV-1
    D. Donovanosis
    E. Lymphogranuloma venereum
19. Which HPV subtypes are responsible for malignancies?
    A. 16 and 18
    B. 13 and 14
    C. 6 and 11
    D. 31 and 33
    E. 26 and 28
20. Which statement is true about recurrence likelihood?
    A. No difference except in HIV where HSV-1 recurs more
    B. No difference except in HIV where HSV-2 recurs more

   C. HSV-1 recurs more often
   D. HSV-2 recurs more often
   E. No difference

21. Gardasil in males is recommended:
   A. To prevent HPV transmission
   B. Only for men with documented HPV
   C. To prevent anal cancer and genital warts
   D. To prevent genital warts only
   E. Only in men > 26 years
22. Reverse transcriptase is characteristic of:
   A. Human immunodeficiency virus (HIV)
   B. Herpes simplex virus (HSV)
   C. Epstein–Barr virus (EBV)
   D. Cytomegalovirus (CMV)
   E. Pox virus
23. HIV is what type of virus?
   A. Single-stranded RNA
   B. Double-stranded RNA
   C. Single-stranded messenger RNA (mRNA)
   D. Single-stranded DNA
   E. Double-stranded DNA
24. The HIV envelope precursor protein gp160 is cleaved into:
   A. gp123 & gp33
   B. gp124 & gp40
   C. gp141 & gp20
   D. gp120 & gp41
   E. gp120 & gp6
25. HIV infects which immune cells?
   A. Macrophages
   B. B cells
   C. CD4+ (cluster of differentiation 4 positive) T cells
   D. CD8+ (cluster of differentiation 8 positive) T cells
   E. Natural killer (NK) cells
26. Initial screening test for HIV is:
   A. Western blot
   B. Immunofluorescence assay (IFA)
   C. Nucleic acid amplification test (NAAT)
   D. Rapid enzyme immunoassay (rapid EIA)
   E. Viral culture
27. Antiretroviral therapy (ART) is recommended for:
   A. Only CD4 <200
   B. Only CD4 <350
   C. Only CD4 <500
   D. CD4 <500 with symptoms
   E. All HIV patients

28. Which factor is NOT linked to HIV seroconversion risk after needle stick?
    A. Recent infection in source patient
    B. Deep needle injury
    C. Visible blood on device
    D. Device used in artery/vein
    E. Patient dying within 2 months
29. Gene polymorphism linked with HIV-associated nephropathy (HIVAN) in African-Americans?
    A. Tyrosine kinase
    B. Antichymotrypsin-1
    C. Apolipoprotein-1 (APOL1)
    D. Tumor necrosis factor-alpha (TNF-α)
    E. Interleukin-10 (IL-10)
30. Which antiretrovirals are linked with urinary tract stones?
    A. Integrase inhibitors
    B. Fusion inhibitors
    C. Protease inhibitors (PIs)
    D. Non-nucleoside reverse transcriptase inhibitors (NNRTIs)
    E. C-C chemokine receptor type 5 (CCR5) blockers
31. What is the best diagnostic test to detect HIV in the acute phase of infection?
    A. Indirect immunofluorescence assay (IFA)
    B. Viral load assay (HIV-1 RNA)
    C. Western blot
    D. HIV-1/HIV-2 serology assay
    E. Rapid enzyme immunoassay (rapid EIA)
32. Which class of medication can have prolonged half-life when combined with protease inhibitors (PIs) and NNRTIs?
    A. Alpha-blockers
    B. 5-alpha reductase inhibitors (5-ARIs)
    C. Beta-3 agonists
    D. Phosphodiesterase type 5 (PDE5) inhibitors
    E. Fluoroquinolones
33. Which genitourinary (GU) cancer is NOT increased in HIV patients?
    A. Prostate cancer
    B. Kidney cancer
    C. Penile cancer
    D. Testis cancer
    E. Kaposi sarcoma
34. Which of the following is a symptom of acquired immunodeficiency syndrome (AIDS)?
    A. Fever
    B. Swollen lymph nodes
    C. Tiredness
    D. All of the above

35. The first AIDS cases were reported in:
    A. USA
    B. France
    C. Russia
    D. None of the above
36. HIV parasitizes:
    A. Macrophages
    B. T-helper cells
    C. K-helper cells
    D. B lymphocytes
    E. Schwann cells
37. HIV can spread through:
    A. Sharing water
    B. Breathing infected droplets
    C. Sharing needles
    D. Kissing
38. How many stages of HIV infection exist?
    A. 4
    B. 3
    C. 2
    D. 1
    E. No stages
39. HIV is thought to have originated from:
    A. Birds
    B. Mosquitoes
    C. Chimpanzees
    D. None of the above
40. HIV belongs to which genus?
    A. Lentivirus
    B. Capripoxvirus
    C. Gallivirus
    D. Papillomavirus
41. Which is NOT a clinical subtype of anal intraepithelial neoplasia in HIV patients?
    A. Bowenoid
    B. Verrucous
    C. Porokeratotic
    D. Leukoplakic
    E. Erythroplakic
42. Immunodeficiency should be suspected when:
    A. Recurrent severe infections
    B. Infections with unusual organisms
    C. Poor response to antibiotics
    D. All of the above
    E. None of the above

43. HIV vaccine development is difficult because virus:
    A. Integrates into T cells
    B. Undergoes reverse transcription
    C. Mutates rapidly
    D. Integrates into many host genes
44. Which is FALSE about HIV-1?
    A. Has M and O subgroups
    B. Prevalent in India
    C. Prevalent in Africa
    D. More infectious
    E. Poor vertical transmission
45. Which is TRUE about HIV-2?
    A. Has M and O subgroups
    B. Prevalent in India
    C. Prevalent in Africa
    D. More infectious
    E. Poor vertical transmission
46. Male-to-female heterosexual HIV transmission risk is:
    A. 2–15 times
    B. 15–20 times
    C. 20–25 times
    D. >30 times
47. HIV transmission via breast milk may be due to disturbance in:
    A. Immunoglobulin A (IgA)
    B. Immunoglobulin M (IgM)
    C. Immunoglobulin D (IgD)
    D. Immunoglobulin G (IgG)
    E. Immunoglobulin E (IgE)
48. HIV window period is:
    A. 2 weeks before antibodies
    B. 6 weeks before antibodies
    C. 10 weeks before antibodies
    D. 15 weeks before antibodies
49. Which is NOT included in World Health Organization (WHO) stage 3 HIV?
    A. Recurrent fever
    B. Weight loss
    C. Brain toxoplasmosis
    D. Oral thrush
    E. Chronic diarrhea
50. Common ocular manifestation of HIV is:
    A. Argyll Robertson pupil
    B. Optic atrophy
    C. Retinitis
    D. Choroiditis
    E. Vitreous hemorrhage

51. Post-HIV exposure prophylaxis (PEP) is effective within:
    A. 24 hours
    B. 48 hours
    C. 72 hours
    D. 2 weeks
52. Pre-exposure prophylaxis (PrEP) protects up to:
    A. 30%
    B. 50%
    C. 70%
    D. 80%
53. Eye fundus in AIDS may show:
    A. Pinpoint hemorrhage
    B. Corneal opacity
    C. Retinal detachment
    D. White exudates
54. Best delivery choice for mother with active genital herpes:
    A. Cesarean section
    B. Intravenous (IV) acyclovir with vaginal delivery
    C. IV acyclovir then vaginal delivery
    D. Vaginal delivery then neonatal acyclovir
55. Reverse transcriptase enzyme in HIV is:
    A. DNA polymerase
    B. Ribonuclease
    C. Both
    D. None
56. During HIV-1 lifecycle:
    A. CD4 binds to p24
    B. gp125 mediates attachment
    C. Integration occurs at specific sites
    D. Herpes co-infection can reactivate HIV
    E. Only infects T-helper lymphocytes
57. Which is FALSE about HIV-1 genome?
    A. gag & env code for structure
    B. pol codes for protease & integrase
    C. tat increases viral protein production
    D. nef downregulates expression
    E. env is highly conserved
58. Which is wrong about immune response to HIV-1?
    A. First antibodies target p24
    B. IgA in saliva detectable
    C. IgM peaks at 3 weeks
    D. Cytotoxic CD8+ cells important
    E. All infected develop antibodies within 3 months

59. Which is TRUE after HIV infection?
    A. Most lymphocytes contain viral RNA
    B. Central nervous system (CNS) damage due to neuronal destruction
    C. Syncytia absent in cultures
    D. Antibodies to gag appear before env
    E. HIV antibodies always remain high
60. Which is TRUE about immune deficit in HIV-1?
    A. Entirely due to CD4 loss
    B. Mediated by Langerhans cells
    C. May improve hepatitis B vaccine response
    D. Cholera vaccine contraindicated
    E. Also involves macrophages
61. Which is TRUE consequence of HIV infection?
    A. B-cell function minimally impaired
    B. Polyclonal gammopathy occurs
    C. Serum IgG reduced
    D. Latent infections not reactivated
    E. Eosinophilia frequent
62. Which is TRUE about Pneumocystis carinii (Pneumocystis jirovecii)?
    A. Is a virus
    B. Only in HIV-positive patients
    C. Major pulmonary cause in HIV
    D. Only infects lungs
    E. Best diagnosed by culture
63. Which is FALSE about cytomegalovirus (CMV)?
    A. Is a herpesvirus
    B. Secreted asymptomatically from cervix
    C. Sexually transmitted
    D. Self-limited in immunocompetent
    E. Rare in homosexual men
64. Which is TRUE about condylomata acuminata?
    A. Only found anogenitally
    B. Only manifestation of HPV in genitalia
    C. Most caused by HPV 6, 11
    D. Always sexually transmitted
    E. Often regress in pregnancy
65. Which is TRUE about penile wart treatment?
    A. Interferon is first-line
    B. Abstinence advised until resolution
    C. Urethroscopy mandatory
    D. Laser under local anesthetic
    E. Trichloroacetic acid (TCA) reveals subclinical HPV
66. Podophyllotoxin paint:
    A. Safe in pregnancy
    B. Effective on sessile warts

C. May treat vulval warts
D. Option for cervical flat warts
E. Must be washed off within 2 hrs
67. Diagnosis of anogenital HPV:
A. Culture is standard
B. Immunoglobulin G (IgG) to L1 capsid diagnostic of recent infection
C. Biopsy mandatory
D. Koilocytes on Pap smear suggestive
E. Perianal warts = anal intercourse
68. Genital warts:
A. First line treatment includes antibiotics
B. Morphology varies by HPV type
C. Only occur after puberty
D. Only in uncircumcised men
E. Treated with acyclovir cream
69. Which is NOT a feature of primary HSV infection?
A. Fever
B. Meningitis
C. Headache
D. Dysuria in women
E. Hepatitis
70. Differential diagnosis of genital HSV excludes:
A. Behcet's disease
B. Lymphogranuloma venereum
C. Reiter's syndrome
D. Stevens–Johnson syndrome
E. Late latent syphilis
71. Which test does NOT reliably confirm HSV?
A. Viral culture
B. Papanicolaou (Pap) smear cytology
C. Electron microscopy (EM)
D. Direct immunofluorescence
72. Which systemic antivirals treat HSV?
A. Alpha interferon
B. Acyclovir
C. Idoxuridine
D. Vinblastine
73. Primary genital HSV infection:
A. Same as "first attack" herpes
B. Cervical infection in 25% of women
C. HSV-1 causes more recurrences
D. May cause urinary retention
E. Rarely with inguinal nodes

74. Reported incidence of neonatal HSV:
    A. Higher in wealthy groups
    B. HSV-2 in >80% cases
    C. Acquired from non-mother source in 1/3
    D. Worse in preterm neonates
75. Which is TRUE about Hepatitis A (HAV)?
    A. Causes chronic liver disease in 1%
    B. Transmitted fecal-oral route
    C. Incubation 6 weeks–6 months
    D. Fulminant failure in 5%
    E. Best diagnosed by EM of stool
76. Which group is NOT at risk of Hepatitis B (HBV)?
    A. Men who have sex with men (MSM)
    B. Intravenous (IV) drug users
    C. Orthopedic surgeons
    D. Screened heterosexual donors
    E. Female sex workers
77. Which marker indicates active HBV replication?
    A. Anti-HBs (hepatitis B surface antibody)
    B. HBeAg (hepatitis B e antigen)
    C. Anti-HBe (antibody to HBeAg)
    D. Anti-HBc IgG (hepatitis B core antibody, IgG class)
    E. Anti-HBc IgM (hepatitis B core antibody, IgM class)
78. Which hepatitis virus is defective and needs HBV?
    A. Hepatitis A (HAV)
    B. Hepatitis C (HCV)
    C. Hepatitis D (HDV)
    D. Hepatitis E (HEV)
79. Most common route of HCV transmission globally is:
    A. Sexual intercourse
    B. Blood transfusion
    C. IV drug use
    D. Breastfeeding
80. Which hepatitis is linked to high mortality in pregnancy?
    A. HAV
    B. HBV
    C. HCV
    D. HEV
81. Which viral hepatitis has no chronic carrier state?
    A. A and E
    B. B and C
    C. D and E
    D. Only A

82. Which hepatitis virus is a flavivirus?
    A. A
    B. B
    C. C
    D. E
83. Best test for early acute Hepatitis C?
    A. Anti-HCV antibody
    B. HCV RNA PCR (ribonucleic acid by polymerase chain reaction)
    C. HCV core antigen
    D. ELISA
84. Which hepatitis has DNA genome?
    A. A
    B. B
    C. C
    D. E
85. Which hepatitis is usually transmitted via shellfish?
    A. A
    B. B
    C. C
    D. D
86. Pegylated interferon is used in treatment of:
    A. HBV
    B. HCV
    C. Both HBV and HCV
    D. HAV
87. Which is TRUE about Hepatitis B vaccine?
    A. Live attenuated vaccine
    B. Given intradermally
    C. Recombinant subunit vaccine
    D. Protective for 2 years only
88. Which hepatitis virus has the shortest incubation?
    A. A
    B. B
    C. C
    D. E
89. Which viral hepatitis lacks an envelope?
    A. A
    B. B
    C. C
    D. D
90. Chronic infection most common with:
    A. HAV
    B. HBV
    C. HCV
    D. HEV

91. Which virus is the cause of molluscum contagiosum?
    A. Herpesvirus
    B. Poxvirus
    C. Papillomavirus
    D. Adenovirus
92. Which virus causes "giant condyloma of Buschke–Löwenstein"?
    A. HPV 6
    B. HPV 11
    C. HPV 16
    D. HPV 18
93. Which is NOT a feature of molluscum contagiosum?
    A. Umbilicated papules
    B. Caused by poxvirus
    C. Self-limited in immunocompetent
    D. Always requires systemic therapy
94. Which is TRUE about Epstein-Barr virus (EBV)?
    A. Causes infectious mononucleosis
    B. Associated with oral hairy leukoplakia in HIV
    C. Associated with nasopharyngeal carcinoma
    D. All of the above
95. Which STI virus is oncogenic?
    A. HSV
    B. HPV
    C. HIV
    D. Molluscum contagiosum
96. Which antiviral is NOT used in HIV therapy?
    A. Zidovudine
    B. Efavirenz
    C. Saquinavir
    D. Amphotericin B
97. The "p24 antigen" is a marker of:
    A. HSV
    B. HPV
    C. HIV
    D. Hepatitis B virus (HBV)
98. Which HIV protein mediates fusion/entry?
    A. gp120
    B. gp41
    C. p24
    D. nef
99. Which HIV drug class prevents integration of viral DNA?
    A. NNRTIs (non-nucleoside reverse transcriptase inhibitors)
    B. NRTIs (nucleoside/nucleotide reverse transcriptase inhibitors)
    C. Protease inhibitors (PIs)
    D. Integrase inhibitors (INIs)

100. Which viral STI is MOST strongly associated with anal cancer?
   A. HSV-2
   B. HPV-16
   C. HIV
   D. HBV

✅ Key Takeaways

- **HSV-2** causes recurrent painful ulcers; PCR is diagnostic.
- **HPV** is linked to genital warts and malignancies; vaccination is preventive.
- HIV requires **CD4 and viral load** monitoring.
- **HBV/HCV** can be sexually transmitted; chronic forms need long-term follow-up.
- Prevention includes **safe sex, screening, and vaccination**.

✅ Answer Key (1–100)

1. D
2. C
3. A
4. C
5. A
6. C
7. C
8. B
9. B
10. D
11. D
12. B
13. D
14. D
15. B
16. C
17. C
18. A
19. A
20. D
21. C
22. A
23. A
24. D
25. C
26. D
27. E

28. E
29. C
30. C
31. B
32. D
33. A
34. D
35. A
36. B
37. C
38. B
39. C
40. A
41. C
42. D
43. C
44. E
45. C
46. A
47. A
48. B
49. C
50. C
51. C
52. D
53. D
54. A
55. C
56. D
57. E
58. E
59. D
60. E
61. B
62. C
63. E
64. C
65. B
66. C
67. D
68. B
69. E
70. E
71. B
72. B

73. D
74. B
75. B
76. D
77. B
78. C
79. C
80. D
81. A
82. C
83. B
84. B
85. A
86. C
87. C
88. A
89. A
90. C
91. B
92. B
93. D
94. D
95. B
96. D
97. C
98. B
99. D
100. B

Explanations (1–100)

1. Herpes simplex virus type 2 belongs to the herpesviridae family, which are double-stranded DNA viruses. It is spherical and relatively large in size (about 180–220 nm). The incorrect option here was that it is a beta herpesvirus; in fact, HSV-2 is part of the *alpha herpesvirus* group, characterized by rapid replication and latency in sensory ganglia.
2. Recurrence in genital herpes is clinically defined by repeated symptomatic outbreaks after the initial episode. A practical definition is when the patient has more than six attacks per year. This is considered clinically significant and often prompts consideration of suppressive therapy.
3. HSV-2 infection increases susceptibility to HIV. Epidemiologic studies consistently show that the risk of HIV acquisition in HSV-2 infected individuals is roughly doubled. The disruption of mucosal barriers and recruitment of activated CD4 cells explains why HSV makes HIV entry easier.

4. Among diagnostic tests, polymerase chain reaction (PCR) is the most sensitive and specific for genital herpes. Viral culture was historically the gold standard, but it is less sensitive, especially in recurrent disease. Tzanck smears and ELISA can be supportive but lack reliability compared to PCR.
5. Neonatal herpes simplex usually manifests in the first month of life. It is acquired during passage through an infected birth canal. Presentation may be limited to skin/eye/mouth lesions, disseminated infection, or CNS disease. Early recognition is critical because untreated neonatal herpes has high mortality.
6. Suppressive therapy for genital herpes is not necessary in every patient. It is particularly indicated in individuals with frequent recurrent episodes that interfere with quality of life. Long-term antivirals reduce recurrence frequency and also reduce transmission risk to partners.
7. Resistance to acyclovir typically occurs when HSV loses thymidine kinase activity, the enzyme needed to phosphorylate acyclovir into its active form. Such strains remain susceptible to *foscarnet*, which acts directly on the viral DNA polymerase without requiring prior activation.
8. An initial non-primary herpes infection occurs when a person acquires one HSV type while already possessing antibodies to the other. For example, a person previously infected with HSV-1 developing their first HSV-2 genital outbreak. Clinically, the course may be less severe than a true primary episode.
9. Relapsing genital herpes is best managed with either episodic oral antiviral therapy or long-term suppressive regimens. A five-day course of oral antivirals is the standard option for an acute relapse, while suppressive courses are reserved for those with frequent recurrences.
10. Genital condylomas are caused most often by HPV types 6 and 11. Histology is only needed for atypical lesions, such as pigmented or ulcerated forms. Lesions at the urethral meatus may require urethrocystoscopy to assess internal involvement. Thus, all listed statements are true.
11. Penile lesions associated with HPV include bowenoid papulosis, giant condyloma, Bowen's disease, and erythroplasia of Queyrat. Balanitis xerotica obliterans is not HPV-related; it is a chronic inflammatory condition, not viral in origin.
12. Bowenoid papulosis is linked to high-risk HPV types, especially type 16. It presents as multiple pigmented papules on the genitalia and is histologically similar to squamous cell carcinoma in situ, though it often regresses spontaneously.
13. The duration after which a patient is considered non-infectious following treatment of condyloma acuminata remains uncertain. Virus persistence can occur despite lesion resolution, and clearance cannot be reliably defined by a fixed timeline. Therefore, the best answer is that the period is unknown.
14. Kaposi's sarcoma is caused by human herpesvirus type 8 (HHV-8). This oncogenic virus promotes vascular tumor formation, particularly in immunocompromised individuals such as those with AIDS.

15. Gardasil is a quadrivalent HPV vaccine that protects against HPV types 6, 11 (low-risk, genital warts) and 16, 18 (high-risk, cancers). This dual coverage makes it useful for preventing both benign and malignant HPV outcomes.
16. Cervarix is a bivalent vaccine directed specifically against HPV types 16 and 18, the high-risk oncogenic strains associated with cervical, anal, and oropharyngeal cancers.
17. HPV vaccination is recommended for both men and women up to age 26 years, ideally before the onset of sexual activity. It is also beneficial for men who have sex with men and immunocompromised individuals.
18. Chancroid (caused by *Haemophilus ducreyi*) often heals spontaneously, but tender suppurative inguinal lymphadenopathy remains. This distinguishes it from HSV or lymphogranuloma venereum.
19. High-risk HPV types 16 and 18 are responsible for the majority of cervical cancers and also implicated in penile, vulvar, vaginal, and anal cancers. Other high-risk types (31, 33, 45) also contribute but less commonly.
20. HSV-2 recurs more frequently than HSV-1 when affecting the genital tract. HSV-1 tends to recur less often because it is more adapted to oral mucosa, whereas HSV-2 has a predilection for the genital area.
21. Gardasil vaccination in males is recommended to prevent both anal cancers and genital warts. It has a role beyond protecting partners, as HPV also directly causes disease in men.
22. Reverse transcriptase is the hallmark enzyme of HIV, a retrovirus. It allows the viral RNA genome to be converted into DNA, which then integrates into the host genome.
23. HIV is a single-stranded RNA virus belonging to the retrovirus family. Its genome requires reverse transcription into DNA to establish infection.
24. The HIV envelope glycoprotein gp160 is cleaved into gp120 and gp41. gp120 mediates binding to the CD4 receptor, while gp41 facilitates membrane fusion.
25. HIV primarily infects CD4 T helper lymphocytes, although macrophages and dendritic cells can also serve as reservoirs. CD4 loss underlies the profound immunosuppression seen in AIDS.
26. The initial screening test for HIV is typically a rapid enzyme immunoassay (EIA). This test detects antibodies (and sometimes p24 antigen in fourth-generation assays) and is highly sensitive. Positive results are confirmed by more specific tests such as Western blot or PCR.
27. Modern HIV guidelines recommend initiating antiretroviral therapy in all patients, regardless of CD4 count or clinical symptoms. Early treatment reduces morbidity, mortality, and transmission. This represents a shift from older practice when therapy was delayed until CD4 counts dropped below certain thresholds.
28. Risk factors that increase the chance of HIV transmission following a needle-stick injury include deep penetration, visible blood on the needle, and placement of the device in a blood vessel. The patient's disease stage matters; acute infection increases transmissibility. A terminally ill patient is not specifically associated with higher risk.

29. HIV-associated nephropathy (HIVAN) is strongly linked to polymorphisms in the *apolipoprotein L1 (APOL1)* gene. These variants are common among African populations and predispose to collapsing focal segmental glomerulosclerosis, a hallmark of HIVAN.
30. Protease inhibitors, a major class of antiretroviral therapy, have been linked with metabolic disturbances including nephrolithiasis. Drugs like indinavir and atazanavir are notorious for causing urinary tract stones, a relevant adverse effect to monitor.
31. During acute HIV infection, antibody tests may still be negative. The most sensitive diagnostic tool is viral load measurement by nucleic acid amplification, which can detect viral RNA before seroconversion occurs. This makes it the best test for early infection.
32. Protease inhibitors and NNRTIs are metabolized by hepatic cytochrome P450 enzymes. When combined with PDE5 inhibitors such as sildenafil, the clearance of the latter is delayed, leading to prolonged half-life and increased risk of adverse effects like hypotension.
33. In HIV patients, certain cancers are more frequent, such as Kaposi's sarcoma, lymphoma, and anal carcinoma. However, prostate cancer has not shown a higher incidence in this population compared to the general public, making it the exception here.
34. AIDS is defined clinically by the development of opportunistic infections or specific malignancies. Symptoms such as fever, lymphadenopathy, and chronic fatigue are common systemic signs. Recognizing these nonspecific features often prompts testing in at-risk individuals.
35. The first recognized cases of AIDS were reported in the early 1980s in the United States. Clusters of Pneumocystis pneumonia and Kaposi's sarcoma in young homosexual men marked the start of the epidemic.
36. HIV primarily parasitizes CD4 T-helper lymphocytes, as well as macrophages and dendritic cells. The progressive depletion of CD4 cells underlies the profound immune dysfunction seen in AIDS.
37. HIV spreads through sexual contact, contaminated blood transfusion, and needle sharing. Casual contact, kissing, or sharing water does not transmit the virus. Needle sharing is a major mode of transmission among injection drug users.
38. HIV progression occurs in three main stages: Acute HIV infection, characterized by high viral load and flu-like symptoms; Chronic HIV infection (also called clinical latency), where the virus multiplies at low levels with few or no symptoms; and Acquired Immunodeficiency Syndrome (AIDS), the most severe stage where the immune system is severely damaged.
39. HIV is believed to have originated from simian immunodeficiency viruses in chimpanzees, which crossed into humans via zoonotic transmission, likely during hunting or butchering of primates in Central Africa.
40. HIV belongs to the *lentivirus* genus of retroviruses. Lentiviruses are characterized by long incubation periods and chronic, progressive disease courses.

41. Anal intraepithelial neoplasia in HIV-infected patients can present as bowenoid, verrucous, leukoplakic, or erythroplakic forms. Porokeratotic lesions are not recognized subtypes in this context.
42. Immunodeficiency should be suspected in patients with recurrent infections, unusual pathogens, prolonged disease, or poor response to standard therapy. These features collectively raise red flags for underlying immune compromise such as HIV.
43. A key challenge in developing an HIV vaccine is the virus's high mutation rate, especially in the envelope genes. This genetic variability allows it to evade immune recognition and neutralizing antibodies, making vaccine development extremely difficult.
44. HIV-1 is the predominant global strain, particularly in Africa. It is more infectious than HIV-2. The statement that it is prevalent in India is incorrect—HIV-2 predominates in West Africa, while HIV-1 dominates elsewhere.
45. HIV-2 is most common in West Africa. It tends to be less transmissible and progresses more slowly than HIV-1. Vertical transmission is also less efficient compared to HIV-1.
46. Heterosexual transmission from male to female is more efficient than female to male. Epidemiologic studies estimate a risk of 2–15 times higher in this direction, largely due to anatomical and mucosal factors.
47. Breast milk transmission of HIV relates to immunoglobulin disturbances, particularly IgA. Reduced protective secretory IgA allows viral particles to persist and transmit during breastfeeding.
48. The HIV window period is the time between infection and detectability of antibodies. It typically lasts about 6 weeks, though modern combined antigen/antibody tests can shorten detection time.
49. WHO stage 3 HIV disease includes chronic diarrhea, weight loss, and oral thrush. Brain toxoplasmosis, however, is categorized as stage 4, not stage 3.
50. Retinitis, especially due to cytomegalovirus (CMV), is a common ocular complication in HIV/AIDS patients. It presents as visual field defects and can progress to blindness if untreated.
51. Post-exposure prophylaxis (PEP) for HIV is most effective when initiated as soon as possible after exposure, ideally within 72 h. Beyond this timeframe, the efficacy diminishes sharply, making early intervention essential.
52. Pre-exposure prophylaxis (PrEP) with drugs like tenofovir/emtricitabine provides significant protection, reducing risk by up to 70–80% when adherence is good. Partial adherence lowers its protective value to around 50%.
53. Fundoscopic findings in AIDS patients often reveal opportunistic infections such as CMV retinitis. Cotton-white spots and white retinal exudates are characteristic, potentially leading to blindness if not treated.
54. For pregnant women with active genital herpes, cesarean delivery is recommended to reduce the risk of neonatal transmission. Vaginal delivery in this context carries a high risk of infecting the neonate.

55. HIV's reverse transcriptase enzyme has dual functions: DNA polymerase activity to convert viral RNA into DNA, and ribonuclease activity to degrade RNA strands. This unique enzyme is a major therapeutic target.
56. During HIV-1's life cycle, gp120 facilitates binding to CD4 receptors, and gp41 mediates fusion. Integration into host DNA occurs at variable, not specific, sites. Herpes virus co-infection can enhance HIV transcription.
57. In HIV-1, *gag* and *env* genes code for structural proteins, while *pol* encodes reverse transcriptase, integrase, and protease. The *tat* gene upregulates transcription, while *nef* downregulates host immunity. The *env* gene is highly variable, not conserved.
58. Early in HIV infection, antibodies appear first against p24 antigen. IgM rises initially, followed by IgG. Specific IgA can also be detected in mucosal secretions. Not all individuals seroconvert within 3 months; rare cases take longer.
59. Following HIV infection, antibodies to core proteins like p24 typically develop before antibodies to envelope proteins. Neurological damage occurs indirectly, via immune activation and toxins, rather than direct neuron destruction.
60. The immune deficit in HIV is not solely explained by CD4 depletion. Macrophages and monocytes are also affected, serving as viral reservoirs and contributing to immune dysfunction. Vaccination responses are impaired, but not entirely absent.
61. B cell function is not spared in HIV; polyclonal activation leads to hypergammaglobulinemia. Serum IgG is often elevated rather than reduced. This contributes to immune dysregulation and increased risk of autoimmunity.
62. *Pneumocystis jirovecii* (previously carinii) is a fungus, not a virus. It causes pneumonia in immunocompromised patients, particularly those with HIV. It is not confined to the lung but manifests predominantly as pulmonary disease.
63. Cytomegalovirus (CMV) is a herpesvirus. It is often transmitted sexually, as well as via blood and saliva. Asymptomatic cervical shedding is common, particularly in immunocompetent individuals. Infection is frequent among homosexual men, making the opposite statement false.
64. Condylomata acuminata are genital warts caused mainly by HPV 6 and 11. They are not restricted to the anogenital area and can appear in extragenital sites. Pregnancy may cause regression or progression, depending on immune status.
65. Management of penile warts includes patient counseling. Abstaining from intercourse while lesions are present helps reduce transmission. Treatments include cryotherapy, imiquimod, and surgical excision; intralesional interferon is not first-line.
66. Podophyllotoxin paint is contraindicated in pregnancy due to teratogenicity. It is effective for external anogenital warts but not for cervical lesions. It must be applied properly, but unlike podophyllin resin, does not need washing off.
67. Biopsy is not always required in HPV diagnosis, but Pap smears showing koilocytes strongly suggest cervical involvement. Culture is not used, and serology has limited diagnostic value. Koilocytosis is a hallmark cytological finding.

68. Genital warts can appear in children, and though sexual abuse must be considered, vertical transmission and non-sexual routes are also possible. They commonly occur at sites of trauma during intercourse and may show varied morphologies.
69. Primary genital herpes simplex virus infection presents with fever, headache, painful genital ulcers, and lymphadenopathy. Hepatitis, however, is not a common feature of primary disease, making it the exception.
70. Differential diagnoses of genital herpes include Behçet's disease, lymphogranuloma venereum, Reiter's syndrome, and Stevens-Johnson syndrome. Late latent syphilis does not mimic acute genital ulcerative disease, so it is not included.
71. HSV diagnosis can be confirmed by viral culture, electron microscopy, or immunofluorescence. Pap smears are not reliable for HSV diagnosis. Viral culture remains a classic gold standard, though PCR is superior today.
72. Effective systemic antivirals against HSV include acyclovir, valacyclovir, and famciclovir. Alpha interferon and idoxuridine are not used systemically. Acyclovir is the cornerstone treatment.
73. Primary genital HSV infection is the true first encounter with the virus. It can involve the cervix in many women, cause urinary retention, and is associated with marked lymphadenopathy. Recurrence is more frequent with HSV-2 than HSV-1.
74. Neonatal HSV is mostly caused by HSV-2. Transmission usually occurs during birth, not postnatally, and is more severe in premature infants. It represents a significant cause of neonatal morbidity and mortality.
75. Hepatitis A virus is transmitted via the fecal–oral route. It causes acute hepatitis but does not result in chronic infection. Fulminant hepatitis is rare. Diagnosis is made serologically, not by electron microscopy.
76. High-risk groups for hepatitis B include men who have sex with men, intravenous drug users, and healthcare workers. Regular blood donors using sterile equipment are not considered high risk, making them the exception.
77. The marker of active hepatitis B replication is the presence of e antigen, which reflects high viral replication and infectivity, whereas surface and core antibodies only reflect immunity or exposure.
78. The defective virus in the hepatitis family is the delta virus, which requires surface antigen from hepatitis B for its assembly and infectivity, making co- or super-infection clinically significant.
79. The most common route of hepatitis C transmission globally today is through intravenous drug use, although transfusion was historically important before routine screening was introduced.
80. Hepatitis E is particularly dangerous in pregnancy, where fulminant hepatic failure and maternal mortality rates rise steeply, especially in the third trimester.
81. Among the hepatotropic viruses, hepatitis A and hepatitis E never progress to chronicity; they cause acute, self-limiting infections, in contrast to B, C, and D.
82. Hepatitis C belongs to the Flaviviridae family of RNA viruses, distinguishing it from hepatitis B, which is a DNA virus in the hepadnavirus family.

83. The earliest diagnostic marker of acute hepatitis C is viral RNA detected by polymerase chain reaction, as serologic antibodies may take several weeks to appear.
84. Of all the hepatitis viruses, only hepatitis B carries a DNA genome, albeit partially double-stranded, while A, C, D, and E are RNA viruses.
85. The classic foodborne outbreaks of hepatitis A often arise from consumption of contaminated shellfish, which serve as a reservoir for fecal-oral transmission.
86. Pegylated interferon is used to treat both HBV and HCV infections. It enhances antiviral immune response and suppresses viral replication, especially in combination with ribavirin for HCV.
87. The hepatitis B vaccine is a recombinant subunit vaccine prepared from surface antigen proteins, given intramuscularly, and provides long-term immunity.
88. The hepatitis virus with the shortest incubation period is hepatitis A, which typically manifests within a few weeks, shorter than the other forms.
89. Both hepatitis A and hepatitis E lack an envelope, which contributes to their environmental stability and fecal-oral transmission patterns.
90. Chronicity is most characteristic of hepatitis C, with the majority of infected individuals developing persistent infection, compared to the lower rates seen with hepatitis B in adults.
91. Molluscum contagiosum is a viral STI caused by a poxvirus, presenting as dome-shaped, umbilicated papules, especially in immunocompromised patients.
92. Giant condyloma of Buschke–Löwenstein is associated with low-risk HPV types 6 and 11, though its locally invasive growth can mimic malignancy.
93. Molluscum contagiosum is usually self-limiting in immunocompetent hosts and does not require systemic therapy, making observation or local treatment sufficient.
94. Epstein–Barr virus causes infectious mononucleosis, is linked with oral hairy leukoplakia in HIV patients, and is oncogenic, being implicated in nasopharyngeal carcinoma.
95. The most strongly oncogenic sexually transmitted virus is human papillomavirus, particularly high-risk types such as 16 and 18.
96. Amphotericin B, while antifungal, is not part of HIV therapy, in contrast to zidovudine, efavirenz, and protease inhibitors, which are integral to antiretroviral regimens.
97. The p24 antigen is an early structural marker of HIV infection, detectable in serum before seroconversion occurs, making it useful in early diagnosis.
98. The viral protein gp41 mediates fusion of HIV with host cells, while gp120 binds CD4 and co-receptors, together ensuring viral entry into lymphocytes.
99. Integrase inhibitors specifically block the incorporation of HIV DNA into the host genome, representing a key antiretroviral class alongside reverse transcriptase and protease inhibitors.
100. Anal cancer is most strongly associated with infection by high-risk HPV type 16, particularly in high-risk populations such as HIV-positive men who have sex with men.

Further Reading

The explanations in this chapter are supported by the following key references:

1. Centers for Disease Control and Prevention. Sexually transmitted infections treatment guidelines, 2021. MMWR Recomm Rep. 2021;70(4):1–187.
2. World Health Organization. WHO Guidelines for the treatment of sexually transmitted infections. Geneva: WHO; 2016.
3. Doorbar J, Quint W, Banks L, et al. The biology and life-cycle of human papillomaviruses. Vaccine. 2012;30(Suppl 5):F55–70.
4. Corey L, Wald A. Genital herpes. N Engl J Med. 2009;361(14):1376–85.
5. Cohen MS, Chen YQ, McCauley M, et al. Prevention of HIV-1 infection with early antiretroviral therapy. N Engl J Med. 2011;365(6):493–505.
6. Stanaway JD, Flaxman AD, Naghavi M, et al. The global burden of viral hepatitis. Lancet. 2016;388(10049):1081–8.

Special Topics in Sexually Transmitted Infections

20

Learning Objectives

- Identify uncommon STI pathogens and their features.
- Apply appropriate diagnostic tools.
- Understand treatment challenges in resistant organisms.
- Examine STIs in special populations (e.g., HIV-positive).
- Recognize need for research and surveillance.

Select the Single Best Answer

1. The causative organism of trichomoniasis is:
   A. *Candida albicans*
   B. *Trichomonas vaginalis*
   C. *Chlamydia trachomatis*
   D. *Neisseria gonorrhoeae*
   E. *Mycoplasma hominis*
2. The commonest symptom of trichomoniasis in women is:
   A. Dysuria
   B. Pruritus
   C. Vaginal discharge
   D. Dyspareunia
   E. Abdominal pain
3. The characteristic discharge in trichomoniasis is:
   A. Thick curdy
   B. Frothy, greenish-yellow
   C. Watery
   D. Bloody
   E. Clear mucoid

M. S. M. Hasan, M. L. Elsaie, *Comprehensive MCQs in Andrology*, Trends in Andrology and Sexual Medicine, https://doi.org/10.1007/978-3-032-20623-7_20

4. The diagnostic method of choice for trichomoniasis is:
   A. Urine culture
   B. Wet mount microscopy
   C. ELISA
   D. Serology
   E. Dark field microscopy
5. The drug of choice for trichomoniasis is:
   A. Fluconazole
   B. Metronidazole
   C. Doxycycline
   D. Erythromycin
   E. Penicillin
6. Pubic lice are caused by:
   A. Pediculus humanus
   B. Sarcoptes scabiei
   C. Phthirus pubis
   D. Trichomonas vaginalis
   E. Candida albicans
7. First-line treatment for pubic lice infestation is:
   A. Ivermectin
   B. Permethrin cream
   C. Fluconazole
   D. Benzathine penicillin
   E. Podophyllin
8. Genital scabies typically presents as:
   A. Vesicles on glans
   B. Burrows and intense itching
   C. Painless ulcers
   D. Condyloma lata
   E. Urethral discharge
9. Fungal balanitis is most commonly due to:
   A. *Trichomonas vaginalis*
   B. *Candida albicans*
   C. *Chlamydia trachomatis*
   D. HSV-2
   E. HPV
10. Risk factors for Candida balanitis include all EXCEPT:
    A. Diabetes mellitus
    B. Immunosuppression
    C. Long-term antibiotics
    D. Poor hygiene
    E. Circumcision
11. Phimosis is defined as:
    A. Inability to retract foreskin
    B. Painful penile erection

C. Curvature of the penis
D. Tight frenulum
E. Urethral narrowing

12. Paraphimosis is:
A. Inability to protract foreskin
B. Painful retracted foreskin stuck behind glans
C. Congenital curvature of penis
D. Infection of glans
E. Hypospadias

13. The most serious complication of paraphimosis is:
A. Dysuria
B. Phimosis
C. Penile gangrene
D. Urethritis
E. Candidiasis

14. Priapism refers to:
A. Painful short erections
B. Prolonged erection >4 h
C. Inability to ejaculate
D. Premature ejaculation
E. Erectile dysfunction

15. The commonest cause of ischemic priapism is:
A. Trauma
B. Sickle cell disease
C. Antidepressants
D. Leukemia
E. Idiopathic

16. Peyronie's disease involves:
A. Infection of foreskin
B. Curvature of penis due to fibrous plaque
C. Congenital urethral narrowing
D. Erectile dysfunction only
E. Inflammation of corpus spongiosum

17. The typical location of Peyronie's plaque is:
A. Corpus spongiosum
B. Corpus cavernosum tunica albuginea
C. Penile urethra
D. Glans penis
E. Frenulum

18. Reiter's syndrome (reactive arthritis) is associated with:
A. HSV
B. *Chlamydia trachomatis*
C. *Treponema pallidum*
D. Candida
E. HPV

19. The classic triad of Reiter's syndrome is:
    A. Arthritis, balanitis, syphilis
    B. Urethritis, arthritis, conjunctivitis
    C. Dysuria, rash, fever
    D. Genital ulcers, conjunctivitis, arthritis
    E. Arthritis, orchitis, dysuria
20. HIV infection is most commonly associated with which malignancy?
    A. Kaposi's sarcoma
    B. Prostate carcinoma
    C. Seminoma
    D. Basal cell carcinoma
    E. Leukemia
21. Neurosyphilis occurs during which stage?
    A. Primary
    B. Secondary
    C. Latent
    D. Tertiary
    E. Early latent
22. Cardiovascular syphilis most commonly affects:
    A. Pulmonary artery
    B. Coronary artery
    C. Aorta
    D. Femoral artery
    E. Carotid artery
23. The commonest cause of orchitis in mumps is:
    A. HSV
    B. Paramyxovirus
    C. Adenovirus
    D. HPV
    E. Enterovirus
24. Cryptorchidism is associated with increased risk of:
    A. Infertility
    B. Testicular cancer
    C. Torsion
    D. All of the above
    E. None of the above
25. The most common testicular tumor in young men is:
    A. Seminoma
    B. Yolk sac tumor
    C. Choriocarcinoma
    D. Leydig cell tumor
    E. Teratoma
26. Tumor marker for seminoma is:
    A. AFP
    B. β-hCG
    C. PSA

D. CEA
E. CA-125
27. Tumor marker for non-seminomatous germ cell tumors is:
A. AFP
B. β-hCG
C. Both A and B
D. PSA
E. None
28. Gynecomastia in males is caused by all EXCEPT:
A. Klinefelter syndrome
B. Cirrhosis
C. hCG-secreting tumors
D. Androgen excess
E. Testicular tumors
29. The most effective prevention of HPV-related genital cancers is:
A. Condoms
B. HPV vaccination
C. Abstinence
D. Screening only
E. Topical treatments
30. Which vaccine is recommended for STI prevention?
A. HPV
B. Hepatitis B
C. Both A and B
D. Syphilis
E. Gonorrhea
31. The mainstay of syndromic STI management is:
A. Treating based on lab results only
B. Immediate treatment of partners
C. Empiric therapy by syndrome presentation
D. Abstinence only
E. Counseling only
32. The WHO guideline emphasizes STI prevention by:
A. Contact tracing
B. Vaccination
C. Condom promotion
D. All of the above
E. None
33. Donovanosis is caused by:
A. *Klebsiella granulomatis*
B. *Neisseria gonorrhoeae*
C. *Treponema pallidum*
D. *Chlamydia trachomatis*
E. Mycoplasma
34. Donovan bodies are seen in:
A. Wet mount
B. Wright-Giemsa stain

   C. Dark field microscopy
   D. PCR
   E. ELISA
35. Chancroid is caused by:
   A. *Haemophilus ducreyi*
   B. *Treponema pallidum*
   C. HSV-2
   D. Klebsiella
   E. Chlamydia
36. The lesion of chancroid is:
   A. Painful ulcer with soft edges
   B. Painless hard ulcer
   C. Vesicular lesion
   D. Wart-like lesion
   E. Papulosquamous lesion
37. Lymphogranuloma venereum is caused by:
   A. *Chlamydia trachomatis* L1–L3
   B. HSV-2
   C. *Treponema pallidum*
   D. Klebsiella
   E. *Haemophilus ducreyi*
38. The buboes of LGV are:
   A. Painful inguinal lymphadenopathy
   B. Painless subcutaneous nodules
   C. Genital warts
   D. Hard chancre
   E. Vesicles
39. Molluscum contagiosum is caused by:
   A. Poxvirus
   B. HPV
   C. HSV
   D. Chlamydia
   E. Mycoplasma
40. The lesion of molluscum contagiosum is:
   A. Vesicle with central depression
   B. Hard chancre
   C. Painful ulcer
   D. Warty lesion
   E. Papule with fluid
41. Scabies mite burrows are commonly found in:
   A. Palms and interdigital spaces
   B. Scalp
   C. Abdomen only
   D. Penis only
   E. Soles only

42. Condyloma acuminata is caused by:
    A. HPV 6 and 11
    B. HPV 16 and 18
    C. HSV
    D. *Treponema pallidum*
    E. Candida
43. The most oncogenic HPV strains are:
    A. 6 and 11
    B. 16 and 18
    C. 31 and 33
    D. 42 and 43
    E. 51 and 52
44. The drug of choice for syphilis is:
    A. Azithromycin
    B. Doxycycline
    C. Benzathine penicillin
    D. Ceftriaxone
    E. Erythromycin
45. Jarisch-Herxheimer reaction occurs after treatment of:
    A. Gonorrhea
    B. Syphilis
    C. Chlamydia
    D. HIV
    E. Candida
46. Chlamydia is best treated with:
    A. Doxycycline
    B. Penicillin
    C. Ciprofloxacin
    D. Metronidazole
    E. Amphotericin
47. The most common site of HPV-related cancer in men is:
    A. Prostate
    B. Penis
    C. Testis
    D. Urethra
    E. Bladder
48. The most common cause of orchitis in children is:
    A. Mumps virus
    B. HSV
    C. HPV
    D. EBV
    E. Adenovirus
49. The gold standard diagnostic test for HIV is:
    A. Western blot
    B. ELISA

   C. PCR
   D. Rapid test
   E. Viral culture
50. The window period for HIV antibody detection is:
   A. 1–2 days
   B. 2–4 weeks
   C. 6–12 weeks
   D. 6 months
   E. 1 year

✅ Key Takeaways

- **Mycoplasma genitalium** is emerging as a cause of urethritis.
- **Donovanosis** causes painless ulceration; diagnosis via Donovan bodies.
- Atypical STIs may be **resistant** and need **targeted therapy**.
- Immunocompromised individuals may have **atypical presentations**.
- Continued vigilance and updated guidelines are critical.

✅ Answer Key (1–50)

1. B
2. C
3. B
4. B
5. B
6. C
7. B
8. B
9. B
10. E
11. A
12. B
13. C
14. B
15. B
16. B
17. B
18. B
19. B
20. A
21. D
22. C
23. B

24. D
25. A
26. B
27. C
28. D
29. B
30. C
31. C
32. D
33. A
34. B
35. A
36. A
37. A
38. A
39. A
40. A
41. A
42. A
43. B
44. C
45. B
46. A
47. B
48. A
49. A
50. C

Explanations (1–50)

1. *Trichomonas vaginalis* is a flagellated protozoan that infects the urogenital tract. Transmission is almost exclusively sexual, and the infection is often asymptomatic in men but symptomatic in women. Recognizing it is important because untreated trichomoniasis can increase HIV acquisition risk and cause adverse pregnancy outcomes.
2. The hallmark of trichomoniasis in women is a foul-smelling vaginal discharge, often accompanied by vulvar irritation, itching, and burning. Dyspareunia and dysuria may also occur. Many cases are asymptomatic, particularly in men, which facilitates silent transmission between partners.
3. The vaginal discharge in trichomoniasis is frothy, yellow-green, and malodorous, distinguishing it from candidiasis (thick curdy) and bacterial vaginosis (thin, gray, fishy odor). The discharge may also cause erythema of the vaginal walls and cervix, sometimes producing the "strawberry cervix" appearance.

4. Wet mount microscopy remains the first-line diagnostic test, showing motile flagellated trophozoites. Although it is inexpensive and quick, sensitivity is limited (50–60%). Nucleic acid amplification tests (NAATs) are more sensitive but less widely available in low-resource settings.
5. Metronidazole is the treatment of choice, either as a single 2 g oral dose or a 7-day regimen. Treating both partners is essential to prevent reinfection. Tinidazole is an alternative in resistant cases. Reinforcement of safe sex practices is also part of management.
6. *Phthirus pubis* (pubic or crab louse) is a parasitic insect that infests pubic hair. Transmission occurs via sexual contact or contaminated bedding. The lice attach to hair shafts and feed on blood, causing itching, irritation, and sometimes secondary infection due to scratching.
7. Permethrin cream or shampoo is first-line for pubic lice infestation. Application should cover the entire body from the waist down. Bedding and clothes must be washed at high temperatures, and partners treated simultaneously. Oral ivermectin is an alternative in resistant cases.
8. Genital scabies is caused by *Sarcoptes scabiei* mites, producing burrows and papules with severe nocturnal itching. Common sites include genitalia, interdigital spaces, and axillae. Transmission is via close skin contact, often sexual, and outbreaks are common in overcrowded environments.
9. *Candida albicans* is the most common cause of fungal balanitis. It presents with erythema, pruritus, white patches, and sometimes curd-like discharge. Risk is higher in diabetics, immunosuppressed individuals, and those with poor hygiene. Diagnosis is usually clinical.
10. Circumcision reduces the risk of balanitis by eliminating moist environments under the foreskin. Risk factors include diabetes, prolonged antibiotic use, and immunosuppression. Recurrence is common if risk factors are not controlled.
11. Phimosis is the inability to retract the foreskin behind the glans penis. It may be physiological in children or pathological due to scarring. Symptoms include difficulty urinating and recurrent balanitis. Severe cases may require circumcision.
12. Paraphimosis occurs when a retracted foreskin becomes trapped behind the glans and cannot be returned. This creates a constricting band that impairs blood flow, causing swelling and pain. It is a urological emergency requiring manual reduction or surgical intervention.
13. The most serious complication of paraphimosis is ischemia and gangrene of the glans penis. If left untreated, vascular compromise can progress to necrosis and possible penile loss. Prompt diagnosis and intervention are essential.
14. Priapism is a prolonged erection lasting more than 4 h, unrelated to sexual stimulation. It can be ischemic (low-flow, painful) or non-ischemic (high-flow, less painful). Ischemic priapism is a urological emergency due to the risk of permanent erectile tissue damage.
15. Sickle cell disease is the most common cause of ischemic priapism worldwide. Sickled erythrocytes block venous outflow, trapping blood in corpora

cavernosa. Other causes include leukemia, trauma, and drugs such as antidepressants or intracavernosal injections.

16. Peyronie's disease is caused by fibrous plaque formation within the tunica albuginea of the penis. This leads to painful erections and penile curvature. It is often idiopathic, though trauma and microvascular injury are contributing factors.
17. The plaques in Peyronie's disease typically occur in the tunica albuginea of the corpora cavernosa. This fibrous scarring prevents uniform expansion during erection, producing curvature, deformity, and erectile dysfunction in some patients.
18. Reactive arthritis (Reiter's syndrome) is strongly linked to *Chlamydia trachomatis* infection. It is an autoimmune response triggered by infection, often appearing weeks after initial urethritis or enteritis. It is a classic example of a post-infectious complication of STIs.
19. The classic triad of reactive arthritis is urethritis, arthritis, and conjunctivitis. Patients may also present with mucocutaneous lesions such as balanitis circi nata and keratoderma blennorrhagicum. It typically affects young men after chlamydial urethritis.
20. Kaposi's sarcoma, an angioproliferative tumor caused by HHV-8, is strongly associated with HIV/AIDS. It presents as red-purple vascular lesions on skin and mucosa. It is an AIDS-defining illness and can involve visceral organs.
21. Neurosyphilis is a manifestation of tertiary syphilis. It may present as tabes dorsalis, general paresis, or meningovascular syphilis. Although more common in late disease, it can occur earlier in HIV-infected patients.
22. Cardiovascular syphilis typically involves the aorta, causing syphilitic aortitis and aneurysm. This occurs decades after untreated infection. Complications include aortic regurgitation and rupture of aneurysms.
23. Mumps orchitis is caused by the paramyxovirus and usually follows parotitis. It affects post-pubertal males and can cause testicular pain, swelling, and infertility due to testicular atrophy.
24. Cryptorchidism (undescended testis) increases risks of infertility, torsion, and testicular malignancy, especially seminoma. Early surgical correction (orchiopexy) is recommended to reduce risks.
25. Seminoma is the most common testicular tumor in young men. It presents as a painless testicular mass. Prognosis is excellent with radiotherapy and chemotherapy.
26. β-hCG may be elevated in seminomas, though AFP remains normal. This distinction helps differentiate seminomas from non-seminomatous germ cell tumors.
27. Non-seminomatous germ cell tumors often raise both AFP and β-hCG. Yolk sac tumors secrete AFP, while choriocarcinomas secrete β-hCG. Mixed tumors may raise both.
28. Gynecomastia can result from Klinefelter syndrome, liver disease, testicular tumors, or hCG-secreting tumors. Androgen excess does not cause gynecomastia; rather, it causes virilization.

29. HPV vaccination (against HPV 6, 11, 16, and 18) prevents most genital warts and HPV-related cancers of the cervix, anus, and penis. It is highly effective when given before sexual debut.
30. Both HPV and hepatitis B vaccines are effective in preventing sexually transmitted viral infections that lead to cancer. They are critical elements of global STI prevention strategies.
31. Syndromic management treats STIs based on clinical presentation without waiting for lab results. This ensures immediate treatment and reduces transmission. Partner treatment is integral.
32. The WHO STI prevention strategy includes contact tracing, condom promotion, and vaccination. A holistic approach combining behavioral, biomedical, and structural interventions achieves the best outcomes.
33. Donovanosis (granuloma inguinale) is caused by *Klebsiella granulomatis*. It presents with painless, progressive ulcerative lesions in the genital region.
34. Donovan bodies, seen on Wright-Giemsa staining, are intracellular inclusions within macrophages, pathognomonic of donovanosis.
35. Chancroid is caused by *Haemophilus ducreyi* and presents as painful genital ulcers with soft, ragged edges. Painful inguinal lymphadenopathy is common.
36. The ulcers of chancroid are painful, in contrast to the hard painless chancre of syphilis. This clinical difference is a key diagnostic clue.
37. Lymphogranuloma venereum (LGV) is caused by *Chlamydia trachomatis* serovars L1–L3. It begins as a transient genital ulcer followed by painful inguinal lymphadenopathy ("buboes").
38. Buboes in LGV are painful inguinal lymph nodes that may suppurate. They often follow unnoticed genital ulcers, making clinical recognition essential.
39. Molluscum contagiosum, caused by a poxvirus, produces dome-shaped papules with central umbilication. It spreads sexually or by close contact.
40. Lesions of molluscum contagiosum are flesh-colored, pearly, umbilicated papules. They are benign and self-limiting but may persist in immunocompromised patients.
41. Scabies burrows are linear lesions caused by female mites tunneling under the skin. Common sites include web spaces, wrists, and genitalia. Nocturnal pruritus is characteristic.
42. Condyloma acuminata (genital warts) are caused by HPV types 6 and 11. They present as soft, cauliflower-like growths on genitalia and perianal skin.
43. HPV 16 and 18 are the most oncogenic strains, strongly associated with cervical, anal, and penile cancers. Vaccination prevents infection with these strains.
44. Benzathine penicillin is the drug of choice for all stages of syphilis, except neurosyphilis where IV penicillin is needed.
45. Jarisch-Herxheimer reaction is an acute febrile reaction after syphilis treatment due to release of treponemal antigens. It is self-limiting.
46. Doxycycline is first-line therapy for uncomplicated chlamydial infections. Azithromycin is an alternative single-dose regimen.
47. HPV-related penile cancer typically affects the glans and prepuce. High-risk strains (16 and 18) are implicated. Circumcision and vaccination are preventive.

48. Mumps orchitis is a post-pubertal complication of mumps virus infection. It causes testicular swelling, pain, and may result in infertility due to testicular atrophy.
49. The Western blot is the confirmatory test for HIV after a positive ELISA. Modern practice increasingly uses PCR and fourth generation antigen-antibody tests for earlier detection.
50. The HIV window period is 6–12 weeks for antibody detection. fourth generation tests detect p24 antigen earlier, reducing the window to ~2–4 weeks.

Further Reading

The explanations in this chapter are supported by the following key references:

1. World Health Organization. Global progress report on HIV, viral hepatitis and sexually transmitted infections. Geneva: WHO; 2021.
2. Centers for Disease Control and Prevention. Sexually transmitted infections treatment guidelines, 2021. MMWR Recomm Rep. 2021;70(4):1–187.
3. Unemo M, Jensen JS. Antimicrobial-resistant sexually transmitted infections. Lancet Infect Dis. 2017;17(8):e235–47.
4. Barbee LA. Preparing for an era of untreatable gonorrhea. Curr Opin Infect Dis. 2014;27(3):282–7.
5. de Vries HJC, Zingoni A, Kreuter A, et al. European guideline on the management of proctitis, proctocolitis and enteritis caused by sexually transmissible pathogens. J Eur Acad Dermatol Venereol. 2021;35(7):1434–43.
6. Mayer KH, Allan-Blitz LT. Epidemiology of STIs in men who have sex with men. Lancet Infect Dis. 2019;19(9):e273–82.

Urethral Discharge Syndrome

21

Learning Objectives

- Recognize symptoms and signs of urethral discharge.
- Differentiate gonococcal vs. non-gonococcal urethritis.
- Choose appropriate diagnostic tests (NAAT, microscopy).
- Implement evidence-based treatment regimens.
- Emphasize partner notification and STI prevention.

Select the Single Best Answer

1. Which of the following is FALSE about vertical sexually transmitted diseases?
   A. Breastfeeding
   B. Transplacental
   C. Contaminated towels
   D. Vaginal delivery
2. Which of the following is FALSE about prosemen?
   A. Physiological discharge
   B. Cowper gland source
   C. Increased with defecation
   D. Scanty amount
3. The prosemen is a risk factor for:
   A. Non-gonococcal urethritis
   B. Prostatitis
   C. HIV infection
   D. None of the above
4. Which of the following is FALSE about prostatorrhea?
   A. Prostatic gland source
   B. Increase with defecation

M. S. M. Hasan, M. L. Elsaie, *Comprehensive MCQs in Andrology*, Trends in Andrology and Sexual Medicine, https://doi.org/10.1007/978-3-032-20623-7_21

   C. Lead to prostatic carcinoma
   D. Physiological discharge
5. The main clue differentiating prosemen from prostatorrhea is:
   A. Type of discharge
   B. The cause
   C. Sexual stimulation
   D. Odor of the discharge
   E. Color of the discharge
6. Which of the following is FALSE about Dhat syndrome?
   A. Whitish discharge
   B. Related to depression and anxiety
   C. Due to wrong beliefs about normal sexual function
   D. Due to congenital abnormalities in male accessory glands
   E. May be associated with hypochondriasis
7. The normal adult vaginal pH is:
   A. 4–4.5
   B. 4.5–5
   C. 5–5.5
   D. 5.5–6
   E. 6–7.2
8. The gray vaginal discharge color indicates:
   A. Cervical infections
   B. Bacterial vaginosis
   C. Gonorrhea
   D. Chlamydia
   E. Normal ovulation
9. The yellow vaginal discharge color indicates:
   A. Vaginal irritation
   B. Hormonal imbalance
   C. Pelvic inflammatory disease
   D. Bacterial vaginosis
   E. Candidiasis
10. Which of the following is FALSE about trichomonas?
   A. Scanty to profuse discharge
   B. Vulvar itch
   C. pH < 4.5
   D. Offensive odor
   E. Associated with the lower abdomen
11. The vaginal discharge odor in bacterial vaginosis is:
   A. Fishy
   B. Non-offensive
   C. Volatile
   D. Acetone-like
12. The microscopic clue cells are most characteristic of:
   A. Vaginal candidiasis
   B. Bacterial vaginosis

C. Trichomoniasis
D. Gonorrhea
E. Mycoplasma infection

13. Hay–Ison criteria of bacterial vaginosis grade 1 indicates:
    A. Epithelial cells only
    B. Lactobacillus predominance
    C. Clue cell predominance
    D. Mixed flora
    E. Gram-positive cocci only
14. Hay–Ison criteria of bacterial vaginosis grade 2 indicates:
    A. Epithelial cells only
    B. Lactobacillus predominance
    C. Clue cell predominance
    D. Mixed flora mainly
    E. Gram-positive cocci only
15. Hay–Ison criteria of bacterial vaginosis grade 3 indicates:
    A. Epithelial cells only
    B. Lactobacillus predominance
    C. Gardnerella predominance
    D. Mixed flora
    E. Gram-positive cocci only
16. Hay–Ison criteria of bacterial vaginosis grade 4 indicates:
    A. Epithelial cells only
    B. Lactobacillus predominance
    C. Clue cell predominance
    D. Mixed flora
    E. Gram-positive cocci only
17. Which of the following is NOT true about *Trichomonas vaginalis*?
    A. Aerobic protozoa
    B. Flagellated
    C. Exclusive adult sexually transmitted disease
    D. Has an undulating membrane
    E. Unicellular
18. Zoon balanitis is a synonym for:
    A. Queyrat's erythroplasia
    B. Plasma cell infiltration
    C. Circinate balanitis
    D. Traumatic balanitis
    E. Balanitis xerotica obliterans
19. Which of the following is FALSE about Zoon balanitis?
    A. Benign condition
    B. Idiopathic
    C. Smooth shiny red-orange plaque
    D. Common in children
    E. Usually solitary in number

20. The whiff test is used in the diagnosis of:
    A. Bacterial vaginosis
    B. Trichomoniasis
    C. Vaginal candidiasis
    D. Mycoplasma infection
21. Vaginal clue cells:
    A. Indicate an underlying gonococcal infection
    B. Are epithelial cells coated with candidal spores
    C. Are never present in the normal vagina
    D. Cannot support the diagnosis of bacterial vaginosis
    E. Are best visualized by phase contrast or dark-field illumination
22. Bacterial vaginosis:
    A. Is associated with overgrowth of *Gardnerella vaginalis*
    B. Does not occur after menopause
    C. Has not been linked to postpartum endometritis
    D. Is strongly associated with cervical intraepithelial neoplasia
    E. Is associated with decreased amine content in vaginal fluid
23. Diagnosis of bacterial vaginosis is supported by:
    A. Thin heterogeneous discharge
    B. Clue cells on Gram-stained smear
    C. Positive amine test after adding HCl
    D. Vaginal pH < 4.5
    E. Marked vulval erythema
24. Bacterial vaginosis may be effectively treated with:
    A. Oxytetracycline
    B. Metronidazole
    C. Ceftriaxone
    D. Fluconazole
    E. Salicylic acid paste
25. Candidal infection of the vagina:
    A. Causes a thin curdy discharge
    B. If asymptomatic, requires treatment
    C. Associated with vaginal pH > 5
    D. May cause superficial dyspareunia
    E. Due to *Candida glabrata* in ~40% of cases
26. The following agents commonly cause vaginitis:
    A. *Candida albicans*
    B. *Mycoplasma hominis*
    C. *Gardnerella vaginalis*
    D. *Neisseria gonorrhoeae*
    E. A+B+C
27. The following conditions predispose to candidal infection EXCEPT:
    A. Pregnancy
    B. Diabetes insipidus
    C. Antibiotic therapy
    D. Hypoparathyroidism

28. All are TRUE about *Trichomonas vaginalis* EXCEPT:
    A. Is a flagellated protozoa
    B. May cause male urethritis
    C. Causes yellow frothy discharge
    D. Cultured on Feinberg-Whittington medium
    E. Best diagnosed by Gram-stained smear
29. The following infectious agents give specific Pap smear appearance EXCEPT:
    A. *Candida albicans*
    B. *Gardnerella vaginalis*
    C. *Trichomonas vaginalis*
    D. *Actinomycosis*
    E. None of the above
30. Which of the following is the most common cause of non-gonococcal urethritis?
    A. *Chlamydia trachomatis*
    B. *Mycoplasma genitalium*
    C. *Ureaplasma urealyticum*
    D. *Trichomonas vaginalis*
    E. *E. coli*
31. A 24-year-old male presents with dysuria and mucopurulent urethral discharge; Gram stain shows intracellular diplococci. The most likely organism is:
    A. *Chlamydia trachomatis*
    B. *Neisseria gonorrhoeae*
    C. *Mycoplasma hominis*
    D. *Trichomonas vaginalis*
    E. *E. coli*
32. Which complication is MOST associated with recurrent gonococcal urethritis in men?
    A. Epididymitis
    B. Orchitis
    C. Proctitis
    D. Chronic prostatitis
    E. Urethral stricture
33. A frothy, malodorous vaginal discharge with strawberry cervix suggests:
    A. *Trichomonas vaginalis*
    B. Bacterial vaginosis
    C. Candida
    D. Gonorrhea
    E. Herpes simplex
34. Which of the following is the gold standard for diagnosis of chlamydial urethritis?
    A. Gram stain
    B. Culture on chocolate agar
    C. Nucleic acid amplification test (NAAT)
    D. Antigen ELISA
    E. Microscopy

35. In candidal vaginitis, the vaginal pH is usually:
    A. < 4.5
    B. 4.5–5
    C. > 5
    D. Variable
36. Which syndrome is characterized by reactive arthritis, conjunctivitis, and urethritis?
    A. Behçet's syndrome
    B. Reiter's syndrome
    C. Stevens-Johnson syndrome
    D. Zoon balanitis
    E. Dhat syndrome
37. Which finding differentiates bacterial vaginosis from other vaginal infections?
    A. Fishy odor on whiff test
    B. High vaginal pH (> 4.5)
    C. Presence of clue cells
    D. All of the above
38. Recurrent vulvovaginal candidiasis is defined as:
    A. 2 episodes per year
    B. 3 episodes per year
    C. 4 or more episodes per year
    D. Persistent infection beyond 1 month
39. Which of the following organisms is NOT sexually transmitted?
    A. *Candida albicans*
    B. *Chlamydia trachomatis*
    C. *Neisseria gonorrhoeae*
    D. *Trichomonas vaginalis*
40. A young male presents with clear mucoid urethral discharge and sterile pyuria. The most likely diagnosis is:
    A. Gonococcal urethritis
    B. Non-gonococcal urethritis due to *Chlamydia*
    C. Candidiasis
    D. Bacterial vaginosis
41. Which drug is first-line therapy for uncomplicated gonococcal urethritis?
    A. Ciprofloxacin
    B. Penicillin
    C. Ceftriaxone
    D. Doxycycline
42. Which drug is first-line therapy for chlamydial urethritis?
    A. Ceftriaxone
    B. Azithromycin
    C. Ciprofloxacin
    D. Clindamycin

43. What is the most common presentation of mycoplasma urethritis?
    A. Asymptomatic
    B. Dysuria and scant discharge
    C. Profuse purulent discharge
    D. Genital ulcer
44. A patient with urethral discharge tests negative for gonorrhea and chlamydia. The next likely pathogen is:
    A. *Mycoplasma genitalium*
    B. *Candida albicans*
    C. *Trichomonas vaginalis*
    D. *E. coli*
45. Which of the following is the most common cause of vaginal discharge overall?
    A. Gonorrhea
    B. Bacterial vaginosis
    C. Candida
    D. Trichomonas
46. "Strawberry cervix" is pathognomonic of:
    A. Candida vaginitis
    B. Trichomoniasis
    C. Bacterial vaginosis
    D. Gonorrhea
47. Which test is most useful for differentiating bacterial vaginosis from trichomonas infection?
    A. Wet mount microscopy
    B. Gram stain
    C. KOH whiff test
    D. Pap smear
48. Which statement is TRUE about physiologic leukorrhea?
    A. Thick and curdy
    B. Associated with burning and itching
    C. Occurs around ovulation without odor or irritation
    D. Always needs treatment
49. Which vaginal infection shows pseudohyphae on KOH mount?
    A. Gonorrhea
    B. Candida
    C. Chlamydia
    D. Trichomonas
50. Which urethral discharge is typically scanty, clear, and worsens in the morning?
    A. Gonorrhea
    B. Chlamydia
    C. Mycoplasma
    D. Physiological

✅ Key Takeaways

- *Neisseria gonorrhoeae* and *Chlamydia trachomatis* are the main pathogens.
- NAAT is the preferred diagnostic tool.
- Syndromic management is often used where lab access is limited.
- Prompt treatment reduces complications and transmission.
- Partner treatment and counseling are essential.

✅ Answer Key (1–50)

1. C
2. C
3. D
4. C
5. C
6. D
7. A
8. B
9. C
10. C
11. A
12. B
13. B
14. D
15. C
16. E
17. C
18. B
19. D
20. A
21. E
22. A
23. B
24. B
25. D
26. E
27. B
28. E
29. E
30. A
31. B
32. E
33. A

34. C
35. A
36. B
37. D
38. C
39. A
40. B
41. C
42. B
43. A
44. A
45. B
46. B
47. A
48. C
49. B
50. B

Explanations (1–50)

1. Vertical transmission refers to infections passed from mother to child. This can occur through the placenta, during vaginal delivery, or via breastfeeding. Contaminated towels, however, are not a route of vertical transmission but rather a fomite-related transmission.
2. Prosemen is a physiological clear discharge, often from Cowper's glands. It is not linked to bowel movements like prostatorrhea. Suggesting that it increases with defecation is incorrect, as this feature characterizes prostatorrhea instead.
3. Prosemen is not a pathological discharge and is not considered a risk factor for sexually transmitted or infectious conditions. It does not contribute to non-gonococcal urethritis, prostatitis, or HIV transmission. Its appearance is benign and related to sexual stimulation.
4. Prostatorrhea is the involuntary loss of prostatic secretions. While it increases with straining during defecation and arises from the prostate, it does not predispose to carcinoma. Associating it with cancer risk is a misconception.
5. The main difference between prosemen and prostatorrhea lies in their triggering factor. Prosemen is associated with sexual arousal, while prostatorrhea often occurs during straining with defecation. The source and mechanism distinguish them clinically.
6. Dhat syndrome is a psychosomatic disorder often found in South Asia. It involves anxiety over semen loss, leading to whitish discharge complaints. It stems from cultural beliefs, anxiety, or hypochondriasis, not from congenital glandular abnormalities.

7. Normal adult vaginal pH is acidic, usually between 4.0 and 4.5. This environment is maintained by lactobacilli producing lactic acid. Higher pH values suggest infection such as bacterial vaginosis or trichomoniasis.
8. Gray vaginal discharge with fishy odor is a hallmark of bacterial vaginosis. This results from overgrowth of anaerobic bacteria such as *Gardnerella vaginalis*. Color alone provides a strong clue when matched with odor and pH.
9. Yellow vaginal discharge is more often associated with inflammatory processes like pelvic inflammatory disease. It can suggest gonococcal or chlamydial infection as well. This differs from the white, curdy discharge of candidiasis.
10. Trichomoniasis typically presents with profuse, frothy, foul-smelling discharge and vulvar irritation. The vaginal pH is usually elevated above 4.5, not below. Hence, suggesting a low pH is inaccurate for this infection.
11. The odor of bacterial vaginosis is characteristically fishy. It becomes more obvious after applying potassium hydroxide during the whiff test. This finding is diagnostic when combined with clue cells and elevated vaginal pH.
12. Clue cells are vaginal epithelial cells covered by bacteria, mainly *Gardnerella*. They are highly specific for bacterial vaginosis. Their presence on wet mount or Gram stain supports the diagnosis strongly.
13. Grade 1 in Hay–Ison criteria reflects normal flora. It shows predominance of lactobacilli with no overgrowth of pathogenic bacteria. This indicates a healthy vaginal microbiome.
14. Grade 2 suggests intermediate flora. It shows reduced lactobacilli with mixed bacterial species but without clear dominance. This stage is neither normal nor fully diagnostic of bacterial vaginosis.
15. Grade 3 indicates abnormal flora. It is characterized by overgrowth of organisms like *Gardnerella* and paucity of lactobacilli. This grade confirms bacterial vaginosis.
16. Grade 4 represents a markedly disturbed flora with only epithelial cells present. It shows total loss of protective lactobacilli. This abnormality predisposes to infection.
17. *Trichomonas vaginalis* is indeed a flagellated, anaerobic protozoan with an undulating membrane. It is sexually transmitted but can occasionally affect prepubertal girls non-sexually. Thus, labeling it "exclusive adult STI" is incorrect.
18. Zoon balanitis is a benign chronic condition of the glans penis. It represents plasma cell infiltration, presenting as shiny reddish-orange plaques. It is non-malignant but often mistaken for premalignant lesions.
19. Zoon balanitis is an idiopathic condition usually in middle-aged to older men. It is not seen in children and typically manifests as solitary shiny lesions. Suggesting childhood prevalence is therefore wrong.
20. The whiff test detects volatile amines released from vaginal discharge in bacterial vaginosis. Adding KOH solution releases a characteristic fishy odor. It is a rapid office-based diagnostic aid.
21. Clue cells are best identified under specialized microscopy like phase-contrast. They are epithelial cells coated with bacteria, not fungal spores. Their presence is a classic marker for bacterial vaginosis.

22. Bacterial vaginosis arises from overgrowth of anaerobes like *Gardnerella*. It is known to occur even after menopause. It has associations with postpartum endometritis, making contrary claims incorrect.
23. Bacterial vaginosis is diagnosed based on the presence of several clinical findings, most notably the presence of "clue cells" on a Gram-stained smear. These cells are vaginal epithelial cells covered in bacteria, giving them a characteristic "clue" appearance under the microscope.
24. Metronidazole is the drug of choice for bacterial vaginosis. It effectively targets anaerobic bacteria including *Gardnerella*. Other antibiotics like tetracyclines or antifungals are not appropriate here.
25. Candidal vaginitis typically presents with thick, curdy discharge and itching. Vaginal pH remains normal or acidic, usually <4.5. It can cause dyspareunia, but *Candida albicans* is the main pathogen, not *Candida glabrata*.
26. Common causes of vaginitis include *Candida albicans*, *Gardnerella vaginalis*, and *Trichomonas vaginalis*. *Mycoplasma* and gonococcus are not typical causes of vaginitis. Hence, only these main three are implicated.
27. Predisposing factors for candidiasis include pregnancy, diabetes mellitus, and broad-spectrum antibiotics. Diabetes insipidus is not recognized as a risk factor. Hormonal and immune influences play a larger role.
28. *Trichomonas vaginalis* is flagellated and sexually transmitted. It causes frothy yellow discharge and can infect males too. Diagnosis relies on wet mount microscopy, not Gram staining.
29. Certain pathogens show typical cytologic findings on Pap smears. These include *Candida* (pseudohyphae), *Trichomonas* (motile trophozoites), and *Actinomyces* (filamentous bacteria). *Gardnerella* is less specific cytologically.
30. The leading cause of non-gonococcal urethritis worldwide is *Chlamydia trachomatis*. It often produces mild, clear discharge. Early diagnosis prevents complications like epididymitis.
31. Gram-negative intracellular diplococci on microscopy are diagnostic for *Neisseria gonorrhoeae*. This is the hallmark finding in acute gonococcal urethritis. It differentiates it from chlamydial infections.
32. Chronic untreated gonorrhea can cause scarring and fibrosis. Urethral stricture is a common long-term complication. This may result in obstructive urinary symptoms.
33. Frothy, green-yellow vaginal discharge with "strawberry cervix" is classic for trichomoniasis. The cervical mucosa appears punctate due to capillary hemorrhages. This finding is almost pathognomonic.
34. NAAT is the gold standard for detecting chlamydia. It is highly sensitive and specific. Culture and antigen detection are less accurate.
35. Vaginal pH in candidiasis usually remains below 4.5. This helps distinguish it from bacterial vaginosis and trichomoniasis, both of which elevate pH. pH measurement is thus a useful bedside test.
36. Reiter's syndrome is a reactive arthritis triad of arthritis, conjunctivitis, and urethritis. It often follows chlamydial infection. It is one of the "seronegative spondyloarthropathies."

37. Bacterial vaginosis differs by its combination of fishy odor, clue cells, and elevated pH. No single feature is sufficient; together they confirm the diagnosis. This makes the syndrome distinct from candidiasis or trichomonas.
38. Recurrent vulvovaginal candidiasis is defined clinically as four or more symptomatic episodes within a year. It suggests host predisposition or incomplete eradication. This condition requires prolonged antifungal therapy.
39. *Candida albicans* is not sexually transmitted, though sexual activity may exacerbate symptoms. It arises from endogenous overgrowth in the vaginal flora. This contrasts with chlamydia, gonorrhea, or trichomonas.
40. Sterile pyuria with urethral discharge is typical of chlamydial infection. Urine cultures are negative, but NAAT confirms the diagnosis. This presentation is a hallmark of non-gonococcal urethritis.
41. Ceftriaxone is the current first-line therapy for gonorrhea due to resistance issues with fluoroquinolones and penicillin. A single intramuscular dose is recommended. Co-treatment for chlamydia is often added.
42. Azithromycin or doxycycline are the preferred first-line drugs for chlamydial infections. Azithromycin is favored for single-dose compliance. Ceftriaxone alone does not treat chlamydia.
43. Mycoplasma urethritis often presents mildly. Many cases are asymptomatic or show scanty discharge with dysuria. This makes it harder to diagnose without molecular tests. While dysuria (painful urination) and a scant discharge can occur with Mycoplasma urethritis, they are not the most common presentation.
44. If gonorrhea and chlamydia tests are negative, *Mycoplasma genitalium* is often the next suspected pathogen. It is increasingly recognized as a cause of persistent urethritis. Treatment may require azithromycin or moxifloxacin.
45. The most common cause of vaginal discharge overall is bacterial vaginosis. It surpasses both candidiasis and trichomoniasis. Its prevalence is linked to disruption of normal lactobacilli.
46. The "strawberry cervix" appearance with punctate hemorrhages is characteristic of trichomoniasis. It is rarely seen with other infections. This sign helps confirm the diagnosis clinically.
47. Wet mount microscopy showing motile trichomonads distinguishes trichomoniasis from bacterial vaginosis. The whiff test and pH help, but direct visualization is most specific. Pap smears are less reliable.
48. Physiologic leukorrhea is a normal increase in vaginal secretions around ovulation. It is clear, non-irritating, and odorless. It does not require treatment.
49. Candidiasis shows pseudohyphae and budding yeast on KOH mount. This microscopic finding is diagnostic. It is absent in bacterial vaginosis or trichomonas.
50. Chlamydial urethritis usually produces scanty, mucoid discharge, often noticed in the morning. This contrasts with gonorrhea, which typically causes copious purulent discharge. The subtle presentation explains its frequent underdiagnosis.

Further Reading

The explanations in this chapter are supported by the following key references:

1. Centers for Disease Control and Prevention. Sexually transmitted infections treatment guidelines, 2021. MMWR Recomm Rep. 2021;70(4):1–187.
2. World Health Organization. WHO guidelines for the treatment of sexually transmitted infections. Geneva: WHO; 2016.
3. Horner PJ, Donders G, Cusini M, et al. European guideline on the management of non-gonococcal urethritis. Int J STD AIDS. 2016;27(11):928–37.
4. Workowski KA, Bachmann LH, Chan PA, et al. Sexually transmitted infections treatment guidelines, 2021. Clin Infect Dis. 2022;74(Suppl 2):S1–S187.
5. Manhart LE, Broad JM, Golden MR. Mycoplasma genitalium: Should we treat and how? Clin Infect Dis. 2011;53(Suppl 3):S129–42.
6. Taylor SN. Management of urethritis. Clin Infect Dis. 2015;61(Suppl 8):S763–9.

MIX
Papier aus verantwortungsvollen Quellen
Paper from responsible sources
FSC® C105338

If you have any concerns about our products,
you can contact us on
ProductSafety@springernature.com

In case Publisher is established outside the EU,
the EU authorized representative is:
Springer Nature Customer Service Center GmbH
Europaplatz 3, 69115 Heidelberg, Germany

Printed by Libri Plureos GmbH
in Hamburg, Germany